Handbook of Trauma
for Southern Africa

Disclaimer

While every effort has been made to check drug dosages in this handbook, it is still possible that errors have been overlooked. Dosages continue to be revised and new side-effects recognized. Oxford University Press makes no representation, express or implied, that the drug dosages in this book are correct. For these reasons, the reader is strongly urged to consult the *South African Medicines Formulary* or the drug manufacturer's printed instructions before administering any of the drugs recommended in this clinical handbook. The authors and the publishers do not accept responsibility or legal liability for any errors in the text or for the misuse or misapplication of material in this work.

Handbook of Trauma
for Southern Africa

Edited by
Andrew Nicol
and
Elmin Steyn

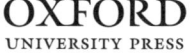

OXFORD
UNIVERSITY PRESS

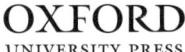

OXFORD
UNIVERSITY PRESS

Great Clarendon Street, Oxford OX2 6DP

Oxford University Press is a department of the University of Oxford.
It furthers the University's objective of excellence in research, scholarship,
and education by publishing worldwide in

Oxford New York

Auckland Bangkok Buenos Aires Cape Town Chennai
Dar es Salaam Delhi Hong Kong Istanbul Karachi Kolkata
Kuala Lumpur Madrid Melbourne Mexico City Mumbai
Nairobi São Paulo Shanghai Taipei Tokyo Toronto

Oxford is a registered trade mark of Oxford University Press
in the UK and in certain other countries

Published in South Africa
by Oxford University Press Southern Africa, Cape Town

Handbook of Trauma for Southern Africa

ISBN 0 19 578080 9 (10 digit, current)

ISBN 978 019578 0802 (13 digit, from 2007)

© Oxford University Press Southern Africa 2004

The moral rights of the authors have been asserted
Database right Oxford University Press (maker)

First published 2004
Second impression 2005

Commissioning Editor: Arthur Attwell
Project managers: Sarah O'Neill/Marian Griffin
Editor: Ethné Clarke
Medical proofreader: Dr Bridget Farham
Designer: Mark Standley
Illustrator: Bronwen Lusted
Indexer: Jeanne Cope

Published by Oxford University Press Southern Africa
PO Box 12119, N1 City, 7463, Cape Town, South Africa

Set in 8,5 pt on 11 pt Minion by RHT desktop publishing cc, Durbanville
Reproduction by RHT desktop publishing cc, Durbanville
Cover reproduction by The Image Bureau
Printed and bound by ABC Press, Cape Town

Contents

Contributors

Professor Steve Beningfield
  Head
  Department of Radiology
  University of Cape Town
  Groote Schuur Hospital
Dr Arthur Bird
  Head
  Western Province Blood
  Transfusion Service
Dr Paul Bischoff
  Maxillo-Facial Surgeon
  Vincent Pallotti Hospital
  Cape Town
Professor Kenneth D Boffard
  Clinical head
  Department of Surgery
  Johannesburg Hospital
  Faculty of Health Sciences
  University of the Witwatersrand
Dr Basil Bonner
  Head
  Emergency Unit
  Milnerton Mediclinic
Dr Douglas Bowley
  Department of Surgery
  Chris Hani Baragwanath
  Hospital
  Faculty of Health Sciences
  University of the Witwatersrand
Dr Gerald Dalbock
  Head
  Cardiocare
  Advanced Life Support Training

  Centre
  Panorama, Cape Town
Professor Elias Degiannis
  Department of Surgery
  Chris Hani Baragwanath
  Hospital
  Faculty of Health Sciences
  University of the Witwatersrand
Colonel Herman J.C. du Plessis
  Head: Department of Surgery
  1 Military Hospital
  Thaba Tshwane
  Pretoria
Dr Jenny Edge
  General Surgeon
  Christiaan Barnard Memorial
  Hospital
  Cape Town
Dr Thomas Eshun-Wilson
  Ophthalmologist
  Opthalmology Department
  Groote Schuur Hospital
Dr Luc Evenepoel
  Anaesthetist
  Cape Town
Professor Johannes Fagan
  Head
  Department of ENT
  Groote Schuur Hospital
  University of Cape Town
Dr Jacques Goosen
  Head
  Trauma Unit

Johannesburg Hospital
Faculty of Health Sciences
University of the Witwatersrand

Dr Rory Harvey
Orthopaedic Surgeon
Claremont Surgical Clinic
Cape Town

Professor Chris Heyns
Head
Department of Urology
Tygerberg Hospital
Faculty of Health Sciences,
University of Stellenbosch

Dr Jonathan Karpelowsky
Department of Surgery
University of Cape Town

Dr Walter Kloeck
Chairman
Resuscitation Council of South
Africa

Professor Jake Krige
Hepatobiliary Surgeon
Groote Schuur Hospital
University of Cape Town

Dr Jerome Loveland
Trauma Unit
Johannesburg Hospital

Dr Pradeep Makan
Orthopaedic & Spinal Surgeon
Vincent Pallotti Hospital
Cape Town

Dr David Marshall
Physician
Groote Schuur Hospital

Dr Lorna Martin
Forensic Pathologist
Department of Forensic
Medicine
University of Cape Town

Dr Roux Martinez
Senior Medical Officer
Christiaan Barnard Memorial
Hospital
Cape Town

Alexia Michaelides
Regional transplant manager
Netcare Cape Region
Christiaan Barnard Memorial
Hospital
Cape Town

Dr Lance Michell
Head
Intensive Care Unit
Groote Schuur Hospital

Dr Curt Minnie
Senior Medical Officer
Trauma & Emergency Unit
Christiaan Barnard Memorial
Hospital
Cape Town

Dr Pradeep Navsaria
Trauma Surgeon
Trauma Unit
Groote Schuur Hospital
University of Cape Town

Dr Andrew Nicol
Trauma Surgeon
Head
Trauma Unit
Groote Schuur Hospital
University of Cape Town

Dr Stephen Oliver
Head
Department of Microbiology
Groote Schuur Hospital
University of Cape Town

Dr Jones Omoshoro-Jones
General Surgeon

Trauma Unit
Groote Schuur Hospital

Dr Frank Plani
Consultant Trauma Surgeon
Johannesburg Hospital Trauma
Unit
Johannesburg

Dr Andre Potgieter
General Surgeon
N1 City Hospital
Cape Town

Dr Jan Pretorius
Critical Care Principal Specialist
Department of Surgery
Faculty of Health Sciences
University of Pretoria

Dr Cleeve Robertson
Director
Emergency Medical Services
Provincial Administration of the
Western Cape

Dr Jonathan Rosenthal
Diving Medical Examiner
Hyperbaric Physician
National Hyperbarics
Claremont Hospital
Cape Town

Professor Rob Scott-Miller
Cardiologist
Groote Schuur Hospital
University of Cape Town

Dr Gordon Siboto
Orthopaedic Surgeon
Department of Orthopaedic
Surgery
Groote Schuur Hospital

Professor Martin Smith
Clinical head
Department of Surgery

Chris Hani Baragwanath
Hospital
University of the
Witwatersrand Medical School

Dr Wayne Smith
Deputy Director
Emergency Medical Services
Provincial Administration of the
Western Cape

Dr Mike Solomons
Orthopaedic Surgeon
Head of the Hand Clinic
Department of Orthopaedics
Groote Schuur Hospital

Dr Elmin Steyn
Trauma and General Surgeon
Head: Trauma Units
Vincent Pallotti Hospital and
Christiaan Barnard Memorial
Hospital
Cape Town

Professor Etienne J Theron
Department of Surgery
Kimberley Hospital

Professor Sandie R Thomson
Department of Surgery
Nelson R Mandela School of
Medicine
University of Natal

Dr Sebastian Van As
Head
Trauma Unit
Red Cross Children's Hospital

Dr Elbie van der Merwe
Head, Burns Unit
Department of Surgery
Tygerberg Hospital
Faculty of Health Sciences
University of Stellenbosch

Dr Fred van der Merwe
 Neurosurgeon
 Christiaan Barnard Memorial
 Hospital
 Cape Town
Dr Johan van der Spuy
 Trauma Surgeon
 Trauma Unit

 Groote Schuur Hospital
Gerrit van Wyk
 Clinical Psychologist
 Director of TraumaClinic®
 Counselling Network
 Cape Town

Foreword

The arrival of a trauma textbook developed specifically for South Africa is long overdue. There has been gradual recognition worldwide that trauma is a disease process in its own right, and not just a nocturnal activity of the young. South Africa has been late in its recognition of Emergency Medicine as a specialty, and trauma is becoming a subspecialty of General Surgery.

South Africa has a unique environment in having not only an epidemic of trauma affecting all aspects of the population, but has an almost unique mix of developed and resource challenged medical facilities. Distances may be large, facilities limited, and expertise in short supply. Despite this, care is often of a high standard, provided by committed pre-hospital and medical personnel.

The foundation of trauma care is the recognition that it is multi-disciplinary and multifaceted; that the efforts of many people make up a team, and that the secret of trauma care, whether on a geographical basis, the Emergency Department, Operating Theatre, Intensive Care Unit, Ward, or in Rehabilitation, is that it is based on a systems approach, with an academic background.

Dr. Steyn and Dr. Nicol have succeeded in weaving together a tapestry of the best and most enthusiastic providers of Trauma Care in South Africa and joined their experience into a handbook with a mission to serve as a guide and reference to those who need it.

K. D. Boffard.
BSc(Hons) MB FRCS, FRCS(Edin), FRCPS(Glas), FACS
Professor and Clinical Head,
Department of Surgery,
Johannesburg Hospital,
University of the Witwatersrand.

Acknowledgements

The contributions of a wide spectrum of people and institutions have made this book possible. It is a well-known fact that a high level of expertise in trauma care has been developed in this country, and a compilation of this experience and wisdom is long overdue.

Although several trauma textbooks are available in the international arena, the challenge for us was to reflect principles of practice applicable to the specific problems we face in Africa and South Africa, where the level and availability of resources vary widely, case loads are overwhelming at times and socio-economic factors affect causes and outcomes. Practitioners in the field of trauma care from all over the country were approached, both from academic and private facilities, in order to provide some form of consensus on the management of trauma in South Africa. We are acutely aware that there are a lot more experts out there, with much to contribute. Unfortunately, not all were available or contactable at the time when this book was commissioned.

This book is meant to provide practical guidelines on both initial and definitive care of trauma victims, not only for the (often unsupervised or inexperienced) doctors practising in rural areas, but also for the many students, interns and surgeons in training who are exposed to trauma victims daily. It may also provide valuable background information to pre-hospital emergency personnel, nurses and other trauma care providers. The handy pocket-size format and brevity of style are intended to make it easily accessible as a quick reference source.

Trauma training is only coming to its right in recent times, particularly with the advent of ATLS® training in South Africa, which has grown significantly over the last 10 years and has made a remarkable contribution to the improvement of initial care of the injured patient. Very few chapters in this book can afford to omit referral to the role of the ATLS® principles in the initial stages of management.

We acknowledge the overwelming importance of prevention of injuries and hope that this book will promote awareness about the importance of prevention, not only of injuries, but also of missed injuries and complications.

Andrew Nicol
Elmin Steyn

Introduction

Etienne Theron

A perspective on trauma in South Africa

In South Africa, trauma accounts for 12–15% of all deaths compared with the global figure of 5.2%. Trauma kills an estimated 65 000 to 80 000 South Africans annually (178–218 per day) while another 3.5 million people seek medical care for non-fatal injuries every year. Intentional injuries and interpersonal violence cause 47% of deaths, while accidents account for 35%. The overall homicide rate of 60:100 000 in South Africa is ten times that of the USA. Fifty per cent of these deaths are due to firearms. Traffic-related deaths (21.4 per 100 000) are significantly higher than those in Australia (9.9) and the UK (3.6).

Abuse of alcohol and drugs is implicated in many injuries and homicides. In 1999, a study from Cape Town showed that 35% of all injured patients had blood alcohol levels above 0.05 g/100 ml. The relationship between alcohol and road traffic accidents is well established worldwide. In South Africa, pedestrians account for 40% of the national traffic deaths. Of adults killed on the road, 72% have blood alcohol levels > 0.08 g/100 ml.

Interpersonal violence includes assaults, domestic violence, child abuse, rape, and violence against women. It most often occurs between friends, intimates, and family members. The prevalence of domestic abuse is difficult to quantify, but 30% of women in South Africa may be physically abused at some time. Women rarely present after the first incident and studies indicate that a woman is assaulted an average of 39 times prior to seeking medical intervention. As with many other aspects of interpersonal violence, alcohol and drugs (e.g. mandrax and marijuana) may complicate the picture.

Trauma in all its hideous forms has a vast impact on the economy of a developing country that can ill afford the millions spent on prevention and management of injury. Trauma teams in and outside hospitals are dedicating time and resources to the resuscitation of thousands of victims of interpersonal violence and high-speed collisions, whilst wards and ICUs are filled with trauma cases. Ultimately, the cost of life-saving treatment, rehabilitation, chronic care, disability grants, and man-hours lost to the economy add up to a shocking R80 million per day.

Training of doctors, nurses, and others at undergraduate level is inconsistent. Most training institutions cannot provide a comprehensive trauma care course in an already overcrowded curriculum. The daily exposure to vast numbers of fresh trauma cases in casualty and emergency departments does, however, afford the junior doctor, nurse, and medic a unique hands-on learning experience. The popular training courses available in South Africa include ATLS (Advanced Trauma Life Support®), and Dip.PEC (Diploma of Primary Emergency Care). These courses are incorporated in the formal training of specialist surgeons and other emergency medicine practitioners. A number of programmes and systems aimed at surveillance, strategy planning, primary prevention, injury control, and capacity building are actively run by government, non-governmental organizations, and private initiative bodies. The CVIP (Crime, Violence, and Injury Lead Programme) of the MRC (Medical Research Council), with its Injury Mortality Surveillance system, is an important role-player in the fight against trauma in all its facets. Surveillance and epidemiological data produced by such systems renders vital information for policy and practice formulation. Prevention programmes, budget motivation, training programmes, and teaching should all benefit from information gleaned from these systems.

The Arrive Alive Road Safety Campaign launched in 1997 reduced traffic deaths by 6.4%, saving 623 lives. Casualty crashes were reduced by 7.9%, resulting in a cost saving of R475.3 million. Law enforcement has had a visible effect on traffic accidents, and violence in the home should diminish once new legislation on domestic violence takes effect. For the future, the weaknesses of poor public awareness and apathy among healthcare workers and administrators should be addressed. Many deficiencies still exist regarding training, public education, and effective law enforcement. The small band of committed enthusiasts should be expanded. Prevention strategies, a change in social behaviour and life-style, together with effective management of the trauma victim, must eventually relieve South Africa of the scourge of trauma.

References and recommended reading

Barclay, G. and Travares, C. 2002. International comparisons of criminal justice. Statistics 2000. From www.homeoffice.gov.uk/rds/pdfs2/losb 502.pdf. (April 2003.)

Department of Transport: Report on Arrive Alive Campaign 2000. www.transport.gov.za/search/arrive alive phase 3 main achievements.

Editorial. Injury and Safety Monitor, June 2002, Vol 1 No 1.

Jacobs, T., Steenkamp, M., Marais, S.1998. Domestic violence against women: A close look at intimate partner violence. *Trauma Review*, Aug, Vol 6, No 2 (MRC).

Matzopoulos, R. Profile of Fatal Injuries in SA, 2000. CVI Lead programme of MRC.

MRC *Trauma Review*, June 2000, Vol 8 No1.

National Injury and Mortality Surveillance System (NIMSS) of MRC. Report 2000 in Injury and Safety Monitor, June 2002, Vol 1 No 1.

National Injury and Mortality Surveillance System. Third Annual Report. Crime, Violence and Injury Lead Programme. 2002. Edited by R. Matzopoulus. http://www.mrc.ac.crome/crime.htm. (October 2003.)

Peden, M. MRC Report. March 2000. Personal correspondence.

Statistics on Violence against Women in South Africa available on http:/www.tricky.org/POWA/Stats.htm. (October 2003.)

WHO Report on Trauma: 1988.

PART 1

Early management of the injured patient

1 Prehospital care

Wayne Smith, Cleeve Robertson

Introduction

All injuries benefit from early appropriate medical care. In Southern Africa, however, most injuries occur among the vast rural population living in remote areas where poverty, scarcity of resources, and poor road and communication infrastructure may lead to delayed emergency medical care. Prehospital emergency care systems of the highest international standards are available in and around all of South Africa's major urban centres, including the sprawling townships in the vicinity of cities and industrial areas. Our emergency prehospital practitioners are skillful and well trained, and often perform their duties in daunting circumstances where personal safety comes second to the life of the patient. Trauma doctors and nurses stand to gain additional insights with knowledge and awareness of prevailing prehospital treatment protocols.

Principles of care in the prehospital phase are essentially the same as in the hospital environment, with some notable differences, namely:

- Circumstances are uncontrolled and varied.
- The environment may be hazardous, requiring specific measures.
- Patients may be trapped in wreckage.
- Resources, such as equipment and staff, may be limited.
- The working area may be dirty or contaminated.
- Mass casualty situations may be present.

Managing an accident scene

Indiscriminate or uncontrolled removal of victims trapped in the wreck of a vehicle may exacerbate injuries. No injured person should be moved until the situation is assessed and, where appropriate, immediate stabilization care administered, unless the lives of the victims or rescuers are in danger.

Scene assessment

The following should be assessed at the scene of an accident:

- Number and type of vehicles
- Extent of damage
- Number of patients and types of injuries
- Hazards present

- Emergency services on the scene (if so, identify yourself to a senior person and offer assistance)

Assistance mobilization

Back-up services need to be mobilized, namely: Ambulance, Traffic, Police, Fire, and Rescue agencies.

The following information will be required by the control room:
- Exact location of accident
- Type of incident
- Hazards present at scene
- Access route to the scene
- Number and severity of casualties
- Emergency services present and required

Hazard control and safety considerations

- Identify and control all hazards to rescuers, patients, and bystanders at the scene.
- Wear gloves, goggles, and visible protective clothing (reflective at night).
- Control and channel or divert traffic flow. Protect the scene from oncoming traffic by utilizing traffic cones and a parked heavy vehicle in a fend-off position.
- Appoint civilian marshals to control the crowd until law enforcement personnel arrive.
- Isolate and evacuate the area until the Fire department arrives and implements HAZ-MAT (hazardous material) procedures.
- Isolate the area with exposed or downed electrical wires until utility services arrive.
- Activate handbrake or place unstable vehicles in gear. Secure and stabilize as best as possible until rescue agencies arrive.
- Note that environmental conditions such as rain, wind, snow, etc. may complicate all activities.
- Use sand to control spilt fuel, have an extinguisher immediately available, and keep cigarettes and open flames out of the area.
- Disconnect the battery to prevent activation of undeployed airbags.

Gaining entry to wreckage to reach trapped victims

Use the quickest and easiest route – usually via doors, windows, or by removing the windshield. The windshield is laminated glass, which is extremely difficult to break through, and may not allow access to the interior.

Immediate patient care

Triage the injured and treat critical patients first. Treatment should be initiated in the wreckage while rescue crews gain access and create space. The primary and secondary survey systems are used to prioritize assessment and treatment, based on the principle that airway (A) problems kill before breathing (B) problems, which in turn kill before circulation (C) problems, followed by neurological injury or disability (D), and environmental or exposure (E) related issues. Defibrillation (D) may be required after assessment of the circulatory status.

First primary ABCDE survey

Assess airway

- Maintain cervical spine (C-spine) alignment.
- Assess level of consciousness and ability to vocalize.
- Clear airway with Magills forceps to remove foreign body, suction to evacuate liquids.
- Apply jaw thrust and insert oropharyngeal airway.
- Prevent aspiration by application of cricoid pressure.

Assess breathing

- Maintain C-spine alignment.
- Ventilate with bag valve mask (BVM) and reservoir with oxygen if breathing is inadequate.
- Add supplementary oxygen by face mask if breathing is adequate.

Assess circulation

- Control external haemorrhage immediately with direct pressure.
- Assess circulation by checking skin, pulse rate and character, and level of consciousness.
- Begin CPR if in cardiac arrest.

Defibrillation

- Assess rhythm.
- Assess for ventricular fibrillation or pulseless ventricular tachycardia.
- Defibrillate if the environment is safe.
- Extricate the patient immediately to allow defibrillation in safety if a fuel spill is present.

Repeat primary survey

Airway

- Maintain C-spine alignment.

- Intubate if necessary.
- Assess tube placement and fix tube securely.
- Apply definitive C-spine control with a rigid cervical collar and extrication equipment.

Breathing
- Ventilate with BVM and reservoir with oxygen if breathing is inadequate.
- Apply supplementary oxygen by face mask if breathing is adequate.
- Monitor oxygen saturation.
- Assess for life threats and manage tension pneumothorax, flail chest, cardiac contusion, massive haemothorax, cardiac tamponade.

Circulation
- Continue CPR if required, administer adrenaline for cardiac arrest.
- Control haemorrhage with appropriate pressure.
- Site large-bore IV lines and initiate fluid replacement.
- Connect ECG leads and check rhythm.
- Serially document blood-pressure readings.

Disability
- Do mini-neurological assessment: GCS, pupillary responses.
- Do cranial nerve assessment: eye movements, facial movements, and sensation.
- Grossly check peripheral nervous system: limb movements and sensation.

Exposure
- Undress victim.
- Prevent hypothermia.
- Splint fractures.

Secondary survey

- Take appropriate history.
- Do head-to-toe examination of head, neck, chest, abdomen, pelvis, perineum, limbs, and back.

Accessing a patient

Methods of access

Mechanical rescue tools are used to gain proper access to patients while medical care is in progress. Techniques employed include:

- Roof removal
- Forced door opening
- Forced front-seat reversing
- Side take-downs
- Dash roll up
- Dash lift
- Direct spreading, ramming, or cross-ramming

Controlled patient release

Use space-making techniques to systematically dismantle the vehicle, with slow release of crush injury. Remove the vehicle from around the patient and not the patient from the vehicle.

When the external pressure and tamponading effect is suddenly removed from limbs trapped for a prolonged period, acute decompensation may occur due to hypotension, hyperkalaemia, myoglobinaemia, acidosis, and uncontrolled haemorrhage. Polytraumatized limbs will suddenly have no external splinting, which will cause additional pain and soft tissue injury.

Monitor all vital signs while disentanglement is taking place. Be prepared to interrupt the disentanglement process in order to stabilize the patient appropriately.

Analgesia is essential for the conscious patient during the extrication process.

Where the patient is in immediate danger from the surroundings or a life-threatening medical condition, immediate release can be initiated. Examples of this include fire, toxic fumes, submergence, hazardous materials spills, uncontrolled civil disturbance or terrorist incident, critical medical conditions, for example cardiac arrest with ventricular fibrillation.

Methods of immediate release include manoeuvring, manipulation, traction, strategic spreading, ramming or cutting, and selective amputation.

Packaging and removal of casualties

Appropriate immobilization and packaging are done with commercially available spinal protection equipment. Proper spinal immobilization should be applied throughout the process.

- Thoroughly secure all tubes and lines.
- Splint all fractures.
- Remove the patient from the wreckage and stabilize further, prior to transport to the nearest appropriate trauma facility.
- Arrange transport via ground or air ambulance.

- Monitor appropriately en route to the receiving facility.
- Notify the receiving facility prior to arrival.
- Appropriate handover and proper record-keeping are essential. This should include the following:
  - name and age of patients
  - mechanism of injury
  - vital signs at scene
  - initial findings on assessment
  - procedures on scene
  - response to treatment given
  - relevant history
  - known allergies.

Scene clean-up and resolution

Once casualties have been evacuated, the scene is rendered safe by containing all hazards and then normal traffic flow can be re-established.

Mass casualty incidents

The principle of mass casualty management is to have a simple system of sorting patients for distribution to appropriate levels of care. Disasters can be defined as events where normal response systems are overwhelmed and extraordinary responses are required.

Disaster types

- Natural: earthquake, fire, flood, tornado
- Technological: chemical, nuclear, biological, or terrorist-instigated incident
- Transport: aircraft, shipping, rail and road-related incident

Phases of disaster management

Prevention

- Environmental risk assessment and analysis with implementation of control measures to prevent or predict occurrence
- Information-gathering and monitoring of high-risk areas

Preparation

- Emergency services, hospitals, rescue agencies, fire departments, law enforcement agencies, local authorities, national and provincial governments, military, etc. need to be prepared.

- Equipment must be stored and ready for logistical support.
- Vehicles must be available.
- Inter-agency letters of agreement must be in place.
- Standardized training for all agencies and groups must be ensured.
- Communication systems must be in place.
- Volunteer corps must be available.
- Established standard operating procedures must exist for callout and mobilization, disaster management, HAZ-MAT management, mass casualty situations, etc.

Response

- Contain, manage, control, and limit progression of the situation.
- Communicate information between agencies and within departments.
- Coordinate all responding resources, agencies, and departments.
- Ensure cooperation between all responding or involved agencies and departments.
- Control all involved staff, vehicles, equipment, patients, etc.
- Recover incurred costs and ensure financial support for victims.

Recovery

Affected communities should be assisted to re-organize and re-build.

Mass casualty plan

Every medical emergency service and hospital emergency department must have a well-rehearsed mass casualty plan. Important elements of the plan are given below.

Example: Mass casualty 'standby' hospital protocol
- Medical, nursing, and administrative coordinators meet and establish a control centre.
- Liaise with ambulance control regarding details and status of incident.
- Start preparing the casualty department for reception of casualties.
- Appoint a medical incident control officer.
- Warn theatres, ICU, outpatient department, X-ray department, etc. about possible mass casualty incident.
- Establish accurate bed status.

Example: Mass casualty 'incident declaration' hospital protocol
- Medical, nursing, and administrative coordinators meet and establish a control centre.
- Liaise with ambulance control regarding details and status of incident.
- Appoint a medical incident control officer.
- Mobilize standby and off-duty staff.
- Clear the casualty department of existing patients and prepare department for reception of casualties.
- Establish a triage point.
- Inform theatres, out-patient department, X-ray department, laboratories, etc. that normal activities must be suspended.
- Ask ICU to clear beds if possible.
- Place blood bank on standby.
- Designate wards for reception of admitted casualties and begin clearing them of existing patients.
- Organize and delegate staff as they arrive.
- Establish accurate bed status.
- Arrange liaison area for press and family.
- Appoint media liaison officer.

Leadership

- Someone must have the delegated authority to declare a mass casualty incident.
- Someone must be in charge.
- There must be a clear chain of command.

Communication

- All communication in and out of the hospital should go through a central communication facility that deals with the mass casualty-related issues only.
- There must be additional communications systems like radio and paging because public and cellular phone systems collapse under the volume of calls during major incidents.
- Communication systems to activate large numbers of staff at once are necessary, for example paging.
- A central mass casualty bureau for the region should track patients and deal with enquiries from relatives in an attempt to relieve the communications load on hospitals.

Space

Space for receiving and treating the different triage categories of patients should be predetermined. Certain wards may have to be cleared to manage the sudden influx of patients.

Personnel

- Personnel should be contactable outside normal hours of work.
- Key personnel should be pre-identified and clearly understand their function.
- There should be a mass casualty personnel plan to ensure that the emergency services can all function at high capacity for the duration of the incident.

Patient identification

A patient identification system should identify each patient as a part of the mass casualty incident and remain with them even if transferred between hospitals.

Catering

Personnel, patients, and family need access to food and liquid refreshments.

Stores

Large volumes of medical and surgical disposables need to be available at short notice.

Public relations and family management

A suitably qualified and experienced person needs to counsel the families of victims and deal with their concerns and their grief.

Security

Person and property need to be protected.

Hospital access

- Access roads must be kept open.
- Parking must be available for arriving staff.

Media liaison

The media must be handled by a liaison officer so that the medical management of patients is not affected.

Triage

Primary triage

Triage or patient sorting is performed in order to ensure the best possible appropriate care for the greatest number of patients within the constraints of available resources.

Triage categories are graded according to priority, or colour coded:

RED, or Priority 1: Stretcher or walking patients with altered vital signs; that is, a decreased level of consciousness or signs of respiratory, cardiovascular, or neurological compromise.

YELLOW, or Priority 2: Stretcher patients with normal vital signs, that is, normal level of consciousness, normal breathing, normal pulse, normal blood pressure.

GREEN, or Priority 3: Walking patients with normal vital signs, that is, normal level of consciousness, normal breathing, normal pulse, normal blood pressure.

BLUE, or Priority 4: Dead patients or those who have no chance of survival.

Secondary triage

RED patients are further triaged according to the ABCs by determining the predominant problem as follows:

Airway compromise has a higher priority than
Breathing compromise has a higher priority than
Circulatory compromise.

This implies that patients with an airway problem are treated before those with breathing or circulatory problems.

On-scene mass casualty management

Providing optimal care to the victims of a disaster or a mass casualty situation requires more than medical management of the injured. Additional problems need to be considered, such as the ongoing risk of further injury to victims and rescuers, the presence of crowds, the optimal integration of all resources and agencies involved, logistics of the site, and issues of leadership. Ideally, a pre-agreed plan of action should be implemented, with all role players fully aware of their duties and chains of command.

An example of the layout of emergency facilities around a disaster area is shown in Figure 1.1 and described below.

Access route: The route of entry into a disaster area is kept open for incoming emergency service vehicles and patrolled by the traffic department. No civilians are allowed on the route.

Egress route: The route of egress out of the disaster area is kept open for outgoing emergency service vehicles and patrolled by the traffic department. No civilians are allowed on the route.

Equipment holding area: This is the holding area for all emergency vehicles, relief staff, and equipment. It is located outside of the outer cordon.

Outer cordon: This is a circular area surrounding or partially surrounding the inner cordon, manned by the traffic department with only emergency personnel allowed beyond this point. All civilians are evacuated out of this area.

Inner cordon: This is a barrier surrounding the incident area, manned by police with only specific emergency rescue personnel allowed beyond this point. Depending on hazards within the incident area, special protective gear and clothing may have to be worn beyond this point. General emergency workers are not allowed beyond this point. Casualties are evacuated from this area to the CCS (casualty clearing station) by appropriately protected rescue personnel. Minimal resuscitation is done within this area due to the hazard risk.

Figure 1.1 Layout of emergency facilities at a disaster scene

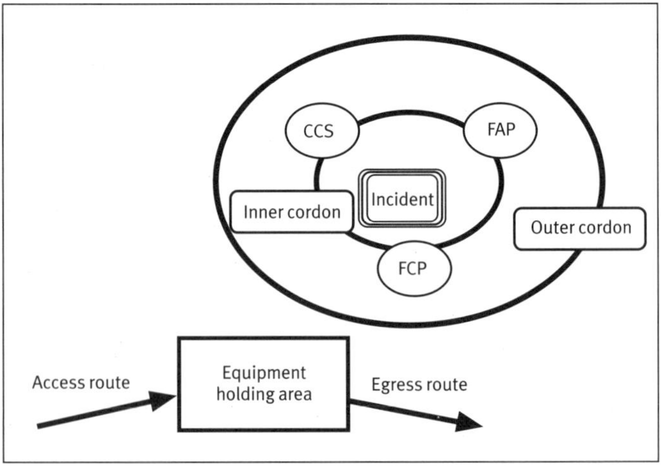

FCP (Forward Control Point): This is the point at which senior managers from emergency medical services, fire, traffic, ambulance, disaster management, police, etc. manage the on-scene co-ordination and control functions. All representatives have dedicated radio communication channels with their respective disciplines and have strict reporting and control structures. Information is shared, decisions made, and tasks delegated between the different departments, agencies, and disciplines at this control point.

FAP (First Aid Point): This is the site where all walking wounded or uninjured persons are managed and documentation done. It should preferably be at a distance from the resuscitation area, to prevent overcrowding. It is manned by paramedic officers and nursing staff.

CCS (Casualty Clearing Station): This is the site where all red- and yellow-code patients are resuscitated, stabilized, and treated prior to loading for transport to hospital. It is manned by doctors, nurses, and paramedics. All resuscitation is undertaken within this area prior to loading. Patients are brought to this area by rescue staff from within the inner cordon.

Loading area: This is the area where ambulances are loaded with casualties and instructions given as to which hospital will receive them. It is located at the edge of the CCS and controlled by the senior ambulance officer.

Temporary morgue: This is the area next to CCS where blue-code patients are kept prior to removal to the state forensic laboratory and morgue.

Pitfalls

- The most dramatic injury is not always the most serious one.
- Hypoxia or head injury leads to an altered level of consciousness, alcohol is to blame only if these two have been excluded.
- All polytrauma patients have a cervical spine injury until excluded clinically and radiologically.
- Sudden shortness of breath mandates exclusion of a tension pneumothorax.
- Both the institution and its sub-units should have individual but co-ordinated disaster plans.
- The role and function of each member of the team should be spelt out and practised at regular disaster practice sessions.
- Pre-prepared checklists covering all facets of the disaster plan should be available, as personnel often include volunteers from other departments, who may need clear guidelines.
- Frequent re-assessment of patients, even after they have been allocated a certain level of priority, should take place, as evolving injury may lead to clinical deterioration.

References and recommended reading

American College of Surgeons, Committee on Trauma. Advanced Trauma Life Support® Course for Doctors (ATLS®). 1997. Student Manual. Sixth edition. Chicago: ACS.

Bronstein, A. C., Currance, P. L. 1994. *Emergency care for hazardous materials exposure.* St Louis: Mosby.

Crippen, David W. Disaster management: Lessons from September 11, 2001. 8th World Congress of Intensive and Critical Care Medicine, Oct/Nov 2001. Australia: Sydney. Medscape/Medline Conference Coverage http//www.medscape.com/conferencedirectory/surgery

Young, A., Van Niekerk, C. F., Mogotlane, S. (eds.) 2003.*Nursing in disaster situations. Juta's Manual of Nursing.* Lansdowne: Juta & Co.

2 Initial assessment

Andrew Nicol

Of all the deaths from traumatic injury, 50% occur in the first two hours after injury. Twenty-five per cent occur within two days, and the remaining 25% within the next two months. The first two hours are crucial in the management of trauma patients to exclude these life-threatening injuries. It is also often the manner in which the initial resuscitation is performed that will dictate the trauma patient's eventual survival.

A management plan is essential in dealing with any injured patient and a step-wise approach is needed to avoid missing any injuries. The patients should be resuscitated according to standard ATLS® recommendations. The correct priorities are to ensure the survival of the patient, treat the individual injuries, and then to provide rehabilitation.

Priority management plan

- Blood precautions
- Survival assessment
- Primary survey:
    - **A** Airway with cervical-spine control
    - **B** Breathing
    - **C** Circulation and arrest of haemorrhage
    - **D** Disability (Neurology)
    - **E** Exposure
- Monitoring, essential X-rays, insertion of tubes, and essential bloods
- Re-assessment of the patient
- Secondary survey (history and full examination)
- Completion of X-rays and further radiological investigations
- Documentation
- Transfer to definitive care

Blood precautions

With the high prevalence of HIV/Aids in the community, it is essential to adopt precautions against possible exposure during the resuscitation. The following should be worn:
- Eyewear
- Water-impervious gown
- Gloves

Survival assessment

In order to make the diagnosis of 'Dead on arrival' (DOA), all of the following must be documented:

- No respiration
- No carotid pulse
- No cardiac activity on ECG (no pulseless electrical activity)
- Fixed dilated pupils
- No life signs in preceding 5–10 minutes
- Core temperature of more than 35 °C

A potential survivor arriving in the emergency department will be a patient with either of the following, despite the fact that there is no respiration, no carotid pulse, and the pupils are fixed and dilated:

- Pulseless electrical activity (PEA)
- Any life signs in preceding 5–10 minutes

It is important in the potential survivor that a full resuscitative attempt is undertaken.

Primary survey

The primary survey is directed at detecting those conditions from which a trauma patient will demise within minutes if not immediately identified and corrected. (Table 2.1.)

Table 2.1 Primary survey and the conditions that immediately affect outcome

Priority	Cause of death
Airway + C-spine protection	Hypoxia (airway obstruction)
	C-spine injury
Breathing	Hypoxia
	Tension pneumothorax
Circulation	Hypovolaemic shock
	Cardiac tamponade
	Aortic rupture
Disability	Head injury
Exposure	Hypothermia

A = Airway and cervical spine protection

- Call for help – another doctor/surgeon/anaesthetist.
- Perform chin lift.
- Perform jaw thrust.
- Remove any foreign debris with a suction apparatus.
- Stabilize the cervical spine with a hard cervical collar. Always presume that there is a C-spine injury until X-rays have excluded this possibility. Maintain the neck in a neutral position. A rolled-up blanket or sandbags can also be placed on either side of the neck to stabilize the cervical spine. If the patient requires intubation, then ensure that the neck is not extended.
- Perform oral intubation if any of the following are present:
  - no breathing
  - cyanosis
  - Glasgow Coma Score (GCS) ≤ 8
  - stridor
  - signs of airway obstruction (use of accessory muscles)
  - extensive facial fractures
  - evidence of an inhalation burn (peri-oral burns)

Use a size 7.0 to 7.5 endotracheal tube (ETT) for an adult female, and a size 7.5–8.0 for an adult male; the tube should be inserted to the 23 cm mark at the level of the teeth. Always confirm that the ETT has been correctly placed by using an ambubag and auscultating the chest for breath sounds. Avoid oropharyngeal airways, particularly in the conscious patient, where placement can induce vomiting and aspiration. Oropharyngeal airways are only of use in preventing an intubated patient from biting on the endotracheal tube.

A cricothyroidotomy should be performed for failed oral intubations. A nasotracheal intubation should not be attempted at this stage, as a base of skull fracture has not been excluded.

B = Breathing

In all polytrauma cases, routinely use a 40% oxygen (O_2) face-mask. If the patient is breathless, consider the following possibilities:

- Tension pneumothorax
- Open pneumothorax
- Haemothorax
- Cardiac tamponade
- Flail chest
- Pulmonary contusion
- Aspiration pneumonia
- Acute diaphragmatic herniation.

A tension pneumothorax is a clinical and not a radiological diagnosis. The patient will be breathless with decreased breath sounds on the affected side and the trachea may be pushed over to the contralateral side. The chest should be decompressed with a 14-gauge needle inserted into the second intercostal space, mid-clavicular line. This should be followed with the insertion of a chest drain.

- A flail chest may not be immediately apparent. The chest should be palpated with both hands to feel for any movement or crepitus.
- Percussion and auscultation of the chest should be performed at this stage.
- If the patient has been intubated, connect to a ventilator. Use the SIMV mode with a tidal volume of 8 ml/kg and a respiratory rate of 12 breaths per minute. Initially use an FiO_2 (inspired oxygen concentration) of 0.1 (100% O_2), but attempt to reduce this down to 0.4 (40% O_2).

C = Circulation and haemorrhage control

The first priority is to stop any bleeding. This may be achieved with direct pressure with abdominal swabs or with digital pressure. A Foley's catheter can be inserted into neck stab wounds and the bulb inflated.

Avoid placing haemostats (arterial clamps) through the wound. Blind placement can result in damage to the underlying structures, particularly nerves. Rather use elevation and pressure.

- Do not use tourniquets except where there has been a traumatic amputation. The problem with tourniquets on the limbs is that the pressure applied is generally not above systolic blood pressure. The tourniquet then cuts off all venous return from the limb but allows forward arterial flow. This will result in venous hypertension and ischaemia distal to the site of the tourniquet.
- Determine the pulse rate and blood pressure. A palpable femoral pulse implies a systolic blood pressure of at least 60 mmHg. If a brachial artery pulse is palpable, then the systolic blood pressure should be in the region of 100 mmHg.
- If the patient is shocked, set up two intravenous lines with a minimum 16-gauge intravenous cannula. Look first for venous access in the antecubital fossa. If this is not possible, attempt cannulation of the external jugular vein provided that there is no concern over a C-spine injury. A saphenous vein cut-down should be the next site attempted. In the resuscitation scenario, this should be performed on the medial aspect of the thigh. The reason for this site as opposed to the ankle, is that the vein is of a larger calibre in this region, and the venous access is less likely to be lost with movement of the limb. In the region of the femoral triangle,

the saphenous vein has numerous larger tributaries that can be damaged in the dissection. If a cut-down fails then try for the internal jugular vein, the subclavian vein, or a femoral vein push-in.

- Flow through an infusion set is governed by Poiseuille's law, which states that:

$$\text{Flow} = \frac{[\,P1 - P2\,]\,.\pi.r^4}{8\,L\eta}$$

Where $[\,P1 - P2\,]$ is the pressure difference between the fluid in the bag and the outflow pressure in the vein; r is the radius of the tubing, L is the length of the tubing and η is the viscosity of the fluid. Halving the radius of a cannula will result in a $16\times$ reduction in flow. (See Table 2.2.)

- The rapid infusion of fluid will require a high-pressure gradient (pressure bag) and an administration set and cannula of wide bore and short length. Ensure that a high-capacity blood administration set is used for resuscitations.

- In shocked patients, administer 2 litres of *warmed* Modified Ringer's lactate as rapidly as possible. If the patient remains shocked, he/she will require emergency blood. In the transient and non-responders to fluid management, always consider whether another cause for shock is present. If the peripheries are warm, this is not hypovolaemic shock. If there is any doubt as to the nature of the shock that is present, then insert a central venous pressure catheter (CVP). Always confirm that the tip of the CVP catheter is in the superior vena cava. If the patient has a low systolic blood pressure but a high CVP reading, this implies that the shock is due to a cardiogenic or neurogenic cause. Look for distended neck veins and auscultate the heart for muffled heart sounds.

- Watch the amount of crystalloid used in the resuscitation area and remember that each litre will drop the haemoglobin level by 1.5 g%.

- In the case of penetrating hypovolaemic cardiac arrest, a thoracotomy and internal cardiac massage is required.

Table 2.2 Flow rates with respect to cannula size

Gauge	Diameter of cannula (mm)	Flow rate ml/minute
14	2.1	330
16	1.7	205
18	1.3	95
24	0.7	20

D = Disability (brief neurological evaluation)
- Perform a quick evaluation of the patient's Glasgow Coma Score.
- Check pupillary size and reaction.

E = Exposure
- Completely undress the patient and prevent hypothermia.

Monitoring, essential X-rays, and tubes

Monitors
The following monitors should be attached:
- Cardiac leads
- Non-invasive blood-pressure cuff
- O_2 saturation meter

Essential X-rays
The essential X-rays to be performed at this stage are those that may dramatically alter the management. In the polytrauma patient, this will consist of a C-spine, chest X-ray (CXR), and pelvis. In a patient with a penetrating chest injury, the only essential X-ray will be a CXR. The remaining X-rays should be obtained only after the secondary survey.

Tubes
- Insert an orogastric tube. A nasogastric tube (NGT) may be inserted if there is obviously no base of skull fracture.
- Insert an urinary catheter (provided there is no blood at urethral meatus). If a urethral injury is suspected, a supra-pubic catheter must be placed.

Bloods
The following are essential blood tests at this point:
- Arterial blood gas (ABG) if ventilated
- Blood glucose on finger-prick
- Haemoglobin
- Cross-match

Reassessment of the patient's condition

Reassess the airway, breathing, and circulation. Ensure that the airway is intact, oxygenation is adequate, and that the blood pressure has normalized. The following sources of blood loss should be considered if the patient remains shocked:
- Haemothorax (exclude on the CXR)

- Ruptured thoracic aorta (look for a widened mediastinum)
- Intra-abdominal injury (perform a diagnostic peritoneal lavage in the unconscious patient or an ultrasound in the resuscitation room)
- Pelvic fracture (look at the pelvic X-ray to exclude)
- Femoral shaft fracture
- Onto the floor from lacerations/incised wounds

Haemostatic surgery may be required at this stage to control blood loss. Control surgery consists of the following:
- Thoracotomy
- Laparotomy
- Pelvic stabilization with an exoskeleton

Secondary survey

History

Obtain a history from the ambulance personnel or family.
Enquire about:
- The time of the accident and the mechanism involved
- Any medication taken by the patient
- Whether the patient has any allergies
- Past medical history of patient
- Whether the patient is pregnant
- The time of the last meal

Examination (head-to-toe)

Perform a complete head-to-toe examination:

Head:	Scalp lacerations	*Abdomen*:	Distention
	Obvious fractures		Tenderness
Eyes:	Hyphaema		Signs of peritonism
	Lens dislocation	*Musculoskeletal*:	
	Foreign body		Contusion
	Penetrating injury		Deformity
	Visual acuity		Tenderness
Face:	Maxillofacial trauma		Palpation pelvic ring
	Mandibular fracture		Thoracic/lumbar
	Dento-alveolar fracture		vertebrae
Nose:	CSF leak		Peripheral pulses
Ears:	Haemotympanum	*Rectal*:	PR examination
	CSF otorrhoea		Blood
Neck:	C-spine tenderness		Anal tone
	Elevated JVP (jugular venous pressure)		High-riding prostate

Chest: Flail segment   *Neurological*:
        Rib fractures (palpate)   Sensation
        Surgical emphysema   Weakness
        Breath and heart sounds   Paralysis

- Examine with hands and eyes. Palpate for rib fractures, subcutaneous emphysema, crepitus, and stability of the pelvis.
- All penetrating neck wounds must be covered with an occlusive dressing. Do not allow the patient to sit up as an air embolism may occur.
- Check for a medic alert bracelet.
- Always log-roll the patient at the end of the secondary survey, whilst maintaining protection of the cervical spine, and look for injury on the back. This is vital to avoid missing any injuries. When the patient has been turned, a rectal examination should be performed.
- A rectal probe should be inserted and the core temperature determined.

Endpoints of the resuscitation
The following parameters indicate that the resuscitation has been completed:
- Normal arterial oxygen saturation
- Normalization of blood pressure and pulse rate
- A urine output of 1 ml/kg/hour
- Normalization of the base excess
- Serum lactate level of less than or equal to 2 mmol/litre

Completion of X-rays and further investigations

Ensure that the patient is haemodynamically stable prior to the patient being transferred to another area for radiological investigations. If the patient requires haemostatic surgery as an emergency, these other investigations (i.e. CT scan of the head) should wait until after the surgery has been performed. Never send an unstable patient out of the resuscitation room unless it is to theatre.
- Complete X-rays of sites of suspected fractures.
- Pregnancy test must be performed in all women aged 12–55 years.
- Perform the following investigations if indicated:
     CT scan
     Angiogram
     IVP (intravenous pyelogram)
     Ultrasound (U/S)
     MRI (magnetic resonance imaging)
     Endoscopy

A 'single shot' IVP can be performed in the resuscitation room. In penetrating renal injuries, where the patient has an acute abdomen, the only information required is whether the patient has a functioning kidney on the opposite side to the injury. This is essential in case a nephrectomy has to be performed. 100 ml of a non-ionic, water-soluble iodinated contrast medium is injected intravenously, followed by an immediate radiograph after injection. A further film can be obtained in five minutes. Obtaining a 'single shot' IVP should not result in a major delay in getting the patient into theatre.

Documentation

It is essential to have accurate documentation of the status of the patient, what has been administered and what has been revealed on X-rays and special investigations. Always note entrance and exit wounds, and the position of any retained projectiles on X-ray. For this purpose a lateral X-ray is required.

Transfer to definitive care

Patients may be transferred to the following areas:
- Theatre for acute abdomen/fixation of fractures
- Admission to ward or an intensive care unit
- Transfer to another hospital. Doctor-to-doctor communication is vital prior to transfer

Commonly missed injuries

The following injuries are frequently missed, so be vigilant:
- Facial fractures
- Cervical spine fractures
- Spinal cord injuries
- Pelvic fracture
- Dislocated shoulder
- Fractured clavicle
- Ruptured bladder
- Hypothermia (always check core temperature if found by side of road)

Pitfalls

The following pitfalls should be avoided:
- Not undressing the patient fully.

- Assuming that a low GCS is the result of intoxication. In the unruly patient with a potential head injury, rather sedate and intubate. This will allow a CT head to be performed. If the CT scan of the head is normal, the patient can be allowed to wake up and be extubated.
- Spinal cord injuries will not develop signs of peritonism.
- Severe head injuries will also not develop an acute abdomen.
- Continuing on and on with resuscitation when surgical control is needed.
- Not turning the patient to look at the back.
- Not obtaining full C-spine views down to T1.
- Misdiagnosing neurogenic shock as hypovolaemic shock. The giveaway is warm peripheries and bradycardia.
- Sedating the head-injured patient without performing a CT scan.
- Attempting resuscitation through small cannulas.
- Sending unstable patients for CT scan or angiography.

Recommended reading

American College of Surgeons Committee on Trauma: Advanced Trauma Life Support® Course for Doctors (ATLS®). 1997. Student Manual. Sixth edition. Chicago: ACS.

Boffard, K. D. (ed.) 2003. Manual of Definitive Surgical Trauma Care. International Association for the Surgery of Trauma and Surgical Intensive Care. London: Arnold.

3 Airway management

Gerald Dalbock

Airway compromise or obstruction is a leading cause of death in severely injured patients. Furthermore, prolonged poor tissue oxygenation causes late complications in survivors, such as sepsis and multiple organ failure.

Causes of airway obstruction

The following are causes of airway obstruction:
- Solid foreign body: food, dentures, broken teeth, etc.
- Liquids: secretions, blood, vomitus, etc.
- Soft tissue swelling: oedema of soft tissues due to inhalation burns, anaphylaxis
- Unconscious states: flaccidity of muscles of tongue and mastication, loss of protective reflexes
- Trauma of airway: facial fracture, laryngeal fracture, etc.

Clinical features of airway obstruction

The following are clinical features of actual or impending airway obstruction:
- Restlessness with agitation
- Depressed level of consciousness with loss of protective reflexes
- Severe facial trauma
- Obstructive sounds: stridor, gurgling, snoring
- Chest wall recessions: suprasternal, supraclavicular, intercostal, sternal, subcostal
- Paradoxical movement of chest and abdomen
- Tracheal tug and use of accessory muscles
- Apnoea
- Cyanosis

Management of airway obstruction

Management of airway obstruction is based on the following principles.

Protect the C-spine

Maintain head and cervical spine in neutral alignment and ask assistant to stabilize the patient's head.

Clear the airway

- Inspect the mouth and pharynx.
- Use a laryngoscope blade as illuminated tongue depressor.
- Use Magill forceps and a rigid suction catheter to remove foreign material.
- Beware of precipitating a cough or gag reflex.

Protect the airway

If the patient has no protective airway reflexes:
- Apply cricoid pressure immediately to prevent aspiration.
- Do not press on thyroid cartilage or tracheal rings, as airway occlusion will occur.

If vomiting occurs:
- Stop cricoid pressure immediately (to prevent oesophageal rupture).
- Log-roll patient into lateral position as a single unit, ensuring C-spine control.
- Remove foreign material from mouth using spatula and suction.

Maintain the airway

- Apply chin-lift or anterior jaw-thrust manoeuvre.
- Do not do a head tilt in a trauma victim.
- If poor or no gag reflex present, insert oropharyngeal airway.
- If poor or no gag reflex present and patient is clenching the jaw, insert nasopharyngeal airway.
- Do not use nasopharyngeal airway if base of skull or facial fractures are suspected.

Assess and manage breathing

If breathing is adequate, administer supplementary O_2 (60–100% using non-rebreather mask at 10–12 ℓ/min).

If breathing is inadequate:
- Use bag valve mask device (BVM) to ventilate the patient.
- Ensure that the reservoir is attached to O_2 flow at a rate of 12–15 ℓ/min for adults.

If the patient is adequately ventilated and oxygenated but airway is not yet secure, intubate the patient.

Table 3.1 Advanced airway management

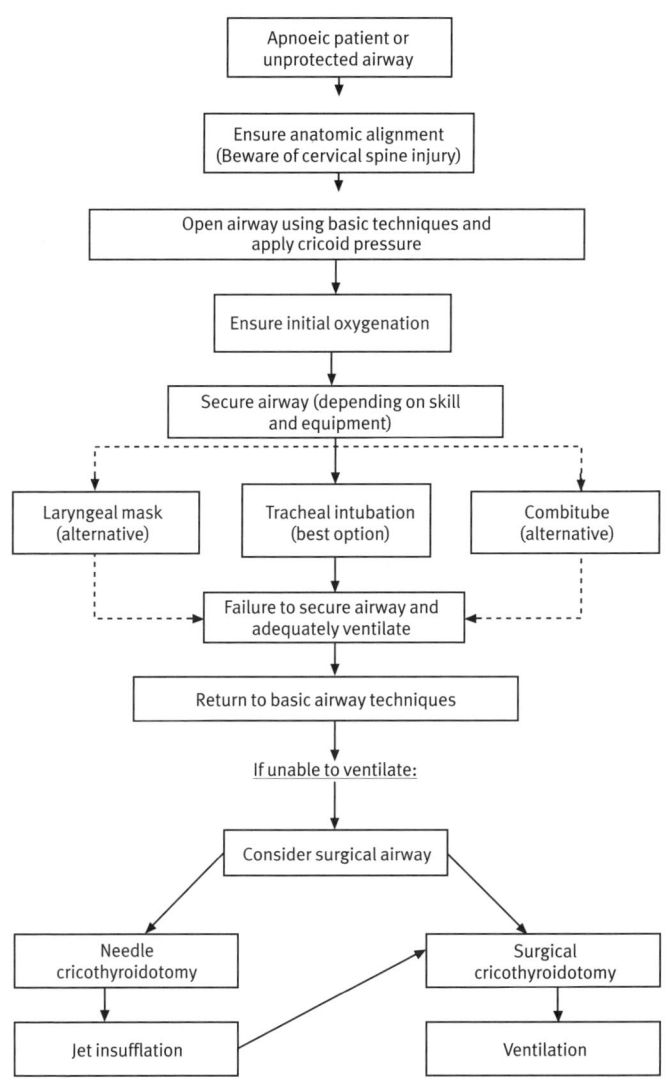

If unable to intubate, consider alternative airway techniques (laryngeal mask or Combitube).

If unable to ventilate and intubate:

- Return to basic airway techniques with BVM ventilation.
- Consider causes: incorrect technique, equipment failure, short neck, total occlusive foreign body airway obstruction, inhalation burns, anaphylaxis with laryngeal oedema, laryngeal carcinoma, facial and airway trauma, infective processes.

If able to ventilate and maintain airway by means of basic airway technique, but airway is not secure, prepare for urgent tracheostomy in theatre. If unable to ventilate at all, because of total airway obstruction, proceed to emergency surgical airway.

Emergency airway

Needle cricothyroidotomy with jet insufflation:
- Can provide oxygenation (but not ventilation) for up to 40 minutes.
- Will need a surgical cricothyroidotomy or tracheostomy to follow.
- CO_2 retention can occur.

Surgical cricothyroidotomy. Surgical cricothyroidotomy is a definitive airway that can be used to ventilate the patient prior to a tracheostomy.

Airway management procedures

Trauma chin lift

- Immobilize the head of the patient to prevent C-spine movement.
- Pull the mandible anteriorly by grasping the chin and lower incisors.

Trauma jaw thrust

- Place hands on either side of the patient's head with patient in supine position.
- Maintain in-line C-spine control with light traction.
- Displace mandible forwards with index and middle fingers.
- Provide counter-pressure by pushing the thenar eminences on the maxillary areas.
- Press thumbs caudally to open the mouth.

Insertion of oropharyngeal airway

- Size: measure from corner of mouth to posterior aspect of angle of mandible.

- Do not insert in conscious patient as gagging, vomiting, and aspiration could occur.
- Displace tongue anteriorly using tongue depressor or laryngoscope blade.
- Suction with catheter and remove solid foreign material with Magill forceps.
- Insert airway along the posterior contour of the tongue.
- Insert to the depth that the flange touches the lips.
- Once sited correctly, remove tongue depressor or laryngoscope blade.
- Check airway patency and breathing.
- Provide supplemental oxygen or ventilate if required.

Insertion of nasopharyngeal airway

Nasopharyngeal airways are uncuffed tubes made of soft rubber or plastic. They are used for intoxicated or semiconscious patients who are jaw

Figure 3.1 Jaw thrust

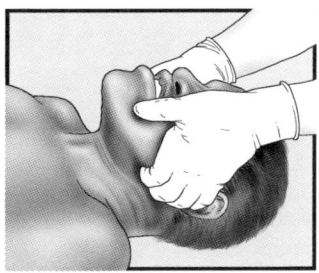

Figure 3.2 Oropharyngeal airway

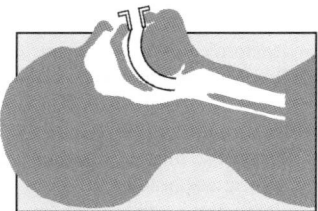

Figure 3.3 Nasopharyngeal airway

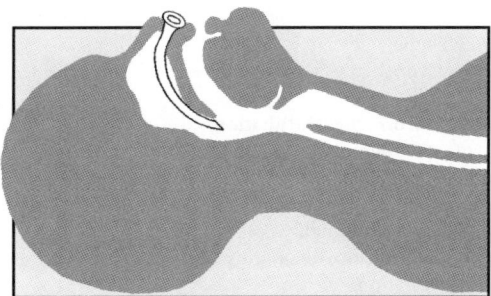

clenching or cannot tolerate an oropharyngeal airway. They are less likely to induce gagging, vomiting, and aspiration. Note the following:

- Do not insert if base of skull fracture is suspected.
- Measure from tip of nose to posterior aspect of angle of mandible.
- Ensure that the diameter of the tube matches the diameter of the patient's little finger.
- Lubricate the tube with water-soluble lubricant.
- Insert the tip of the airway into one nostril close to the midline along the floor of the nose.
- Note that the airway must be directed posteriorly until the tip is in the pharynx.
- Never force the airway in.
- Check airway patency and breathing.
- Provide supplemental oxygen or ventilate if required.

Endotracheal intubation

Indications

- Cardiorespiratory arrest
- Apnoea
- Airway compromise or obstruction
- Unconscious states: GCS ≤ 8
- Anatomical disruption of airway
- Respiratory failure with need for elective ventilation

Benefits of intubation

- *Airway*: definitive airway control and protection from gastric inflation, regurgitation, and aspiration.
- *Breathing*: control of ventilation, inspired O_2 concentration and tidal volume.
- *Circulation*: improved cardiac output if CPR is required, as asynchronous compression/ventilation technique can be used.
- *Drugs*: adrenaline, atropine, lignocaine, and naloxone can be administered via ET tube.
- *Evacuation*: bronchial secretions can be effectively suctioned.

Preparation for orotracheal intubation

- Ensure adequate ventilation and oxygenation using basic airway techniques.
- Ensure that there is a cardiac output; if not, initiate CPR.
- Maintain C-spine immobilization.
- If patient is unconscious, maintain cricoid pressure to prevent regurgitation and aspiration.

- Attach ECG monitor and pulse oximeter.
- Ensure adequate pre-oxygenation.
- Site IV line (time permitting).
- Check laryngoscope handle and batteries.
- Connect appropriate laryngoscope blade and check that bulb is working. Curved blade for adults (size 3–4), straight blade for infants (size 0–1).
- Choose appropriate endotracheal tube:

Newborn	± 2.5–3.5 mm internal diameter
Infant	± 4 mm internal diameter
2 year old	± 5 mm internal diameter
>2 years	($1/4$ age in years) + 4 = mm internal diameter
Adult female	± 7–7 $1/2$ mm internal diameter
Adult male	± 8–8 $1/2$ mm internal diameter

- On average the external diameter of the tube must match the patient's little finger.
- Do not use cuffed tubes in children younger than 8–10 years of age.
- If a cuffed tube is used, check the functionality of the cuff and the one-way valve.
- Deflate the cuff prior to intubating.
- Place an introducer inside the tube to stiffen it if necessary.
- Ensure that the tip of the introducer does not protrude through the tip of the tube because laryngeal injury will result. Introducer should be lubricated with saline for ease of removal.
- Have an assistant maintain in-line C-spine control.
- Remove oropharyngeal airway and false teeth (if not already done).
- Most patients can be safely intubated with small doses of midazolam or etomidate as sedation.

Technique of orotracheal intubation
- Grasp the laryngoscope in the left hand.
- Insert the laryngoscope blade into the right-hand side of the patient's mouth. Beware of lacerating the lower lip between the blade and lower teeth.
- Guide the blade along the curvature of the tongue while displacing the tongue to the left.
- If any secretions are present, suction under direct vision. Remove solid material with Magill forceps.
- For curved blade: when the epiglottis is visualized, slide the tip of the blade into the vallecula anterior to the epiglottis.
- For straight blade: when the epiglottis is visualized, slide the tip of the blade posterior to the epiglottis.

- Displace the laryngoscope antero-superiorly at a 45-degree angle, lifting the tongue and mandible forward. Do not use the upper teeth as a fulcrum, as dental damage will occur.
- Identify the vocal cords and gently pass the tube through the open cords into the trachea.
- Note depth of tube – vocal cord marker at cords and upper end of cuff ± 1.5–2 cm below cords.
- Inflate the cuff with enough air to provide an adequate seal. Do not over inflate, as tracheal necrosis will occur.
- Remove laryngoscope from mouth and connect bag valve device to universal connector to ventilate patient and check tube placement.
- Ventilate and observe chest clinically to check equal chest expansion bilaterally.
- Auscultate chest and epigastrium with a stethoscope to assess proper tube placement.
- Check tube placement using end tidal CO_2 or oesophageal detector device.
- If tube is correctly placed, secure and tie the tube in place to prevent dislodgement.
- Place oropharyngeal airway next to endotracheal tube, to act as a bite block.
- Pass orogastric or nasogastric tube to decompress the stomach and prevent diaphragmatic splinting.
- Check oxygen saturation, pulse oximetry, and heart rate to assess clinical status.

NB: Intubation should not take longer than 30 seconds in an apnoeic

Figure 3.4 Laryngoscope placement

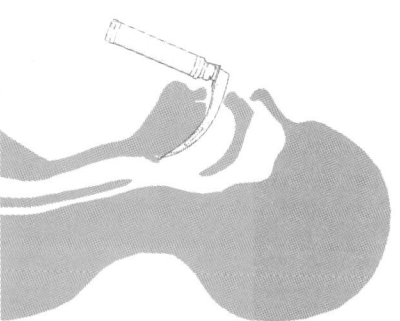

Figure 3.5 View of cords

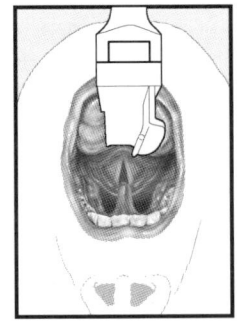

patient. If the intubation is taking too long, ventilate the patient between attempts. The patient should not be apnoeic for longer than 30 seconds at a time.

- A chest X-ray may be useful post-intubation.
- The tube placement must regularly be re-assessed, especially after moving the patient.

Nasotracheal intubation

Nasotracheal intubation is indicated only for patients who are breathing spontaneously, and contraindicated in the presence of severe midface fractures and skull-base fractures.

- Perform C-spine control, pre-oxygenation, and equipment check as for orotracheal intubation.
- Spray nasal passage with anaesthetic and a vasoconstrictor.
- Place lubricated tube into nostril and gently advance slightly upward (past inferior turbinate) and then posteriorly into the nasopharynx.
- As the tip of the tube moves down the pharynx, listen to the sound of breathing via the tube. At the point where airflow is most prominent, wait for inspiration, and then advance tube rapidly through the cords.
- Inflate cuff, ventilate and oxygenate, check placement position and secure the tube, as for orotracheal intubation.

Complications of endotracheal intubation
Take note of the following complications:

- Fracture of incisor teeth
- Damage to root of tongue
- Intubation of right main bronchus
- Oesophageal intubation
- Tube size too large with subluxation of arytenoid cartilage
- Perforation of larynx with introducer
- Avulsion of vocal cords
- Oral or nasal mucosal tears
- Tube size too small with air leak or increased resistance to airflow
- Overinflation of cuff causing tracheal necrosis
- Underinflation of cuff causing aspiration
- Obstruction of tube due to secretions
- Kinking of tube
- Unintentional extubation
- Laryngospasm
- Bradycardia
- Exacerbation of spinal injury
- Vomiting with aspiration

Sudden deterioration of the intubated patient.
Always think of DOPES:

D   Displacement into right main bronchus or oesophagus
O   Obstruction due to mucus, blood, kinked tube, etc.
P   Pneumothorax or tension pneumothorax
E   Equipment failure or tube that is too small
S   Stomach: gastric distension with diaphragmatic splinting

Rapid sequence induction

This technique is not without risk and the user must be trained in the technique. It is indicated in a patient who requires a secure airway and is difficult to intubate because of uncooperative behaviour (head injury, hypoxia, hypotension, or intoxication).

Technique

- Check all drugs and equipment.
- Attach ECG monitor and pulse oximeter.
- Establish IV line.
- Pre-oxygenate patient with 100% oxygen. Ventilate if ventilation is inadequate. Assistant applies cricoid pressure if patient is unconscious.
- Protect the cervical spine and maintain in-line C-spine control.
- Premedicate with atropine and analgesic spray if appropriate.
- Give a sedative agent to provide sedation/hypnosis, e.g. thiopentone, midazolam, ketamine, etomidate, etc. (consider indications/contra-indications).
- Follow induction immediately with a muscle relaxant, e.g. succinyl-choline 1.0 mg/kg IV.
- When the patient is sufficiently relaxed, intubate and inflate the cuff. Cricoid pressure must be applied until the cuff is inflated.
- Treat bradycardia during intubation (if vagally induced) with 0.5 mg atropine IV (use smaller doses for children).
- Check tube position and if correctly placed, tie it in while ventilating.

Laryngeal Mask Airway (LMA)

An LMA is an adjunctive airway device composed of a tube with a cuffed mask-like projection at the distal end. With proper cleaning and storage, the LMA may be re-used. The LMA is available in a range of pediatric and adult sizes. It is useful in situations where appropriate positioning of the patient for endotracheal intubation is impossible.

Figure 3.6 Positioning of the Laryngeal Mask Airway (LMA)

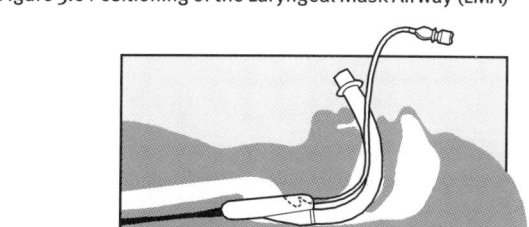

Technique of insertion

- The LMA is introduced into the pharynx and advanced until it 'seats itself', i.e. resistance is felt as the distal portion of the tube with its cuff locates in the hypopharynx.
- There is no need for laryngoscopy with cord visualization during insertion.
- Once 'seated', the cuff is then inflated, which creates a seal around the laryngeal opening.
- The distal opening of the tube is now located above the glottic opening, providing a clear secure airway.

Oesophageal-tracheal double lumen airway (Combitube)

This is an invasive double-lumen airway with two inflatable cuffs that is inserted blindly. Assessment of the location is then made and the patient is ventilated through the appropriate external opening. One lumen has a distal open end with a cuff similar to an endotracheal tube. The second lumen ends blindly above the first lumen cuff but has ventilation side holes at the hypopharyngeal level. It has a large pharyngeal cuff proximally.

The device should not be used in patients:

- Younger than 16 years of age
- Where there is an intact gag reflex
- With known oesophageal disease
- With recent ingestion of caustic substances

Insertion of the double lumen airway (Combitube)

- Blindly insert the tube until the alveolar markers on the tube are aligned with the front teeth.
- Using a large syringe, inflate the pharyngeal cuff with ± 100 ml of air. The cuff should seat itself in the posterior pharynx behind the hard palate.
- Using a small syringe, inflate the distal cuff with ± 15 ml of air.
- The device will generally be located in the patient's oesophagus (80% of insertions).
- Ventilate through the longer oesophageal tube (the air will exit through the side holes). If auscultation of breath sounds is positive and gastric insufflation is negative, continue ventilating. Assess for adequate chest movement.
- If auscultation of breath sounds is negative, and gastric insufflation is positive, the tube has been placed in the trachea. Immediately change the ventilation device to ventilate via the shorter tracheal connector.
- Re-auscultate to confirm adequate ventilation.
- Once ventilation is adequate, secure the tube by tying it in place.

Needle cricothyroidotomy

Needle cricothyroidotomy with jet insufflation through the cricothyroid membrane can provide a temporary means of oxygenating a person with complete or partial airway obstruction. This may be necessary after failed attempts at definitive airway care and an inability to ventilate the patient using basic techniques. The patient can be successfully oxygenated for up to 40 minutes. While this is being done, equipment and staff can be arranged for more advanced invasive airway procedures.

Figure 3.7 Double lumen airway (Combitube)

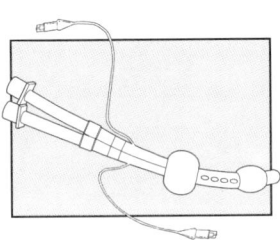

Figure 3.8 Placement of the double lumen tube

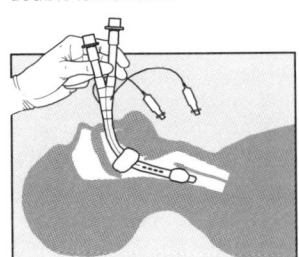

Needle cricothyroidotomy technique
See chapter on emergency surgical procedures.

Surgical cricothyroidotomy

Surgical cricothyroidotomy with ventilation through the cricothyroid membrane can provide a means of ventilating a person with complete or partial airway obstruction.

This could be necessary after failed attempts at definitive airway care and an inability to ventilate the patient using basic techniques. While this is being done, equipment and staff can be arranged for more advanced invasive airway procedures.

Surgical cricothyroidotomy technique
See chapter on emergency surgical procedures.

Oxygen delivery devices

Nasal cannula

A nasal cannula is a low-flow system to provide inspired oxygen when the patient is breathing spontaneously.
- Percentage inspired O_2 depends on flow rate and patient's tidal volume.
- At 1 l/min, it provides 24% O_2.
- Increasing the O_2 flow by 1 l/min will increase the inspired oxygen concentration by approximately 4% to a maximum of 44% at 6 l/min.

Simple face mask

The simple face mask delivers 40–60% oxygen at flow rates of 6–10 l/min.

Face mask with oxygen reservoir

The face mask with oxygen reservoir delivers 60–100% oxygen at flow rates of 6–10 l/min.

Venturi mask

The mask accurately controls the proportions of inspired oxygen. It is useful in patients with chronic hypercarbia and moderate hypoxemia.

Principles of ventilatory assistance

Ventilatory volumes with BVM ventilation

Tidal volume for adults is 10–15 ml/kg if ventilating with room air. If 100% oxygen is used, reduce tidal volume to 6–8 ml/kg.

Ventilation rate with BVM ventilation

- Inspiratory time:

Infant	1 second
Child	1–1$^1/_2$ seconds
Adult	1$^1/_2$–2 seconds

  If the patient is intubated, shorter inspiratory times can be used.
  Ventilatory rate:

Infant	30–60 breaths per minute
Toddler	24–40 breaths per minute
Preschooler	22–34 breaths per minute
School age	18–30 breaths per minute
Adolescent	12–16 breaths per minute
Adult	12–16 breaths per minute

  Expiratory time should be at least equal to inspiratory time. Preferably the expiration should be twice the length of inspiration.

Co-ordination of ventilation with chest compressions

- If CPR is being done on the patient and a definitive airway has not yet been placed to secure the airway, compressions and ventilations *must* be synchronized.
- Do not ventilate while doing chest compressions, as the air will enter the oesophagus causing gastric distension with regurgitation and aspiration.
- Once the airway has been secured with a cuffed endotracheal tube, asynchronous ventilation and chest compressions can be done, and the cardiac output generated will improve.

BVM ventilation with 100% oxygen

- If ventilation with 100% oxygen is desired, a reservoir bag must be attached to the room air port at the rear of the bag. If this is not done, the patient will receive 40–60% oxygen only.
- The wall oxygen flow rate must be such that the reservoir bag is constantly distended.
- This requires a flow rate of ± 12–15 ℓ/min for an adult male at normal tidal volumes and ventilation rate.

Adult ventilator settings immediately after intubation

- SIMV (synchronized intermittent mandatory ventilation) is the most versatile mode if available.
- Respiratory rate at 12–16 depending on pCO_2.
- Tidal volume 7–10 ml/kg (lean body weight).
- FiO_2 initially 0.1 (100% O_2), adjust down as soon as possible.
- PEEP (positive end-expiratory pressure) +3 to +5 cm H_2O.

Pitfalls

Oropharyngeal airway

- Inappropriate placement could push tongue back and occlude airway.
- Vomiting or laryngospasm could be precipitated in conscious patients.
- Wrong size tube may abut against the tongue or push epiglottis over the larynx.
- The oropharyngeal airway does not protect against aspiration.

Nasopharyngeal airway

- Incorrect insertion will injure nasal mucosa with subsequent haemorrhage.
- Vomiting and laryngospasm may be precipitated.
- The nasopharyngeal airway does not protect against aspiration.
- Too long an airway may enter the oesophagus with subsequent gastric insufflation.

Laryngeal Mask Airway (LMA)

Although the LMA does not ensure absolute protection against regurgitation and aspiration, it provides better protection than bag valve mask ventilation on its own.

Bag-valve-mask ventilation

- Failure to check equipment prior to use: check bag and valves. Check mask sizes and cuffs.
- Pressure relief valves (pop-off valves): if pop-off valve is present, note the pressure limit and know how to activate or deactivate the valve. If chest is not moving while ventilating and the valve is venting, close the valve and ventilate the patient.
- Excessive resistance to ventilation may be due to tube obstruction, developing pneumothorax, tension pneumothorax, bronchospasm,

pulmonary oedema, displaced tube, lung pathology, patient fighting ventilation, etc. Find the cause and treat appropriately.

- Inadequate mask seal while ventilating: best to use two persons to ventilate; one to maintain airway (jaw thrust with oropharyngeal airway inserted), keep spine in neutral alignment and seal the mask to the face, and the second person to squeeze the bag – ensuring delivery of appropriate tidal volumes – while applying cricoid pressure.

- Not maintaining and protecting victim's airway: if the patient is unconscious and a definitive airway has not yet been placed, use an oropharyngeal airway, jaw thrust, and apply cricoid pressure. Place a definitive airway, i.e. endotracheal tube, laryngeal mask, or Combitube as soon as possible.

Recommended reading

Guidelines 2000 for cardiopulmonary resuscitation and emergency cardiovascular care. Supplement to *Circulation*, Vol 102, Number 8, Aug 22, 2000.

PALS Provider Manual, Pediatric Advanced Life Support course, American Heart Association, 2002.

4 Shock and fluid therapy

André Potgieter

Shock can be defined as a state of inadequate cellular perfusion and oxygenation, leading to anaerobic metabolism and acidosis. If left untreated, progressive shock will lead to cell damage, organ failure, and death. The treatment of shock should therefore aim to correct cellular oxygenation and re-establish aerobic metabolism, and not merely to improve measured blood pressure.

This chapter will focus on types of shock associated with trauma patients.

Classification of shock

Hypovolaemic:
 Haemorrhagic shock
 Plasma/extracellular fluid loss
Cardiogenic:
 Myocardial infarction
 Myocardial contusion
Distributive:
 Septic shock
 Anaphylactic shock
 Neurogenic shock
 Acute adrenal insufficiency
Obstructive:
 Mediastinal compression
 Cardiac tamponade
 Tension pneumothorax
Other:
 Air embolism

Physiological parameters of circulation

Cardiac output (CO)

- Cardiac output is determined by preload (PL), afterload (AL) (impedance), heart rate (HR), and cardiac contractility.

  $CO = HR \times SV$ (stroke volume)

   $= 60/min \times 75\,ml$

   $= 5\,litres/min$

- CO should be optimized as part of achievement of optimal oxygen delivery.
- CO is measured by a thermodilution technique utilizing a Swan-Ganz catheter. This is seldom required in the acutely injured patient.
- Normal values:

Right atrial pressure RP (CVP)	2–8 mm Hg
Right ventricular pressure (RVP)	S: 20–30 mmHg, D: < RAP
Pulmonary artery pressure (PAP)	S: 20–30 mmHg
	D:5–15 mmHg
Pulmonary capillary wedge pressure (PCWP)	2–12 mmHg. Must be diastolic
Cardiac output (CO)	4–6 litre/min
SvO_2 (venous oxygen saturation)	65–75%

Preload

Preload is an estimate of ventricular end-diastolic volume (EDV), and is equivalent to end-diastolic pressure (EDP). The central venous pressure (CVP) is the EDP of the right ventricle (RV) and is dependent on the EDV of the right ventricle. Similarly, the pulmonary capillary wedge pressure (PCWP) is the EDP of the left ventricle (LV), and is representative of the EDV of the left ventricle.

According to the Starling curve, maximal CO (or SV) is achieved at an optimal filling pressure (PCWP) of about 18 to 22 mmHg. The higher the filling pressure (PCWP), the higher the EDV.

As the heart is a functional unit between right and left side, the CVP and PCWP are linked and changes will occur simultaneously. Therefore, an increase in preload should lead to an improved cardiac output.

Generally, a low CVP reflects a low intravascular volume and will be accompanied by low PAWP and low preload.

> This volume/pressure relationship is valid in the absence of valvular disease, pulmonary hypertension, intracardiac shunt, cardiac tamponade, etc. and is not applicable in LV ischaemia, infarction, severe sepsis and cardiomyopathy. Should a right to left heart discordance be present, the CVP measurement would not allow accurate prediction of PCWP.

Afterload

Afterload (AL) refers to the left ventricular wall tension required to overcome the resistance (impedance) to the ejection of blood from the ventricle during systole. This outflow impedance is in fact the systemic vascular resistance (SVR).

SVR = (MAP-CVP) × 80 = 800–1 200 dyne.sec/cm
SVR is the vascular tone, i.e. the degree of vasoconstriction or vasodilatation in the peripheral circulation.

Cardiac contractility

- Cardiac contractility is an indication of the ability to pump blood from the ventricle.
- It is a measure of the velocity and power of myocardial fibre shortening during systole.
- The Frank-Starling curve describes the relationship between the optimal stretch length of a muscle fibre, and the power of contraction.
- As EDV determines the lengthening (or stretch) of the muscle, volume (CVP/PACWP) can be substituted for length. Optimum volume therefore equates to optimum contractility of the muscle.
- Contractility is difficult to measure since the afterload has a direct impact as well. Indirect methods include ejection fraction (echocardiography or radio-isotope) and calculation of the LVSW (left ventricular stroke work).
- To improve contractility:
  Increase preload
  Reduce afterload
  Add inotropic support

Oxygen delivery (DO_2)

- Factors that influence the delivery of oxygen to the cell are haemoglobin (Hb), arterial oxygen saturation (SaO_2), arterial partial pressure of oxygen (PaO_2), heart rate (HR), preload (PL), afterload (AL), and contractility.
- DO_2= CO × CaO_2 x 10 = 900–1 000 ml/min
  CaO_2 = arterial oxygen content = (Hb × 1.37 × SaO_2) + (0.003 × PaO) = 22 ml/dl.
- SaO_2 (arterial oxygen saturation), PaO_2 (arterial partial pressure of oxygen), and Hb (haemoglobin) are obtained from the blood gas profile.

Cellular absorption of oxygen (VO_2)

- To determine if DO_2 is adequate to satisfy tissue needs, an independent measure of cellular absorption of oxygen (VO_2) is helpful.
- VO_2 = CO x (CaO_2–CO_2) × 10
  Where CO_2 = mixed venous oxygen content in blood returning to the heart = (Hb × 1.37 × SvO_2) + (0.003 × PvO_2) = 250 ml/min
- PvO_2 and SvO_2 are obtained from blood drawn from a pulmonary Swan-Ganz catheter.
- Thus: DO_2–VO_2 = 750 ml/min: which is the O_2 reserve under normal conditions.

O₂ Supply and demand balance

$CaO_2 - CvO_2 = C(a-v)O_2 = 4-6$ ml/dl.

Assessment of the shocked patient

Assessment of the shocked patient follows the ABC system as with all injured patients:

- Establish a secure airway while protecting the cervical spine. Profoundly shocked patients may require endotracheal intubation.
- Examine the chest, assess breathing for signs of haemothorax or tension pneumothorax, check for rib fracture and significant blunt chest trauma, obtain a chest X-ray, arterial oxygen saturation, and arterial blood gas profile. Place intercostal drainage tube if required.
- Assess circulation: pulse rate, skin- and cerebral perfusion, blood pressure, etc., and control external bleeding if present.
- Obtain vascular access by rapidly inserting two large-bore cannulas (≥16 gauge) into the cubital fossae, provided there is no proximal fracture. Saphenous vein cutdowns, intra-osseous needles or large-bore high-flow central (femoral, jugular, or subclavian) venous catheters may be useful if the upper limbs are not accessible. Secure well.
- Administer 2 litres of warmed Ringer's lactate rapidly. Pressure-pump warming devices can deliver 1–2 litres fluid or blood per minute if required. Monitor ECG, pulse, blood pressure, oxygen saturation, and urine output.

Table 4.1 Haemodynamic profiles of different types of shock

Type of shock	Pulm. art. wedge pressure (PAWP)	Cardiac output (CO)	Systemic vascular resistance (SVR)
Cardiogenic	↑↑	↓	↑
Hypovolaemic	↓	↓	↑
Distributive: Septic Neurogenic Anaphylactic	↓ or N	↑, N, ↓	↓
Obstructive: Tamponade Tension pneumo Pulm embolus	↑ ↑, N, ↓ ↓, N	↓ ↓ ↓	↑ ↑ ↑

- Categorize the patient as a responder, transient responder, or a non-responder, according to the response to IV fluid administration. This will assist with the diagnostic and therapeutic decision-making process.

Normalization of peripheral perfusion, pulse, and blood pressure will indicate that the bleeding has stopped, whereas patients who respond transiently may have ongoing blood loss.

The primary and secondary surveys are completed with specific attention to potential sites of bleeding, such as the adominal, thoracic, or pelvic cavities, as well as non-haemorrhagic reasons for shock, such as quadriplegia, cardiac tamponade, or myocardial contusion. Oliguria may be from prerenal, intrarenal, or postrenal (obstructive) causes.

Haemorrhagic and hypovolaemic shock

These are the most common causes of shock in the trauma patient and if progressive and untreated, they will lead to cell death and multi-organ failure.

Pathophysiology

- Hypovolaemic shock is due to loss of blood, plasma, or extracellular fluid.
- The physiological response to shock is tachycardia, vasoconstriction, venoconstriction, redistribution of blood flow, and narrowed pulse pressure, due to sympathetic and adrenergic discharge.
- As compensatory mechanisms fail with ongoing volume loss, blood pressure falls, oxygen delivery decreases and lactic acidosis results.
- Eventually, cell membrane integrity is lost and sodium and water shifts into cells. Further depletion of cellular ATP leads to cell death and organ failure.

Management

Haemorrhagic shock is treated rapidly with the following measures:

- Control external bleeding.
- Administer two litres of warmed Ringer's lactate as a bolus. If there is a poor response, administer a further 2 litres warmed crystalloid or colloid solutions while obtaining blood.
- Obtain the most appropriate blood products available; fully cross-matched fresh whole blood is best, but is seldom available; fully cross-matched packed red cells are the best alternative type; specific packed red cells are mostly available; O Rh negative blood is for absolute emergencies.
- Involve the surgeon early.

- Identify non-responders immediately and treat surgically for exsanguinating haemorrhage with resuscitative laparotomy or thoracotomy.
- Rule out neurogenic or cardiogenic causes of shock.
- Note that transient responders usually allow physical examination and diagnostic investigations to determine the bleeding site, but then usually require surgical intervention.
- Improve cellular oxygenation (DO_2) by optimizing preload, afterload, cardiac output, contractility, heart rate, Hb, SaO_2, PaO_2, CaO_2.
- Note that increasing the Hb from 9 g% to 11.5 g% increases oxygen delivery by 30%, while increasing PaO_2 from 8 to 12 kPa increases oxygen saturation by only 7%.
- Prevent lactic acidosis and loss of body heat.
- Replenish fluid deficit with crystalloids, or with appropriate electrolytes in cases of depletion. The ratio of crystalloids to colloids should be 3:1.
- Use adjuncts to manage bleeding from open-book type pelvic fractures – the MAST suit, external compression garment (Pelvigrip), sling, or external fixator.
- Note that the MAST suit application carries the risk of a drop in cardiac output due to an increase in peripheral resistance, time delay to definitive treatment, and compartment syndrome of the legs.
- Use autotransfusion devices, especially for thoracic bleeding in the emergency unit, and for bleeding from elsewhere during surgical procedures.
- Note that indiscriminate laparotomy is not indicated in cases of closed pelvic fracture and severe bleeding. Consider the option of interventional radiology and embolization.

If indicated, perform resuscitative emergency department thoracotomy, with cross-clamping of the lower thoracic aorta and open cardiac massage. This may be useful for the patient in refractory shock, in order to get to the operating room for definitive surgical control of the bleeding. This procedure carries a high mortality. See chapters on damage control and vascular injuries.

Permissive hypotension

Much more evidence is now available on the controversial topic of permissive hypotension. The current trend is to limit fluid administration until the bleeding has been controlled. 'Evolving evidence suggests that aggressive fluid resuscitation prior to haemostasis leads to additional bleeding through hydraulic acceleration of haemorrhage, soft clot dissolution and dilution of clotting factors. Aggressive pre-operative fluid infusion is still

Table 4.2 Categorization of the degree of blood loss (ATLS®)

Class of shock	% Blood loss	Volume loss (ml)	Pulse rate	Blood pressure	Pulse pressure	Respira-tion/min	Urine ml/kg/hr
I	15	750	< 100	N	N	14–20	1
II	30	750–1 500	> 100	N	↑	20–30	< 1
III	40	2 000	> 120	↓	narrowed	30–40	< 0.5
IV	> 40	> 2 000	> 140	↓	narrowed	> 35	< 0.25

considered appropriate for unconscious patients without palpable blood pressure or for those with controllable haemorrhage (e.g. isolated head or extremity injury). However, the latest recommendations are to limit or delay intravenous fluid resuscitation pre-operatively in those with uncontrollable haemorrhage (e.g. those with penetrating torso injuries) even if they are hypoperfusing' (Fowler & Pepe, 2002).

Recommendations for the treatment of trauma victims in the prehospital setting are:
- Cannulation should take place en route.
- Only two attempts at cannulation should be made.
- Transfer should not be delayed by attempts to obtain access.
- Entrapped patients require cannulation on scene.
- Normal saline is recommended.
- 250 ml boluses may be titrated against the presence or absence of a radial pulse (Greaves et al. 2002).

Cardiogenic shock

Pathophysiology
- Myocardial dysfunction, as a result of heart muscle injury, restriction of ventricular filling, or diminished venous return, leads to cardiac output failure.
- Cardiac contusion is caused by blunt trauma to the chest, and is manifest by hypotension, ECG changes, arrythmias, and cardiac enzyme elevation. Myocardial infarction may be coincidental to the trauma, and will present in much the same way.
- Cardiac tamponade or tension pneumothorax are caused by mechanical factors and culminate in a reduced cardiac output. See the chapters on blunt and penetrating chest trauma.

Management

- Cardiogenic shock is treated with a careful fluid challenge, preferably while on CVP monitoring, to increase the preload. Afterload reduction may require nitrates, and inotropes may be necessary to increase the cardiac output.
- PCWP measurement with Swan-Ganz catheterization is occasionally required, and will rise sharply with a fluid challenge, with a simultaneous drop in cardiac output.
- Constant ECG monitoring for arrythmias is essential, especially in the first 24 hours post injury. Beta-blockade may be necessary.
- Cardiac tamponade may require echo-cardiographic diagnosis, but is usually clinically diagnosed on the grounds of hypotension, muffled heart sounds, distended neck veins, and a narrowed pulse pressure. Pericardiocentesis is a temporary but life-saving procedure, but does carry risks, and is not always successful. Surgery will be required.
- Tension pneumothorax is a clinical diagnosis, based on unilateral absent breath sounds, hyperresonance on percussion and tracheal deviation to the contralateral side. Treatment is immediate drainage, by needle or tube thoracostomy.

Inotrope effects: Dobutamine	↑ LVSW + ↓ SVR + ↑↑PR
Adrenaline	↑LVSW+↑SVR + ↑Coronary flow
Dopamine	↑LVSW+↑SVR+↑PR

Neurogenic shock

Pathophysiology. Neurogenic shock usually follows spinal cord injury, and is the result of loss of sympathetic vascular tone, leading to vasodilatation and hypotension. The pulse pressure is wide, the skin is dry and warm, and urine output may be normal.

Management

- Treat as for hypovolaemic shock, with a fluid challenge.
- Consider small doses of vasopressors if the hypotension persists, and the patient is oliguric or poorly perfused, centrally or peripherally. This is not indicated in the asymptomatic patient.
- Investigate the possibility of the presence of ongoing bleeding.
- Monitor CVP, as this may be helpful to prevent fluid overload.

Vasogenic (distributive) shock

Pathogenesis. Septic shock is rarely present in the initial 24 hours post-injury. Early septic shock presents with peripheral vasodilatation, increased cardiac output, and increased oxygen consumption. Patients may be relatively hypovolaemic. They soon develop multi-organ failure and death results.

Management
- Identify the cause of the infection, treat surgically if indicated, and obtain microbiological sensitivity and treatment guidelines.
- Administer the correct antibiotics.
- Optimize fluid balance, invasive monitoring is very helpful.
- Use vasopressors as required for persistent hypotension.

The crystalloid-colloid debate

It is important to understand the physiology and patient requirements in order to decide on the appropriate fluid and electrolyte management.

Crystalloids are cheap, readily available, easy to use, and safe. Colloids are more expensive and have more side-effects. Although less colloid is needed for equivalent volume effect, no class I or II evidence is available to confirm better survival with colloids. Balanced salt solutions have a half life of 20 min in circulation while gelatin remains 4–6 hrs and hetastarch up to 24 hrs in the circulation.

Hypertonic saline is a promising but potentially dangerous resuscitation fluid. Several randomized trials suggest that patients resuscitated with hypertonic saline survive longer, provided that it was given early as the initial therapy. Currently consensus dictates that hypertonic saline is best used in the management of head injuries. Hypertonic saline may be more effective when mixed with a small amount of an oncotically active molecule such as dextran. However, the response to trauma, pain, and various neuro-endocrine and hormonal pathways leads to salt and water retention following the insult. In addition, patients with cardiac or renal disease have a limited ability to excrete sodium and are susceptible to fluid overload.

Resuscitation and rapid replacement of fluid are best accomplished by a solution similar to extracellular fluid (ECF), i.e. relatively high in sodium, low in potassium, and without glucose. Ideal fluids are 0.9% NaCl, Ringer's lactate, and Plasmalyte B®. Ease of use dictates that the first two (in plastic bags) are preferred to Plasmalyte B, which is produced in a glass bottle.

The debate on the choice of crystalloid or colloid remains unanswered. Colloid solutions are supposed to remain in the intravascular compartment, whereas crystalloid solutions are distributed throughout the ECF.

Although crystalloid replacement requires three times the intravascular volume deficit, it is still favoured because of its cheapness, safety, and availability.

Colloids reverse shock more rapidly and with less volume. However, pulmonary oedema due to over-treatment is a potential threat. In addition, colloids are expensive and carry certain risks namely:

- Infection – plasma solutions
- Coagulation and cross-match difficulties – gelatins, dextrans and starches
- Allergic reactions – all.

The rationale for colloid solutions is based on the size of intercellular pores and membrane gates. These apertures are about 45 000 D in size and allow free movement of small molecules. Bigger molecules are restricted and do not pass through easily. Most colloid solutions like fresh frozen plasma (FFP), stabilized human serum (SHS), albumin, gelatins have molecules larger than 45000 D. The starch products (hetastarch, pentastarch) vary from 150 000 D to 450 000 D. Some molecules remain in circulation between 3–9 times longer but can still be transported across membranes or leak out through damaged membranes. There is concern about accumulation of such molecules in the interstitium with resultant persisting oedema. For the present, crystalloids appear to be the cheaper, safer, and easier to use fluid for resuscitation purposes.

Blood loss is managed by transfusing of blood and blood products and coagulation is corrected by using the appropriate plasma products. Blood substitutes like perfluorocarbons and bovine haemoglobin (Hemopure®) have several potential advantages, but have not gained widespread use. No cross-matching is necessary, disease transmission is not an issue, and shelf-life is extended. Haemoglobin substitutes include bovine haemoglobin and diaspirin cross-linked haemoglobin.

Intravenous fluid therapy

Aims

Fluid therapy is aimed at:

- Replacing intravascular volume
- Maintaining cardio-vascular homeostasis
- Maintaining renal function
- Maintaining normal body fluids and electrolytes

Types of intravenous fluids

Blood and blood products
Whole blood
Packed red cells
Fresh frozen plasma
Stabilized human serum
Cryo-precipitate
Platelets
Specific factors
Haemoglobin substitutes

Crystalloids
Resuscitation fluid
Rehydration fluid
Maintenance fluid
Replacement solutions
Special purpose fluids
Parenteral nutrition mixtures
Other types

Colloids
Dextran 40 10% in sodium chloride 0.9%
Dextran 70 6% in sodium chloride 0.9%
Mannitol 20%
Gelatine solutions (Gelofusine®, Haemaccel®)
Starch products (Haesteril® , Pentastarch®, Voluven®)

Crystalloid solutions
Resuscitation fluids. These fluids contains water, Na$^+$ and Cl$^-$ and are basically iso-osmolar.

They are required to treat shock where a loss of sodium and water occurs from the plasma to the interstitium.

Types:
- 0.9% sodium chloride
- Ringer's lactate
- Balanced electrolyte solution (Balsol® or Plasmalyte B®)
- 0.9% NaCl + 5% Dextrose
- Ringer's lactate + 5% Dextrose

Rehydration fluids. Dehydration occurs with diminished water intake and/or excessive loss of water.

It presents with marked thirst, dry mucous membranes, diminished urine output, and urine concentration.

Types of solutions:
- General rehydration
- Dextrose 5%
- $^1/_2$ Dextrose Darrows (paediatric)

Maintenance fluids. Requirements depend on basic metabolic rate and this is altered by shock, major trauma, multi-organ failure, burns, etc. Normal daily water requirement = 2 500 – 3 000 ml/day.

Types of fluid:
- Maintelyte5%®
- Electrolyte no 2®
- Neonatalyte® (paediatric)

Replacement fluid. This is used to correct existing body fluid deficits and replace ongoing losses, e.g. gastric drainage.

Types of fluid:
- General replacement solution
- 5% Dextrose Darrows (paediatric)

Special solutions
- Sodium bicarbonate 4.2%
- Sodium chloride 0.45%
- Sodium chloride 5%
- Sodium chloride 0.45% + 5% Dextrose

The third-space effect

This effect occurs due to tissue damage where isotonic fluid is lost from the functional body compartments to non-functional ones. It remains seques-trated in the interstitium for days, causing oedema.

Replacement guidelines
- Minimal derangement – no replacement required
- Minor trauma   –1–2 ml/kg/hr
- Moderate trauma   –2–4 ml/kg/hr
- Major trauma   –4–6 ml/kg/hr

Pitfalls

- Not recognizing early signs of shock: tachycardia, narrowed pulse pressure, confusion, and oliguria.
- Not maintaining intravascular volume in obstructive shock.
- Not recognizing that the initial approach to septic shock, neurogenic shock, and cardiogenic shock is fluid therapy.
- Not recognizing that intravascular volume must be optimized before loop diuretics are used in patients with oliguria.
- Positive end-expiratory pressures (PEEP) and positive-pressure ventilation (PPV) affect the interpretation of these values.

References and recommended reading

Fowler, R., Pepe, P. E. 2002. Fluid resuscitation of the patient with major trauma. *Current Opinion in Anaesthesiology,* April, 15:173–178.

Greaves, I., Porter, K. M., Revell, M. P. 2002. Matter for debate – Fluid resuscitation in pre-hospital trauma care: A consensus view. *Journal of the Royal College of Surgeons Edinburgh,* April, 47:2, 451–457.

Shoemaker, W. C., Appel, P. L., Kram, H. B. et al. 1998. Prospective trial of supranormal values of survivors as therapeutic goals in high-risk surgical patients. *Chest,* 94:1176.

5 Blood transfusion therapy

Arthur Bird

Blood transfusion is a vital component in the management of the trauma victim. Indications for transfusion must, however, be present, as blood is expensive and there are inherent risks attached.

Indications for blood components in trauma

- Restore O_2 carrying capacity and blood volume after massive haemorrhage (whole blood).
- Restore O_2 carrying capacity once blood volume has returned to normal (red-cell concentrate).
- Correct defective haemostasis (fresh frozen plasma, cryoprecipitate, platelet concentrate).
- Improvement of colloid oncotic pressure (possible role for albumin, stabilized human serum).

Blood components available

Whole blood (WB)
- Total volume approximately 525 ml
- Consists of 63 ml anticoagulant +465 ml WB
- Final haematocrit (Hct) ±0.4 l/l (40%)
- Final haemoglobin (Hb) concentration ±120 g/l (12 g/dl)

Red cell concentrate
- Total volume ±310 ml (includes 100 ml SAGM – a metabolic rejuvenation solution containing saline, adenine, glucose, and mannitol)
- Final Hct ±0.65 l/l (65%)
- Final Hb concentration 200 g/l (20 g/dl)

Fresh frozen plasma (FFP)
- Volume ±260 ml
- Contains all coagulation proteins normally present
- Recommended dosage 10–15 ml/kg body weight

Cryoprecipitate
- Volume ±8 ml

- Contains in concentrated form; Factor VIII/Von Willebrands factor, fibrinogen, fibronectin, Factor XIII
- Usual practice is to pool 10 units to obtain total dose of fibrinogen of 2 g

Platelet concentrate
- Volume ±50 ml
- Platelet dose per pack $6-8 \times 10^{10}$
- Adult dose is 5–6 bags pooled (rough guide is 1 unit per 10 kg body weight)

Correct procedure for the administration of blood components

The following procedure should be followed when administring blood components:
- Ensure correct identification and verification of the patient and the blood unit. This includes clear specimen and request form labelling.
- Check that the unit is cold (for red cell components); that it has not expired (the Blood Bank will obviously check this but a recheck should always be done); that there is no abnormal appearance (haemolysis/frothing); and that a cross-match appropriate to the component has been done.
- Note that the aseptic technique should be meticulous when setting up a transfusion as blood is a good culture medium for bacteria.
- Observe patient at onset of transfusion for a minimum of 10 minutes and preferably for the first 30 minutes.
- With the exception of normal saline for infusion, no medications or other fluids should be added to blood components.

Adverse reactions

Adverse reactions consist of:
- Acute haemolytic reaction
- Delayed haemolytic reaction
- Bacterial contamination
- Anaphylactic reactions
- Transfusion-related acute lung injury (TRALI)
- Febrile reactions (without haemolysis)
- Allergic reactions

A number of adverse effects have been documented; in the trauma setting the acute reactions are the most relevant.

Acute haemolytic reaction

An acute haemolytic reaction is a rare but life-threatening event and is the result of a clerical or administrative error, most frequently in the ward or in theatre. It follows the administration of ABO-incompatible blood.

Signs and symptoms

The signs and symptoms are usually abrupt and occur within minutes after the infusion begins; heralded by tachycardia, fever, flushing, pain at the site of infusion, loin pain, chills, dyspnoea, chest pain, followed by signs of shock and later, disseminated intravascular coagulation (DIC). Abnormal bleeding and hypotension may be the only signs in an unconscious patient. Haemoglobinuria may also be observed.

Management

- Stop the transfusion.
- Change the administration set.
- Start crystalloid infusion to promote diuresis.
- Send specimen, bag and blood-giving set to Blood Bank with report.
- Check ECG, electrolytes, and coagulation profile.
- Monitor urine output.
- Consult the Haematology department immediately.

Delayed haemolytic transfusion reaction

Delayed reaction is usually the result of undetected antibodies in the patient's serum. It tends not to be life-threatening and occurs some days after the transfusion.

The reaction may be accompanied by fever and a mild jaundice but sometimes the only evidence is a failure of the haemoglobin level to be maintained.

Bacterial contamination

Bacterial contamination is very rare but with rapid onset; chills, fever, abdominal cramps, hypotension, vomiting, diarrhoea, and renal failure.

Management

It requires immediate cessation of transfusion, change of filters and tubing, and immediate aggressive sepsis management. The mortality rate is high.

Anaphylactic reactions

These reactions are extremely rare. They are usually due to antibodies to IgA immunoglobulins.

Signs and symptoms
These are typical of any anaphylactic reaction, often with marked gastro-intestinal symptoms.

Treatment
This is the same as for any anaphylactic reaction – adrenaline, steroids, dopamine, etc. Patients should be followed up to check the immunoglobulin profile.

Transfusion-related acute lung injury (TRALI)

TRALI may cause severe pulmonary symptomatology – the result of leucoagglutinins in the donor's plasma.

Signs and symptoms
These are dyspnoea, fever, and hypotension. Signs of bilateral pulmonary oedema usually occur within four hours of transfusion.

Management
This consists of oxygen and ventilatory support.

Febrile reactions (without haemolysis)

This is not a life-threatening reaction and usually begins within 1–2 hours after the start of the transfusion.

The fever is often accompanied by headache, myalgia, chills, tachycardia, and hypertension.

Management
- Stop the transfusion
- Administer anti-pyretics
- Further transfusions should probably be with leucocyte-depleted components since the cause is usually recipient leucocyte antibodies.

Allergic reactions

Allergic reactions are caused by allergens to plasma proteins.
They are usually mild with itching, urticaria, and erythema.

Management

Stopping the transfusion and administering antihistamines is the recommended management.

Massive transfusion

Definition. A massive transfusion consists of:
- Transfusion of > 30 ml/kg of blood at a rapid rate
- Infusion of a minimum of 10 units within a short period of time
- Replacement of at least one blood volume within 24 hours

Complications of massive transfusion

Manage the complications of massive transfusion as follows:
- *Fluid overload* – monitor patient carefully with CVP, ECG, and urine output.
- *Central hypothermia* – warm blood in designated blood warmer if blood is to be administered rapidly.
- *Bleeding/coagulopathy* – monitor platelet count, INR, partial thromboplastin time, and fibrinogen. Administer platelet concentrates, FFP, or cryoprecipitate according to clinical signs and abnormal tests.
- *Citrate intoxication* – as citrate is normally metabolized rapidly, it is difficult to develop significant hypocalcaemia (citrate binds to calcium) and the routine administration of calcium chloride in massive transfusions is not recommended and has led to significant hypercalcaemia. Ionized calcium measurements are ideal.
- *Hyperkalaemia* – older banked blood has higher levels of potassium than freshly donated blood. The use of the freshest blood available is recommended, together with ECG monitoring and electrolyte checks.
- *Acidosis* – rapid resuscitation and the use of fresh blood are recommended.

In general, the use of fresh blood avoids some of the complications; however, blood banks do not have limitless supplies of this and therefore it is important to monitor the patient. It is axiomatic that the stoppage of further losses is critical.

Autotransfusion

Autotransfusion of the patient's own shed blood has the attraction of guaranteed compatibility and the freedom from allogeneic transfusion-transmitted disease.

It is safe to use in the following circumstances:
- Stab wounds
- Gunshot wounds
- Blunt trauma, even with fractured ribs

Contraindications

Autotransfusion should not be considered under the following circumstances:
- Left lower chest-penetrating injuries
- Potential bowel contamination
- Established coagulopathies
- Haemothoraces > 8 hours old

For auto-infusions using haemothorax blood, the Sorenson apparatus can be used. There is a danger of activated clotting factors contaminating the collection and the cost of the apparatus needs to be factored in. A convenient way of using the Sorenson apparatus is to add 1 000 units of heparin to a chest drain bottle containing normal saline (not water). This should be performed when the clinical circumstances or the chest X-ray appearance suggest a large haemothorax.

For larger autotransfusions from abdominal or other surgery, the Haemonetics Cell Saver can be used; the danger of a coagulopathy occurring is minimized, since the blood is washed and resuspended in saline. It is relatively expensive to set up and ideally requires dedicated personnel to do so. It is really only cost-effective if 3–4 units of blood can be salvaged.

Coagulopathies in trauma patients

In essence, the main pathology is that of disseminated intravascular coagulation, complicated sometimes by the dilutional effects of massive transfusion.

Pathophysiology of DIC

The main trigger factors for DIC are:
- Severe tissue destruction (crush injuries, burns)
- Sepsis and infections
- Hypoxia and prolonged shock
- Liver dysfunction
- Hypothermia
- Some snake venoms
- Obstetric emergencies, such as abruptio placentae and amniotic fluid embolism
- Malignancy

Figure 5.1 Main events leading to the clinical picture of DIC

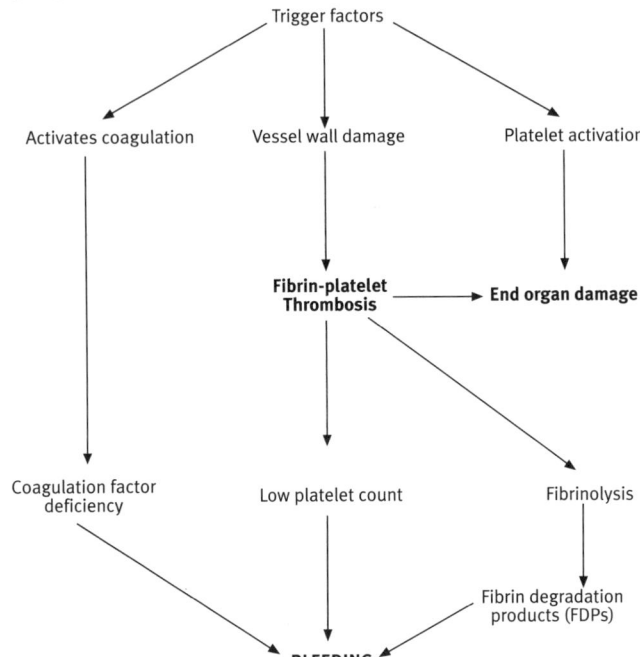

It must be remembered that the picture of DIC is often further complicated by the activation of the complement and kinin pathways and their relative systemic effects.

Diagnosis

The diagnosis of DIC relies on recognizing:

- The clinical trigger factors
- The presence of diffuse bleeding from the skin and mucous membranes
- Associated organ dysfunction following thrombosis and systemic effects of kinin and complement activation

Laboratory confirmation can usually be obtained by measuring the platelet count, INR, PTT, fibrinogen, and FDPs.

Management of DIC

This consists of:

- Prevention: avoid trigger factors such as sepsis, hypothermia, etc.
- Restore blood volume and replace haemoglobin.
- Administer platelets if the platelet count is low and active bleeding is present.
- Give FFP if the clotting factors are depleted.
- If fibrinogen levels drop below 0.5 g/ℓ with active bleeding, cryoprecipitate is recommended.
- Heparin probably has no place in trauma-associated DIC and should be reserved for chronic DIC states or where there are prominent thrombotic signs.

Blood substitutes

Currently in South Africa, there is only one licensed blood substitute, namely Hemopure®, which is a purified haemoglobin solution extracted from bovine haemoglobin. The trials were conducted in patients undergoing elective surgery so it is not clear what role Hemopure® can play in trauma resuscitation. Presumably if blood is not available at the original resuscitation site it may be useful in providing a bridging treatment until blood is available. It has a relatively short half-life and is extremely expensive.

Guidelines on the surgical use of blood products

- If a patient presents in hypovolaemic shock with obvious massive blood loss – give emergency blood.
- Do not allow the Hb to drop below 8 g/dl in a resuscitation – remember that each litre of crystalloid will drop the Hb by 1.5 g/dl. It is imperative to watch closely the amount of crystalloid being administered.
- For every 4 units of blood give 1 FFP (as a rule).
- For every 4 litre of blood loss, administer a random pack of platelets.

Pitfalls

- Continuing with the resuscitation and blood replacement when urgent haemostatic surgery is required.
- Failing to ensure that all blood is warmed to prevent hypothermia.
- Medication must not be added to blood components.

Recommended reading

Clinical guidelines for the use of blood products in South Africa. Edited by Directors of the South African National Blood Service. 2001.

6   Emergency procedures

Elmin Steyn

The basic practical skills required to manage life-threatening injuries are relatively easy to learn and include the following: endotracheal intubation and surgical airway access techniques, the ability to safely and correctly insert a chest drain, peripheral vascular access via cut-down or venipuncture, central venous catheter placement for central venous pressure (CVP) monitoring or as an additional high-flow line, and diagnostic peritoneal lavage for very specific indications.

It is wise to acquire these skills through practical training on simulators, models, and in the animal laboratory or mortuary, if available and appropriate. The Advanced Trauma Life Support® programme offers optimal opportunities for this. When the clinical need arises, there is often no time for lengthy teaching sessions, nor is it the time for inexperienced clinicians to practise new skills without supervision.

Surgical airway techniques

Endotracheal intubation skills are discussed in detail in the chapter on management of the airway in the trauma patient. The chapter deals with orotracheal intubation, nasotracheal intubation, and placement of oral- and nasopharyngeal airway devices, as well as ventilatory techniques with bag valve mask devices. Surgical airway techniques will be discussed here.

Needle cricothyroidotomy

Needle cricothyroidotomy with jet insufflation through the cricothyroid membrane can provide a temporary means of oxygenating a person with complete or partial airway obstruction. This may be necessary after failed attempts at intubation and an inability to ventilate the patient using basic techniques. The patient can be successfully oxygenated for up to 40 minutes. While this is being done, equipment and staff can be arranged for more advanced invasive airway procedures.

Needle cricothyroidotomy technique
- Assemble equipment needed: 14 G catheter over needle, 10 ml syringe and jet insufflation device or a Y-connector connected to oxygen tubing.

- Place patient in supine position, with in-line immobilization of the neck.
- Identify landmarks of the cricothyroid membrane.
- Attach syringe to catheter over needle.
- Clean area with alcohol swab or cleaning solution.
- Hold catheter over needle plastic base between thumb and index finger of instrumentation hand.
- Support instrumentation hand on underside of mandible.
- Pull skin tight across cricothyroid membrane between thumb and index finger of other hand.
- Hold the catheter over needle with the bevel facing upward and place needle tip in midline of cricothyroid membrane.
- Aim needle in a caudal direction at 45-degree angle relative to the trachea.
- Insert needle through skin and membrane under controlled circumstances.
- Advance needle forward at 45-degree angle while drawing back on syringe. Air returning into the syringe suggests tracheal placement.
- Hold metal needle stable at a 45-degree angle and advance the plastic cannula into the trachea.
- Withdraw the metal needle.
- Attach the insufflation adaptor or Y-connector to the end of the cannula and connect to oxygen tubing.
- Insufflate at 1:4 second ratio using high-flow oxygen (8–10 ℓ/min).
- Note that insufflation requires occlusion of the side hole of the adaptor for 1 sec allowing 100% O_2 to enter the trachea. The side hole is then uncovered for 4 sec, allowing no airflow into the trachea.
- Repeat 1 sec insufflation with 4 sec 'exhalation' cycle.
- Secure catheter in place.

Remember: CO_2 retention will occur, as the patient is not being ventilated.

Surgical cricothyroidotomy

Surgical cricothyroidotomy with ventilation through the cricothyroid membrane can provide a means of effectively ventilating a person with complete or partial airway obstruction. This may be necessary after failed attempts at intubation and an inability to ventilate the patient using basic techniques.

Surgical cricothyroidotomy technique

- Assemble equipment required: scalpel blade and handle, size 5–7 cuffed ET-tube (endotracheal tube or tracheostomy tube), bag valve mask device connector, and bag valve device.
- Position patient in supine position. If C-spine injury is suspected, do not extend the neck!
- Identify landmarks of the cricothyroid membrane.
- Clean area with alcohol swab or cleaning solution.
- Pull skin tight across membrane between thumb and index finger.
- Make a 1–2 cm horizontal stab incision though skin and cricothyroid membrane, preventing injury to the posterior wall of the trachea by monitoring the depth of the blade.
- Continue to pull skin tight across membrane between thumb and index finger of other hand while removing scalpel blade from incision.
- Insert artery forceps into horizontal incision with instrumentation hand while continuing to stabilize skin across membrane.
- Open artery forceps tips in horizontal plane to enlarge incision.
- Close artery forceps tips and rotate tips through 90 degrees.
- Open artery forceps tips in vertical plane to enlarge incision.
- Insert ET-tube into trachea through incision between artery forceps tips.

Figure 6.1 Surgical cricothyroidotomy technique: criothyriod membrane

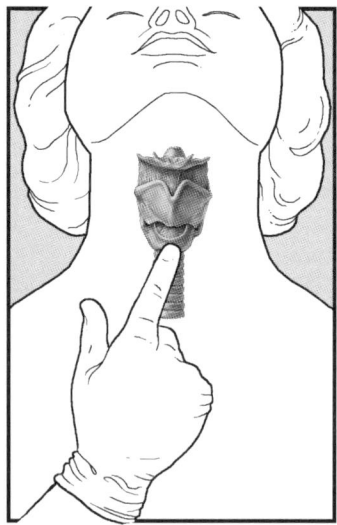

- Check that tube is in trachea and sited correctly, then inflate cuff.
- Attach bag valve device and ventilate patient.
- Auscultate chest to assess correct position of tube while ventilating.
- Tie tube in securely.

Risks and complications of surgical cricothyroidotomy
- Creating a false passage in the soft tissues of the neck
- Bleeding and aspiration of blood
- Injury to oesophagus and posterior tracheal wall
- Injury to vocal chords or recurrent laryngeal nerve
- Subglottic stenosis or laryngeal stenosis

Chest drainage

Needle decompression (thoracentesis)

This procedure is done as emergency management of a clinically diagnosed, life-threatening tension pneumothorax. Needle decompression converts a tension pneumothorax to an ordinary pneumothorax, which, although not an emergency, still requires definitive management.

Technique of needle decompression
- Identify the signs of tension pneumothorax: absent breath sounds, ipsilateral hyperresonance on percussion, distended neck veins, and (late) tracheal displacement to the contralateral side.
- Identify and prepare the side and site where the needle is to be inserted: the second intercostal space, in the mid-clavicular line, and clean with an alcohol swab.
- Avoid injuring the intercostal neurovascular bundle that runs deep to the inferior border of the rib above.
- Insert a 14 G intravenous cannula at right angles to the skin through the chest wall, guiding it over the superior border of the rib below, until the sound of decompression is heard.
- Withdraw the needle and tape the cannula in position.
- Prepare to place a standard intercostal drainage tube in the fifth intercostal space at the anterior axillary line.
- Obtain a chest radiograph.

Complications of needle decompression
- Lung laceration
- Pneumothorax
- Haemorrhage

Placement of chest drains

Intercostal drainage tubes are placed to drain a pneumothorax or haemothorax. Sterile surgical technique should be strictly adhered to, as infective complications, although rare, could lead to considerable morbidity and prolonged hospital stay.

Technique of chest drain placement

- Confirm the side of pathology clinically and radiologically.
- Prepare a sterile tray with instruments, alcohol-containing cleaning solutions, needle, syringe, gauze swabs and 3/0 nylon skin suture. Fill a drainage bottle with 300 ml of sterile water, and connect the sterile underwater drainage tube system.
- Place the patient in a supine or semi-sitting position, with the elbow flexed and the hand behind his/her head to open up intercostal spaces. Protect the C-spine at all times if indicated.
- Prepare the skin over a wide area of the lateral chest wall, and drape with sterile towels.
- Infiltrate skin, subcutaneous tissue, and rib periosteum with 10 ml of 1% lignocaine in the fifth intercostal space, anterior axillary line (lateral to and in line with the nipple).

Figure 6.2 Technique for insertion of chest drain

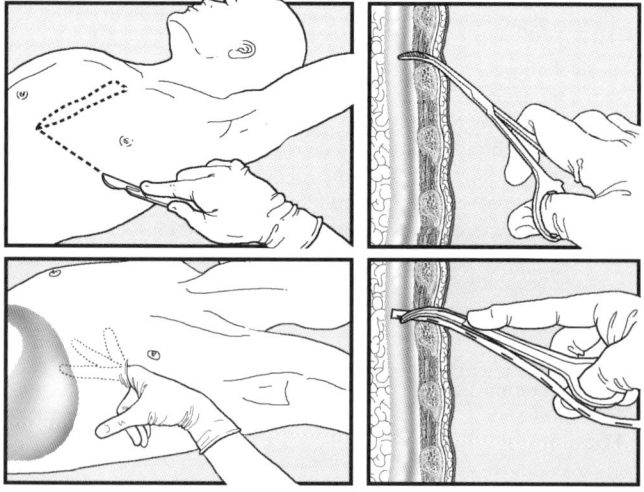

- Make a 2 cm horizontal incision through the skin.
- Dissect bluntly through the chest-wall muscle layers with a small curved artery forceps, keeping close to the superior margin of the rib below.
- Puncture the pleura and stretch open with the instrument.
- Insert a small finger to ascertain that the pleural space has been entered.
- Insert the tube drain with the sharp end of the stylet pulled back from the distal opening, or with a large artery forceps stabilizing the tip of the tube. Clamp the proxial end.
- Advance the drainage tube posteriorly and cranially.
- Connect the proximal end to silicone tubing and the underwater drainage bottle. The pleural contents should be seen draining down the tube or bubbling in the bottle.
- Place a purse string suture close to the wound (2–3 mm from the wound edges, to prevent eversion of the wound margins after closure).
- Fix the tube drain to the skin in such a way that the suture can be unravelled later and pulled together to close the wound.
- Cover the drain entrance wound and secure the drain to the skin.
- Obtain a chest radiograph.

Risks and complications of chest drain placement

- Injury to thoracic or abdominal organs: lung, heart, diaphragm, liver, spleen, vessels
- Empyema or superficial wound infection
- Injury to intercostals nerve or vessels
- Surgical emphysema originating from chest drain wound
- Incorrect position, displacement, dislodgement, kinking, or disconnection from underwater drainage bottle
- Persistent pneumothorax, clotted haemothorax

Central venous line placement

Central venous access is routinely obtained via the internal jugular, subclavian or femoral veins. As with all invasive procedures, attention should be paid to sterility, and anatomical landmarks. The risks of air embolism, infection and injury to adjacent structures are avoided by correct technique. Always maintain in-line immobilization of the cervical spine during these procedures, and follow up with a chest radiograph.

As a general principle, the Seldinger guidewire technique is used, as it has less complications than catheter-over-needle or catheter-through-needle systems. Short, wide, single or double lumen catheters are best for rapid fluid resuscitation (such as the 8F Swan-Ganz sheath introducer), while the long narrow multi-lumen catheters are suitable for CVP measurement and maintenance fluid administration.

Figure 6.3 Accessing the internal jugular vein

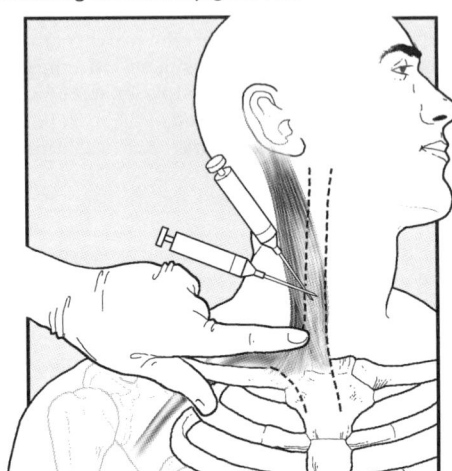

Cannulation of the internal jugular vein

Access to the internal jugular vein may be very difficult in the trauma patient, due to measures to protect the C-spine.

The internal jugular vein is accessed as follows:

- Place the patient in a supine head down position, to prevent air embolism. Protect the C-spine if indicated.
- Identify the triangle between the sternal and clavicular heads of the sternocleidomastoid muscle and the medial third of the clavicle.
- Clean the skin with an alcohol-containing solution and drape the area with sterile towels.
- Infiltrate the centre of the triangle with local anaesthetic.
- Introduce the needle into the centre of the triangle, and advance distally, parallel to the sagittal plane, and at a 30 degree posterior angle to the frontal plane, while aspirating. The internal jugular vein is usually found at a depth of 1–2 cm, do not exceed a depth of 4 cm, as the risk for pneumothorax exists.
- When blood flows freely into the syringe, advance the guidewire, while keeping an eye on the ECG monitor to note any disturbances of rhythm.
- Remove the needle and advance the dilator over the guidewire after slightly enlarging the skin puncture wound with a scalpel blade.
- Remove the dilator and advance the catheter over the guidewire.

- Connect the catheter to the intravenous line, and lower the vaculitre bag slightly to observe the drainage of blood into the tubing. Hang the bag up immediately.
- Fix the catheter to the skin with a 3/0 prolene suture, and place a sterile dressing over the area.
- Obtain a chest radiograph.

Other approaches to the internal jugular vein
- The vein can be approached by inserting the needle at the medial aspect of the midpoint of the sternomastoid muscle, and advancing the needle at an angle of 30–45 degrees with the frontal plane.
- The needle can be inserted at the lateral aspect of the sternomastoid muscle, at a point one-third of the distance from clavicle to mastoid, aiming for the sternal notch. The needle is advanced at a 45 degree angle to the border of the muscle and at a 45 degree angle to the frontal plane.

Cannulation of the subclavian vein

In the injured patient, access to the subclavian vein is easier than the internal jugular vein, but take care not to rotate or extend the neck, until possible C-spine injuries have been ruled out.

Figure 6.4 Accessing the subclavian vein

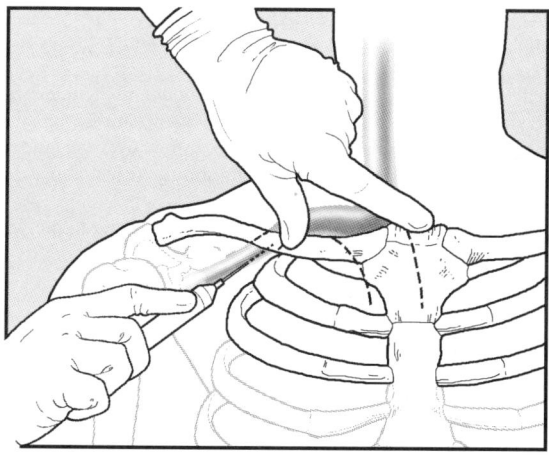

Figure 6.5 Femoral venipuncture

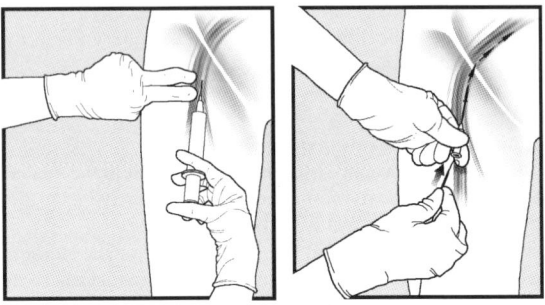

The subclavian vein is accessed as follows:
- Place the patient in a supine head-down position to prevent air embolism. Protect the C-spine if indicated.
- Surgically clean and drape the chest wall and neck near the clavicle.
- Introduce local anaesthetic to the subcutaneous tissues below the clavicle.
- Place the needle 1 cm below the junction of the medial third and the middle third of the clavicle.
- Advance the needle while applying suction and keeping the needle and syringe parallel to the frontal plane.
- Direct the needle to a point at a depth of 1 cm to the suprasternal notch, advancing the needle over the first rib and under the head of the clavicle.
- When blood flows into the syringe, introduce the guidewire while observing the cardiac monitor for rhythm disturbances.
- Remove the needle, dilate and place the cannula over the guidewire as described above. The tip of the cannula should be just above the right atrium.
- Connect the catheter to the tubing and fix the catheter to the skin after testing for backflow of blood.
- Obtain a chest radiograph.

Cannulation of the femoral vein

Femoral vein cannulation provides safe and easy emergency vascular access.
- Place the patient in a supine position, and prepare the skin with an alcohol-based solution, drape with sterile towels.

- Palpate the femoral artery; the vein lies directly medial to the artery. Inject local anaesthetic to the area.
- Introduce the large-calibre needle directly over the femoral vein, advancing slowly in a proximal and posterior direction, parallel to the artery, with gentle suction on the syringe.
- The fingers of the other hand should continue to palpate the arterial pulse.
- When blood flows freely into the syringe, introduce the guidewire while preventing air embolism.
- Remove the needle, place the dilator followed by the intravenous catheter. Connect to IV line.
- Fix the catheter to the skin and dress the area.
- Obtain chest and abdominal radiographs to confirm the position of the catheter.

Risks and complications of central venous cannulation

- Pneumothorax
- Hydro- or haemothorax
- Subclavian artery injury
- Air embolism
- Endotracheal tube cuff perforation
- Venous thombosis
- Catheter fragment embolization
- Infection, local or systemic
- Phrenic nerve or brachial plexus injury
- Chylothorax
- A–V fistula
- Dysrhythmia

Management of air embolism

Air embolus occurring during placement of a central venous catheter presents as sudden onset of acute cardiac output failure. There will be a drop in blood pressure and clinical signs of decreased peripheral and cerebral perfusion. A continuous murmur may be heard over the heart. Jugular veins may be distended.

Treatment includes turning the patient onto his/her left side, administering 100% oxygen and aspirating the air from the right atrium with the same central line.

Intra-osseous infusion access

When percutaneous peripheral venous access cannot be obtained in children under the age of six years, intra-osseous infusion provides emergency resuscitation until intravenous lines can be placed.

- Place the patient in a supine position, with support under the knee of an uninjured limb. The knee should be in approximately 30 degrees of flexion, with the heel resting on the bed or stretcher.
- Prepare and drape the skin at a site 1–3 cm below the tibial tubercle, on the antero-medial aspect of the proximal tibia. Infiltrate with local anaesthetic.
- Introduce a short, large-calibre bone-marrow aspiration needle, or a short 18 G spinal needle with a stylet, at a 90-degree angle through the skin and periosteum, with the bevel directed away from the epiphyseal plate.
- Adjust the direction of the needle in a direction away from the epiphyseal plate, at a 45 to 60-degree angle with the tibia (see diagram in Figure 6.6).
- Advance the needle with a twisting motion through the cortex, into the bone marrow.
- Remove the stylet and aspirate with a saline-filled syringe: bone marrow should be obtained.
- Flush the needle with saline: there should be free flow with no swelling of the subcutaneous tissues.
- Connect the needle to a high-flow IV line and advance the needle until it is securely lodged in the bone.

Figure 6.6 Intra-osseous needle placement

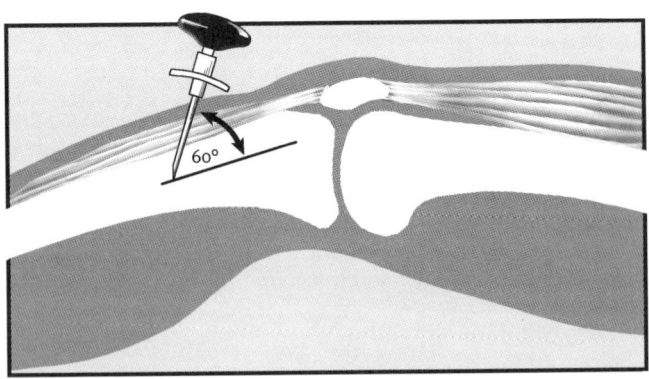

- Dress and tape the needle. Replace with peripheral venous lines as soon as practically possible.

Risks and complications of intra-osseous needle placement
- Injury to joint, epiphyseal injury, neuro-vascular injury
- Infection
- Haematoma, compartment syndrome

Saphenous vein cutdown

Rapid and safe peripheral vascular access can be obtained in patients with unsuitable upper limb veins. The saphenous vein is very consistent in its location and can be found at a point 1.5 cm anterior and proximal to the medial malleolus.

Technique of saphenous vein cutdown
- Prepare a sterile tray with size 11 and 15 surgical blades, three small curved artery forceps, fine-toothed forceps, fine non-toothed forceps, fine dissecting scissors, needle holders, 3/0 absorbable suture ties and 4/0 nylon skin suture.
- Clean the area above the ankle of a non-injured limb with alcohol swabs and drape with sterile towels.
- Infiltrate with local anaesthetic.
- Make a 2 cm transverse incision crossing the course of the vein at a point 1.5 cm above the medial malleolus, extending through the dermis into the subcutaneous tissue.
- Bluntly dissect out the vein by spreading the curved artery forceps parallel to and close to the vessel wall. Press the tips of the artery forceps under the vessel and gently spread until 2–3 cm of the vessel has been dissected free.
- Pass two ligatures under the vein and place gentle traction on the proximal ligature. Ligate the distal vein and place gentle traction on the suture.
- Create an opening in the vein by incising with the smallest scalpel blade through no more than half its diameter. Alternatively the scissors can be used to cut obliquely into the vessel. Be sure to cut cleanly into the lumen.
- Dilate the opening slightly with a small artery forceps, and insert a large intravenous cannula without needle into the vein.
- Connect the intravenous administration tubing to the cannula, and tie the proximal and distal ligatures gently around the cannula.
- Close the skin around the cannula with interrupted nylon sutures, dress, and tape securely.

Risks and complications of saphenous vein cutdown
- Thrombophlebitis
- Haematoma
- Infection
- Delayed wound healing

Diagnostic peritoneal lavage (DPL)

Diagnostic peritoneal lavage is indicated in situations where clinical examination of the abdomen is unreliable to determine the presence of intra-abdominal injury, and ultrasound or CT scan is unavailable or impractical. It is a relatively fast and sensitive test for patients with blunt abdominal injury or stab wounds to the anterior abdomen (98% sensitive for intraperitoneal bleeding, with 2% false-positive and 2% false-negative rates). It is useful for unstable patients who are unconscious, sedated,

Figure 6.7 Saphenous vein cutdown procedure

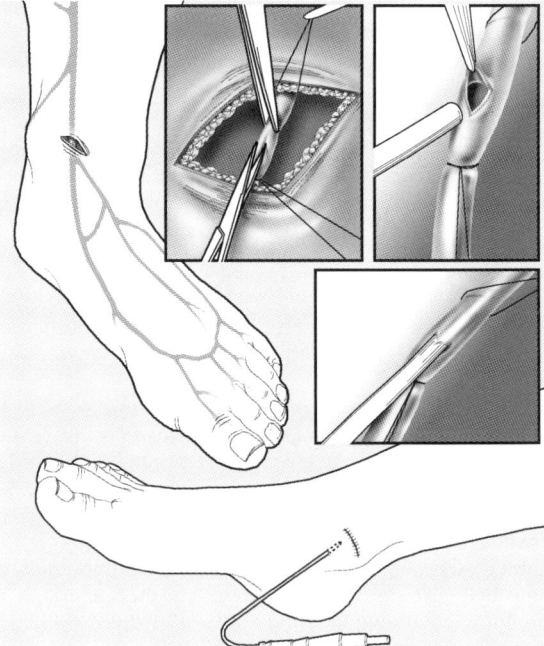

anaesthetized, or who have sustained spinal chord injury. DPL is also used to verify an abnormal ultrasound investigation, or if the ultrasound examination is normal in the presence of clinical signs suggestive of intra-abdominal injury. A negative lavage does not exclude retroperitoneal injuries, isolated hollow viscus perforation, or diaphragmatic injury.

DPL is considered positive if gross blood is aspirated immediately on insertion, or if microscopic evaluation of (unspun) peritoneal fluid obtained after infusion of 1 litre of Ringer's lactate shows red cells >100 000/mm³, white cells > 500/mm³, or the presence of particulate matter, bacteria on Gram staining, bile, or raised amylase levels. Not all laboratories are familiar with appropriate techniques for peritoneal lavage fluid assessment, and local facilities and circumstances should be taken into consideration.

Alternatives to DPL are diagnostic ultrasonography, computed tomography (CT scan), and diagnostic laparoscopy.

It must be remembered that DPL changes subsequent examination and investigational findings, and should preferably be performed by (or in consultation with) the surgical team who will eventually take care of the patient.

DPL should only be performed by suitably skilled persons. An absolute contraindication to DPL is the presence of clear indications for laparotomy. Relative contraindications include previous surgery, pregnancy, obesity, coagulopathy, and significant pelvic fractures.

Techniques of DPL

The open technique is probably safer, but requires surgical instruments and skills. The closed technique requires a commercially available catheter over guidewire kit.

Both techniques require bladder and gastric catheterization for decompression. This is followed by surgical preparation of the whole abdominal wall (as for laparotomy). Local anaesthetic is injected in the midline, one third of the distance from umbilicus to pubic symphysis.

For the open technique, a vertical incision is made, 3–4 cm in length, down to the sheath.

The fascial edges are elevated by two forceps, clamps or sharp-ended towel clips and a small incision is made to the peritoneum. A peritoneal dialysis catheter is inserted into the pelvis, and the wound is sutured.

If gross blood is not obtained, allow 1 litre of warm Ringer's solution to run into the peritoneal cavity.

After 5–10 minutes the fluid is drained by placing the vaculitre bag on the floor. A fluid sample is sent for microscopic examination.

The closed technique requires the elevation of the abdominal wall on both sides of the midline, and careful insertion of the needle attached to a syringe, through skin, subcutaneous tissue and the sheath, where moderate resistance will be felt. The needle is inserted approximately 1 cm into the peritoneal cavity.

The flexible end of the guidewire is then inserted through the needle, and the needle is withdrawn.

A small incision is made at the site of the entrance wound, and the peritoneal lavage catheter is inserted over the guidewire. The guidewire is then removed and an attempt is made to aspirate blood or fluid. If blood is not immediately obtained, proceed with infusion of warm Ringer's solution as described above.

Dress and close wound, and secure catheter.

Risks and complications of DPL
- Intestinal perforation with peritonitis
- Haemorrhage, causing a false-positive finding
- Bladder, retroperitoneal, or solid organ injury
- Wound infection

Figure 6.8 Open technique of DPL

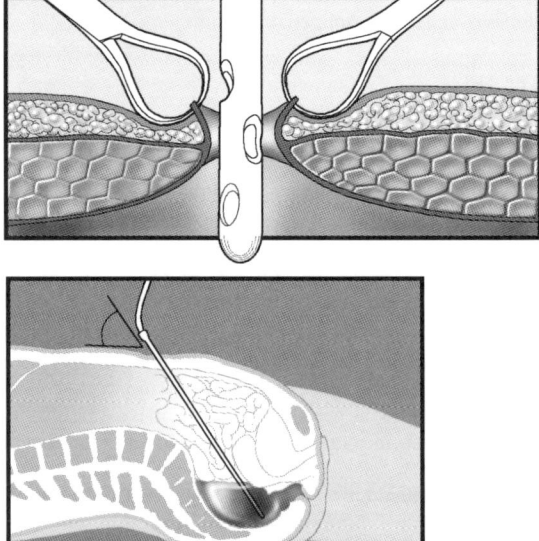

Pitfalls

- Not observing sterile surgical techniques when placing invasive lines and catheters.
- Not being adequately trained or prepared when attempting to do emergency procedures.
- Not controlling the distal end of the guidewire at all times when placing central venous catheters with the Seldinger technique.
- Not checking for blood push-back before running fluids into a central venous catheter.
- Not obtaining radiological confirmation of the position of the central venous catheter, as well as after unsuccessful placement attempts.
- Performing a DPL for the wrong indications.

Recommended reading

American College of Surgeons Committee on Trauma, Advanced Trauma Life Support®. 1997. *Program for Doctors. Student manual.* Sixth edition. Chicago: ACS.

Collicott, P. E. 1991. Initial assessment of the trauma patient. In E. E. Moore, K. L. Mattox, D. V. Feliciano (eds.) *Trauma.* Second edition. East Norwalk: Appleton and Lange, 119.

Moore, F. A., Moore, E. E. 2002. Trauma resuscitation. In D. W. Wilmore, et al. (eds.) *ACS surgery: Principles and practice.* New York: WebMD Corporation.

Nwariaku, F. E. 1999. Catheters and tubes. In F. E. Nwariaku and E. Thal (eds.) *Parkland trauma handbook.* Second edition. London: Mosby.

7 Pain management

Luc Evenepoel

Pain relief for the injured patient is generally agreed to be of vital importance. The risk of significant side-effects from inappropriate analgesic administration, however, can be deleterious, or even disastrous. The aim therefore, is to keep the patient comfortable, not necessarily pain free, by optimizing drug safety and efficiency.

Assessment of pain

Guidelines for assessing pain in patients are as follows:
- Awake and oriented patients can be asked to rate their pain from 0 to 10, 0 being no pain and 10 the worst pain imaginable. Most patients, even children, can easily do this. This is also a good tool to evaluate the effect of the analgesics administered, most patients being relatively comfortable and satisfied when they come down to a score of 5 or less.
- Pain tolerance is very individual: the pain of an identical injury can be rated $^8/_{10}$ by one patient, but only $^4/_{10}$ by another.
- Intoxicated and confused patients, and those with a depressed level of consciousness, cannot reliably communicate their own pain. Do not withhold analgesia, but be cautious, opioids may further depress respiration and consciousness.

Analgesics

The three main groups are opioids, non-steroidal anti-inflammatory drugs (NSAIDs), and local anaesthetics. To keep this text concise, finer details have been omitted, but can easily be found in any pharmacology manual.

Opioids

Pain tolerance varies, and the analgesic effect of opioids can differ ten-fold between individuals. These two factors make it difficult to predict a universally effective opioid dose.

Morphine
- Morphine is still the reference opioid: very effective, widely available, and cheap.

- The onset of analgesic effect is after 3–5 minutes, peak analgesic effect after 10–20 minutes, duration of action 3–4 hours (6 hours in the elderly).
- Its effects and side-effects described here are also relevant to the other opioids.
- It is preferably given intravenously (IV). Intramuscularly (IM) injected morphine does not have a reliable uptake in injured patients, due to relatively poorly perfused muscle. The analgesic effect and side-effects can therefore be delayed for many hours, consequently respiratory depression may occur insidiously.
- The traditional adult total dose of 0.1–0.3 mg/kg is a rough guideline, and depends on the severity of injury, pain tolerance, and the patient's individual opioid sensitivity.
- Give morphine in increments of 0.01–0.02 mg/kg IV every 5–10 minutes. This will allow easy titration of the opioid against its effect. The respiratory rate should stay above 14 breaths/min.
- For a 60 kg adult, give boluses of 0.5–1.5 mg IV every 5–10 minutes.
- Prepare this dilution as a mixture of 1 mg/ml or 0.1 mg/ml for easy administration:
  10 mg morphine (1 ml) in 9 ml sterile water (or 0.9% saline or 5% dextrose) equals 1 mg/ml.
- Onset of effect and side-effects are predictable: blood pressure drops within 2–5 minutes, maximum respiratory depression occurs within 7 minutes, peak analgesic effect occurs within 10–20 minutes.
- Start the opioid titration during the initial resuscitation and ensure that the patient is comfortable before any painful examinations, manipulation, or transport are attempted.
- The analgesic effect of morphine lasts about 4 hours. Prescribe regular follow-up doses every 4 hours, rather than on demand only. (Pethidine lasts only 2–3 hours.)
- Neonates and small children are especially sensitive to the respiratory depressant effect of opioids. Recommended total doses are therefore smaller than for adults:
  younger than 3 months: 0.025 mg/kg
  3 to 12 months: 0.05 mg/kg
  older than 12 months: 0.1 mg/kg
- Note that injured children are generally anxious, which contributes negatively to their pain perception. A small amount of an anxiolytic like midazolam (Dormicum®) 0.1 mg/kg orally or IV in increments, in combination with the opioid, can be useful.
- For children, dilute 10 mg morphine (= 1 ml) to 100 ml: this makes a concentration of 0.1 mg/ml. Administer 0.1–0.3 ml/kg IV of this mixture every 5–10 minutes. Neonates are very sensitive: use small increments.

Side-effects of opioids

Hypotension. Because of histamine release, even small amounts of morphine may cause a drop in blood pressure in hypovolaemic patients. Halve the dose, and wait long enough in between the increments to ensure the blood pressure remains stable. Note that elderly patients are especially prone to hypotension.

Respiratory depression. The risk is vastly enhanced in patients who have ingested alcohol, benzodiazepines, barbiturates, or other central nervous system depressants. Titrate to effect and watch for side-effects. Do not administer morphine for head-injured patients, where respiratory depression leads to hypercapnia, cerebral vasodilation, and increased intracranial pressure. If the patient is on ventilatory support, this becomes irrelevant.

Central vs peripheral respiratory depression
Opioids are central respiratory depressants, whereas patients with rib fractures and abdominal injuries are peripherally depressed, due to pain from the rib fractures or abdominal wound.

Administration of morphine to patients with rib fractures will improve their breathing, oxygenation, and ventilation, provided there is no concomitant head injury or other contraindication for opioid use.

Pethidine

Pethidine has some anticholinergic properties, like a mild positive chronotropic effect.

- This is especially attractive in small children because they depend mainly on heart rate to maintain their cardiac output.
- Do not give to elderly patients because it can make them very confused.
- Avoid with renal impairment (accumulation and toxicity).
- The duration of effect is 2–3 hours, not 6 hours as it is commonly prescribed.
- The recommended dose is 1–1.5 mg/kg.

Tilidine (Valoron®)

- Tilidine is well absorbed when given sublingually or intranasally, but should not be given IV.
- The duration of action is 4–6 hours.
- Adult dose: 50–100 mg.
- Paediatric dose: 1–9 years: 1 drop per year of age + 2 drops
                    10 years and older: max 10 drops (= 25 mg)
- Do not give to children less than one year old.

Tramadol (Tramal®)

- Tramadol is the preferred analgesic for spontaneously breathing head-injured patients, as it has very little respiratory depressant effect.
- Titrate to effect, ±5 mg/kg every 5 minutes, until the patient is comfortable.

Sufentanyl (Sufenta®)

- Sufentanyl is less widely available in the trauma unit, more expensive and shorter acting (1–1.5 hours).
- It is quicker in onset of effect and side-effects (1–5 minutes) than morphine, and therefore more efficient to titrate IV.
- It is much more cardiovascularly stable than morphine.
- Because of its relatively short duration of action, it is most suitable for patients who will undergo surgery within 1 or 2 hours.
- One ampoule of 2 ml contains 10 µg sufentanyl. Titrate IV with increments of 0.02–0.04 (g/kg every 2–5 minutes, i.e. 1.25–2.5 µg (0.25–0.5 ml) per bolus for a 60 kg adult.

Codeine (e.g. DF118®)

- Codeine is popular among neurosurgeons to treat pain in head-injured patients.
- Codeine is a weak analgesic, but is less respiratory depressant. Tramadol remains an attractive alternative.

Opioids are certainly the first choice analgesic in the severely injured patient. However, one must not forget the non-chemical contribution to a patient's comfort: splinting and immobilization, as well as reassuring words, a calm composure, holding the patient's hand, etc. They all contribute to the same goal, and decrease opioid requirements.

Non-steroidal anti-inflammatory drugs (NSAID)

Examples of these drugs are: Aspirin, diclofenac (Voltaren®), ibuprofen (Brufen®), naproxen (e.g. Naprosyn®), ketorolac (Tora-Dol®), etc. and the newer cyclo-oxygenase (COX-2) selective inhibitors: mefloxicam (Mobic®), the coxibs (Celebrex®, Vioxx®).

- They act mainly via a peripheral anti-prostaglandin effect.
- Some textbooks also classify paracetamol in this group. It works via a central anti-prostaglandin effect.
- They are good analgesics against moderate pain, especially musculo-skeletal pain.

- They are not indicated in severely injured patients due to risks of renal impairment, bleeding tendencies, and gastric mucosal damage.
- The onset of effect is at the earliest only after 30 minutes.
- The synergistic effect of NSAIDs and opioids allows the dose of opioid to be decreased by up to 40%. However, this effect becomes apparent only after about 5 hours, and is not relevant in the acute trauma setting.
- Do not combine different NSAIDs and do not exceed the recommended dose. They have a ceiling effect, which means that beyond a certain dose, the analgesic effect does not increase, but the side-effects do. Many pharmaceutical preparations contain a NSAID, and combinations such as a paracetamol-ibuprofen-codeine preparation (Myprodol®) with diclofenac should be avoided.
- The route of administration is irrelevant: the analgesic effect is the same, whether a similar dose is administered IV, orally, intramuscularly, or rectally. The oral route is preferred.
- The side-effects are systemic and therefore also independent of the route of administration, i.e. the effect on the gastric mucosa is the same whether the NSAID is administered orally, rectally, or parenterally. An exception is aspirin: besides its systemic effects, it also has a local caustic effect on the gastric mucosa. Intramuscular diclofenac can form sterile abcesses and cause local pain for weeks afterwards.
- The side-effects of NSAIDs can be devastating in the severely injured patient. Hypovolaemia, hypotension, and the adrenergic response to trauma divert blood from 'non-essential' organs like kidneys and stomach. Additionally, circulating myoglobins add to the burden of the kidneys. The NSAID anti-prostaglandin effect causes further vasoconstriction and decreased blood flow to those organs, significantly increasing the risk for renal failure or stomach ulceration. These complications may cause late fatalities.
- The new, COX-2 selective NSAIDs are safer for the stomach, but not for the kidneys.
- Because of the serious side-effects and relatively little analgesic effect in the severely injured, one should never give NSAIDs to these patients. Reserve these drugs for the stable, normovolaemic, normotensive patient with minor or moderate injuries.

Paracetamol
- Paracetamol is an effective analgesic against mild or moderate pain.
- It relies on a central anti-prostaglandin effect.
- Recent evidence has shown that it has a peripheral anti-thromboxane effect as well, which may cause gastric ulceration.
- It has a synergistic effect with opioids and NSAIDs. Therefore, combining paracetamol with opioids can reduce the opioid requirements by 25%.

- Never give paracetamol to somebody who has ingested alcohol. Just 1 000 mg (2 tablets) with alcohol can cause severe and even fatal liver damage.

Local anaesthetics

Table 7.1 gives some guidelines for the use of various local anaesthetic drugs.

Safety aspects of local anaesthetic use

- Ropivacaine is a new local anaesthetic with lower cardio- and neuro-toxicity. Whether this is clinically relevant remains to be proven. It has inherent vasoconstrictive properties, adding adrenaline does not change its clinical effect.
- Levobupivacaine is an enantiomer of bipuvacaine and is cardio-vascularly much safer. The duration of effect is slightly longer than bupivacaine.
- The duration of effect and risk for toxicity is partly dependent on the vascularity of the injected area. Never exceed the recommended dose with intercostal blocks, as the local anaesthetic is rapidly absorbed from this very vascular area. This quick absorption also shortens the

Table 7.1 Local anaesthetic agents

Local anaesthetic agent		Maximum recommended dose	Onset of analgesia	Duration of analgesia	Recommend dilution for analgesia
Lignocaine	Without adrenaline	3 mg/kg	5–10 min	1–2 hours	0.5–1%
	With adrenaline 1:200 000	7 mg/kg	5–10 min	3–5 hours	0.5–1%
Bupivacaine (Macaine®) Levobupiva-caine (Chirocaine®)	Without adrenaline	2 mg/kg	5–20 min	8–14 hours	0.25%
	With adrenaline 1:200 000	3.5 mg/kg	5–10 min	10–16 hours	0.25%
Ropivacaine (Naropin®)			5–15 min	6–12 hours	2–3.75 mg/ml i.e. 0.2–0.375%

duration of effect. The use of adrenaline-containing preparations here is recommended.

- Never use local anaesthetics with adrenaline in end-organs like fingers, toes, nose, penis, lips. The vasoconstriction may lead to necrosis.
- The thinner a nerve fibre, the easier it is blocked by the local anaesthetic. Pain is transmitted by very thin nerve fibres, much thinner than fibres for pressure, touch or motor power, therefore dilutions as mentioned in Table 7.1 are more than sufficient for pain relief. Use 0.9% sodium chloride to prepare the dilution, not sterile water or 5% dextrose.
- Toxic side-effects are rare if the maximum recommended doses are respected and one takes care to avoid intravascular injections (aspirate regularly while injecting). Early signs are a dull feeling around the lips, anxiety, or excitement, which may quickly progress to tremors, twitching, convulsions, and total central nervous system collapse.
- Cardiovascular side-effects may follow or precede those of the central nervous system: bradycardia, hypotension, collapse.
- Treatment consists of intravenous fluids, ventilatory support, and anticonvulsants if necessary: thiopentone 1–3 mg/kg or a benzodiazepine like midazolam (Dormicum®), increments up to a total maximum of 0.1 mg/kg, or diazepam (Valium®), increments up to a total maximum of 0.015 mg/kg.
- It is mandatory to establish intravenous access prior to doing any but the smallest nerve block, and to have resuscitative equipment immediately available.

Useful and easy nerve blocks in the trauma unit

If the pain of trauma is related to the distribution of one or a few nerves, a nerve block is the most effective way of analgesia, and obviates the need for other pain killers (and the risk of their side-effects).

The most reliable way to do a successful block, is obviously to inject the local anaesthetic close enough to the nerve. Know the anatomy, paraesthesia indicates success. However, do not 'poke around', because with any block, there is the risk of nerve damage, which may be permanent or very uncomfortable for the patient for months afterwards. You can argue: no paraesthesia, no anaesthesia, but also: no paraesthesia, no dysaesthesia! If paraesthesia is obtained, withdraw the needle slightly before injecting to avoid the risk of intraneural injection. When injecting in the right spot, often the patient will feel a dullness or 'something' going down in the direction of the distribution of the nerve. If you cannot obtain paraesthesia, and you are sure to be in the right spot, inject fanlike.

In small compartments, use small volumes (e.g. finger and wrist block) to avoid the risk of neural and arterial compression.

Digital block

- Fingers and toes are innervated by a ventral and dorsal branch running on each side of the digit.
- The injection can be made at the web space at the base of the finger, where the skin is loose. Inject from dorsal to ventral, 1 to 1.5 ml per side is sufficient.
- Alternatively, insert the needle just proximal of the metacarpal or metatarsal head, injecting as you progress from dorsally to ventrally.
- Palpate the area next to the needle to feel the inter-metacarpal or inter-tarsal space fill up. Two millilitres per space is sufficient.
- This block will also affect the adjacent side of the next finger.

Intravenous block (Bier's block)

- This block relies on the spread of local anaesthetic through the venous system of an exsanguinated limb.
- Obtain intravenous access on the healthy arm.
- Then insert an intravenous cannula in the dorsum of the hand, or as

Figure 7.1 Digital block

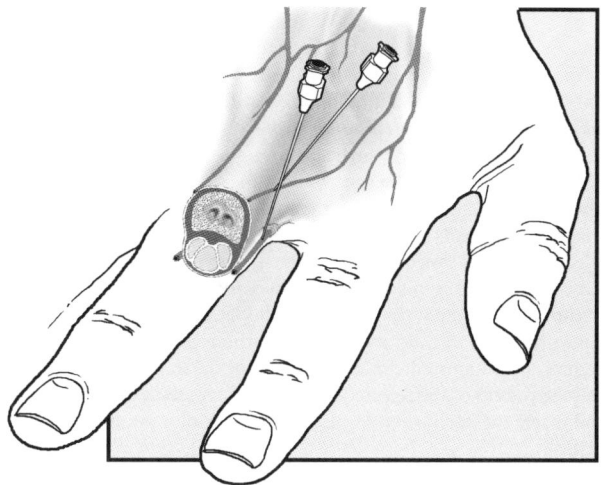

distally as possible, on the injured arm. Do not go too proximal or the block will not work.

- Now exsanguinate the arm by winding a tight elastic bandage around it (Esmarch), or if the arm is too painful, by letting the patient elevate it for 3–4 minutes.
- Inflate a tourniquet on the upper arm to 120–150 mmHg above the systolic pressure.
- Remove the bandage and inject 30–40 ml of lignocaine 0.5% intravenously in the injured arm. Wait 10 minutes for effect.
- To improve comfort, use a double tourniquet on the upper arm, inflating the proximal one first, switching over to the distal one when the patient starts experiencing tourniquet pain. Procedures longer than 1 or 1.5 hours are for this reason not well tolerated.
- After the surgery, simply deflate the tourniquet and the sensation will return again in a few minutes. Do not omit to infiltrate the wound with local anaesthetic during surgery.
- Deflation of the cuff is safe as from 20 minutes after injection of the lignocaine. Never use any local anaesthetic other than lignocaine for Bier's block.
- This block can also be performed on the leg, but the volume of local anaesthetic has to be increased to 50–80 ml, which is often close to a toxic dose. Inflate the tourniquet to a slightly higher level, 150–180 mmHg above the systolic pressure.

Intercostal blocks

- An intercostal block is a useful block to take away the pain of rib fractures or insertion of an intercostal drain.
- The intercostal nerve can be blocked at the costal angle, one hand's breadth lateral from the spinous process.
- For this the patient has to sit, lie prone, or lie on the contra-lateral side. The arm is brought to the front to keep the scapula out of the way.
- The block can also be done in the mid-axillary line, because the local anaesthetic spreads anteriorly and posteriorly over several centimetres, affecting all the branches of the nerve. This approach allows the patient to be supine, and seems to be the most comfortable.
- Do not connect the syringe to the needle yet, but fill the hub of the needle with a drop of fluid, e.g. local anaesthetic. Should the pleura accidentally be punctured, this drop will be sucked in.
- Palpate the rib of the selected intercostal nerve. Pull the skin cranially, and insert the needle perpendicular to the skin or aiming slightly cranially.
- When the needle tip has made contact with the rib, walk the needle tip

caudally until it slides underneath the rib. Carefully advance the needle another 3 mm. A 'click' will be felt when the needle tip passes through the external intercostal muscle.

- Connect the syringe and inject 3–5 ml of local anaesthetic with adrenaline.
- The risk for a pneumothorax is relatively small (1 in 500), and for clinically significant pneumothorax, which requires drainage, only 1:1000.
- Local anaesthetic is rapidly absorbed from this very vascular area, with the risk of toxicity.
- The effect of an intercostal block usually does not last much longer than 6–8 hours, after which it can be repeated.
- For multiple rib fractures, it is better to call an anaesthetist to insert an epidural or para-vertebral block, with an indwelling catheter, to maintain analgesia for several days.

Interpleural block

- Instilling local anaesthetic between the visceral and parietal pleura can be easily done through an intercostal drain, but this is unfortunately not very effective pain relief for rib fractures. It does work well, however, to provide temporary pleural analgesia for the pain caused by the tip of the drain, which is otherwise very difficult to treat.
- Inject about 20 ml of 0.125% bupivacaine with adrenaline or 2 mg/ml ropivacaine as proximal as possible into the intercostal drain, and clamp the drain for about 15 minutes to prevent it all running out again.
- The effect will last 2–4 hours, after which it can be repeated.
- Work on a maximum safe dose of bupivacaine 2 mg/kg and ropivacaine 3.5 mg/kg every 4 hours.

Figure 7.2 Needle placement for intercostal nerve block

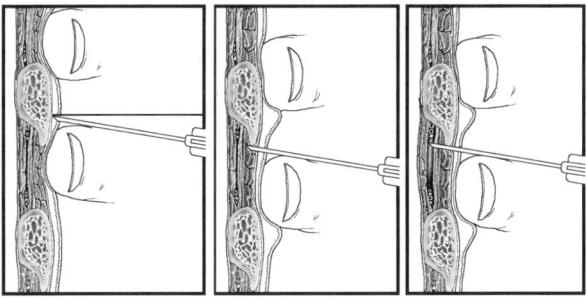

Infiltrating wound edges

This procedure is very easy, and should be routinely done when a wound is sutured or debrided.

Injecting a fracture haematoma

This procedure was popular at one stage but should be avoided because a closed fracture is converted to an open one, with the subsequent risk of sepsis.

Other blocks

- There are many very effective blocks to completely relieve pain: thoracic epidural or paravertebral block for rib fractures, lumbar epidural block for pelvis or leg injuries, lumbar plexus block or femoral nerve block for injuries to the upper leg, sciatic nerve block for the lower leg, interscalene brachial plexus block for shoulder pain, infraclavicular or axillary plexus block for the arm.
- Call upon an anaesthetist to perform one of them as soon as the patient is stabilized.
- An indwelling catheter can be placed, to provide pre-, intra-, and many days of post-operative pain relief.

Pain management recommendations

Practical pain control solutions for various injuries include the following:

Regional nerve block for trauma
An elderly patient with a neck of femur fracture can be rendered pain free with a femoral nerve plexus block, and will not need any opioids. By infusing local anaesthetic postoperatively through the indwelling nerve block catheter, pain relief can be maintained, and opioids further avoided, minimizing side-effects, such as the often cumbersome mental confusion.

Severe multiple injuries

- Titrate IV morphine, but keep the increments small because of the risk of hypotension.
- For the patient going to theatre within an hour or two, sufentanyl is a cardiovascularly more stable option.

Head injuries

- Administer IV increments of tramadol.
- If there are no other injuries, and the patient is stable, NSAID with paracetamol might be sufficient, or added to the tramadol.
- Codeine may cause less respiratory depression, but is a less effective painkiller.
- Morphine can safely be given if the head-injured patient is on ventilatory support.

Minor or moderate injuries

- Administer NSAID with paracetamol; the preferred route is oral.
- If this is not sufficient, add an oral opioid (e.g. tilidine drops or tablet) or if there is intravenous access, titrate morphine IV until the patient is comfortable.

Elderly patients

- Be careful with opioids, these patients are extra sensitive.
- Never use pethidine as the elderly become confused, and there is risk of accumulation and toxicity due to decreased renal function.
- If possible, use the approach with nerve blocks as described above.

Hypoventilation

The patient who is hypoxic due to hypoventilation from chest or abdominal injuries, requires morphine. It will decrease the pain and improve the breathing.

Rib fractures

- The main problem here is pain, call the anaesthetist for a thoracic epidural or paravertebral block.
- Intercostal blocks are fine, but do not last long and will have to be repeated.
- Ventilation for multiple rib fractures can often be avoided if excellent pain relief is provided.

Dislocations

- To reduce dislocations some muscle relaxation is required, which can be obtained with benzodiazepines (centrally acting muscle relaxants).
- Use increments of midazolam (Dormicum®) 0.02 mg/kg every 3–5 minutes.

- If really necessary, small increments of an opioid can be added, but keep monitoring for respiratory depression after the reduction: when the pain has gone, the side-effects of the drugs come to the fore.

Children

- Anxiolysis with a small amount of a benzodiazepine (midazolam) will aid pain relief.
- Be careful with opioids in children less than one year old: use half or quarter dose, see above.
- The anti-cholinergic properties of pethidine have a positive chronotropic effect, which is beneficial for small children.

Nerve block

- Local anaesthetics can render the patient pain-free, obviating the need for other analgesics.
- Be careful not to damage any nerves when doing a block.

Pain medication for patients on discharge

- The first three days, use a NSAID in combination with paracetamol.
- Avoid codeine preparations as they may cause constipation, especially in the elderly.
- After three days, continue with paracetamol, if necessary topped up with a NSAID.

Pain killers that should be stocked in all trauma units

- *Opioids:* morphine IV, pethidine IV, tramadol IV and p.o, tilidine drops and tablets.
- *NSAIDs:* diclofenac p.o. and rectally, one of the coxibs p.o.
- *Local anaesthetics:* lignocaine, bupivacaine with and without adrenaline, and/or ropivacaine (it is not necessary to stock both bupivacaine and ropivacaine).

Pitfalls

- Withholding opioids from patients with rib fractures for fear of respiratory depression.
- Giving NSAIDs to polytrauma patients, which could lead to renal failure.
- Not giving an opioid intravenously to the severely injured.
- Not prescribing regular follow-up medication.

Recommended reading

Gibbon, C. J., et al. (eds.) South African Medicines Formulary. 2003. Sixth edition. South African Medical Association, Health and Medical Publishing Group. Pinelands. Dept Pharmacology, Faculty of Health Sciences, University of Cape Town.

8 Cardiopulmonary resuscitation

David Marshall, Walter Kloeck,
and Rob Scott-Millar

The diagnosis of cardiorespiratory arrest is made when there are no palpable carotid pulses, heart sounds are absent, and there is no spontaneous respiration. It is essential that the underlying cause is identified and corrected. In the case of hypovolaemic cardiac arrest due to penetrating trauma, a thoracotomy is performed early with internal cardiac massage.

Basic principles

The basic principles for cardiopulmonary resuscitation are:
- Perform a 'Primary survey':
  Airway
  Breathing
  Circulation
- Perform rapid evaluation, identification, and treatment of life-threatening conditions.
- Continue with reassessment throughout resuscitation.

Causes of cardiopulmonary deterioration

Deterioration can be caused by the following:
- Severe central neurological injury with secondary cardiovascular collapse.
- Hypoxia secondary to respiratory arrest resulting from neurological injury, airway obstruction, large open pneumothorax, or tracheo-bronchial injury.
- Direct and severe injury to vital structures, such as the heart, aorta, or pulmonary arteries.
- Underlying medical problems or other conditions that led to the injury, such as sudden ventricular fibrillation (VF) in the driver of a motor vehicle or a victim of an electric shock.
- Severely diminished output from tension pneumothorax or pericardial tamponade.
- Exsanguination, leading to hypovolaemia and severely diminished oxygen delivery.

- Injuries in a cold environment complicated by secondary severe hypothermia.

Management

Airway

The indications for intubation include:
- Respiratory arrest or apnoea
- Respiratory failure
- Shock
- Severe head injury
- Inability to protect airway
- Thoracic injuries – flail chest, pulmonary contusion
- Airway obstruction
- Injuries associated with potential airway obstruction (e.g. crushing facial or neck injuries)
- Anticipation of the need for mechanical ventilatory support (inhalation burn)

The airway should be cleared of all debris, false, and broken teeth. If head or neck trauma is a possibility, then ensure that the cervical spine has been stabilized. A jaw thrust and chin lift should be performed without extending the neck. Generally orotracheal intubation should be performed. Avoid nasotracheal intubation in the presence of maxillo-facial injuries. Confirm tube placement clinically and on chest X-ray (CXR). A cricothyroidotomy is indicated if there is an obstructed upper airway and orotracheal intubation is not possible.

Breathing/Ventilation

- Provide high concentrations of oxygen.
- Check for breath sounds – a unilateral decrease may suggest a haemothorax or pneumothorax. A tension pneumothorax may develop after sealing of an open pneumothorax and decompression may be needed.
- Beware of pumping the stomach full of air and causing massive regurgitation – deliver the breaths slowly, apply cricoid pressure, and consider inserting a nasogastric tube after intubation. In the presence of maxillo-facial injuries, nasogastric tubes may migrate intracranially, therefore place with caution, or insert orogastrically.

Circulation

If no signs of circulation (check carotid pulse) then:

- Commence chest compressions at 100 per minute – if the trachea is not intubated the ratio of compressions to ventilations is 15:2. Once the trachea has been intubated, chest compressions at a rate of 100 per minute should continue uninterrupted and ventilation should be continued at roughly 12 breaths/min.
- Attach an ECG monitor to check the cardiac rhythm. Ventricular tachycardia (VT) or VF possibly occurred first causing loss of consciousness – defibrillate immediately if pulseless.
- If a patient has a hypovolaemic cardiac arrest an open thoracotomy is advised with internal cardiac massage.

Pulseless cardiac rhythms include the following.

1 *Pulseless Electrical Activity (PEA-previously called Electro-Mechanical Dissociation) and asystole*

Look for and correct the following potentially reversible causes (5 'H's and 5 'T's):

The 5 'H's are

- Hypovolaemia
- Hypoxia
- Hypothermia
- Hyper-/hypokalaemia
- Hydrogen ion imbalances (acidosis) and other electrolytes

Figure 8.1 ECG showing ventricular tachycardia (VT)

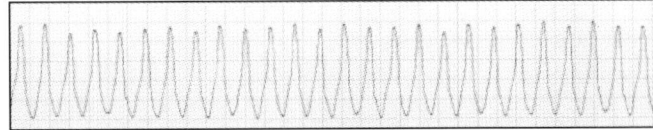

Figure 8.2 ECG with ventricular fibrillation (VF)

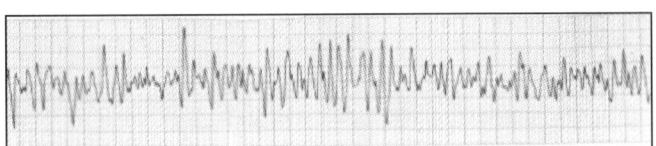

The 5 'T's are
- Tension pneumothorax
- Tamponade (cardiac)
- Thrombo-emboli (cardiac or pulmonary)
- Toxins
- Therapeutic disturbances

2 *Ventricular fibrillation (VF) and pulseless ventricular tachycardia (VT):*
- Treat with immediate defibrillation (200 J, 200 J, 360 J).
- IV adrenaline is typically administered to increase systemic vascular resistance when treating these arrhythmias but is usually ineffective in severe untreated hypovolaemia.
- Look for and correct the ten potentially reversible causes listed above.

Drug treatment

The following drug treatment is indicated:
- Adrenaline 1 mg every 3 minutes is recommended during all cardiopulmonary resuscitation attempts. Give intravenous (IV), but if no IV access is available, then down the tracheal tube (2 mg diluted with 10 ml saline). Intra-osseous injection may be performed in a child less than six years of age (e.g. intratibial). If one has performed a thoracotomy, give directly into ventricular chamber as a last resort (but *not* into the ventricular muscle).
- If VF or pulseless VT is the primary rhythm and defibrillation is unsuccessful, then consider an amiodarone 300 mg IV push, followed by an amiodarone infusion if successful.
- Atropine 1 mg IV every 3 minutes is indicated for PEA (pulseless electrical activity) associated with a bradycardia, as well as for asystole, up to a maximum of 3 mg (0.04 mg/kg).
- Sodium bicarbonate 1 mEq/kg IV is indicated if the patient is hyperkalaemic or has a pre-existing metabolic acidosis, or after every 10 minutes during a prolonged resuscitation attempt. Do *not* give bicarbonate in the presence of respiratory acidosis.

Open thoracotomy

Open thoracotomy does not improve outcome in out-of-hospital blunt trauma, but can be lifesaving with penetrating chest trauma or hypovolaemic cardiac arrest. Whilst volume expansion is in progress, prompt emergency thoracotomy will allow:
- Direct cardiac massage

Figure 8.3 Internal cardiac paddles

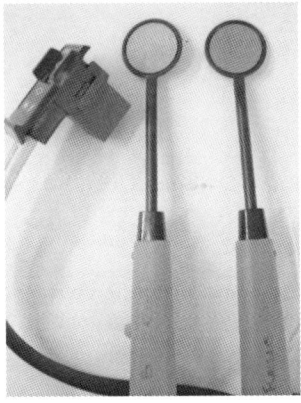

- Surgical procedures as indicated (control of haemorrhage, aortic cross-clamping)
- Defibrillation with internal paddles (start with 10 J, go up to 20 J)
- Administration of adrenaline into the ventricular chamber

Adequate resuscitation may be impossible in the presence of severe uncontrolled haemorrhage and urgent surgical exploration with haemostatic control is indicated in these conditions.

Pitfalls

- Hypovolaemic cardiac arrest due to penetrating trauma will require a thoracotomy and internal cardiac massage.
- Always attempt to identify and correct the *cause* of the cardiac arrest.

Recommended reading

Guidelines 2000 for Cardiopulmonary Resuscitation and Emergency Cardiovascular Care: International Consensus on Science. *Circulation*, 102(8):1–403.

9 Radiology

Steve Beningfield

The objective of imaging in trauma is to facilitate the prompt, efficient, and cost-effective management of the injured patient by providing pertinent and timely information on the state of the patient's body. Imaging frequently requires that the patient be removed from the intense observation and care of the resuscitation team in return for a more accurate idea of the problems to be overcome. Careful monitoring of potentially unstable patients is vitally important throughout the imaging procedure.

The three acute lethal enemies of the trauma patient are head injury, bleeding, and cardiorespiratory problems. In an attempt to pre-empt these, precedence is given to the early imaging triad of chest, pelvis, and lateral cervical spine radiographs.

Apart from the diagnostic imaging service, the radiological therapeutic options that are available for use at all stages of the trauma patient's course are increasing.

Trauma imaging modalities

X-rays/radiographs

Plain X-ray imaging is most commonly performed using film cassettes and chemical film processors, introducing unavoidable delays in the availability of images. Newer solid-state digital radiography devices offer direct image acquisition with the production of computer images in seconds rather than minutes.

Tomography

Tomography relies on the mechanical motion of the tube-detector assembly to blur out irrelevant areas, permitting clearer views of the plane of interest. Although computed tomography (CT) has largely replaced tomography, it retains an important role for imaging in-plane horizontal fractures or displacements.

Contrast studies

By introducing iodine or barium-containing radio-opaque fluids under X-ray visualization, more information about body spaces and visceral interiors can be obtained.

Fluoroscopy

Image intensifiers coupled to video monitors allow real-time radiographic visualization and X-rays of the interior of the body and its function, usually aided by radio-opaque contrast media.

Urography

This includes intravenous pyelography (IVP), based on renal excretion of intravenously injected iodinated contrast medium. Also included are cystography (contrast medium introduced into the bladder), and urethrography (contrast medium used to fill the urethra).

Sinography

Sinography is generally used in the follow-up of trauma cases, to delineate the course and nature of sinuses and fistulae by means of iodinated contrast material injected under fluoroscopy.

Computed tomography (CT)

Conventional CT

This CT is based on mathematical reconstructions of X-ray beams passed radially through the body. CT provides excellent detail in cross-sectional views of the body, usually in the axial plane. Bone, soft tissue, blood, fat, and gas are all very well demonstrated. Interventional procedures under CT guidance are also possible. The addition of an intravenous iodinated contrast medium bolus during scanning greatly facilitates detection of normal and abnormal vascular structures, as well as enhancement of parenchymal and pathological tissues. Orally or rectally administered contrast agents can also be beneficial.

Spiral/Helical computed tomography

The technical advances of slip-ring technology and simultaneous table movement during scanning allow the acquisition of continuous cylinders of high-quality data, rather than discrete, interrupted cross-sectional slices. The greater resultant speed significantly improves the depiction of the phases of injected intravascular boluses of iodinated contrast medium.

Multibeam helical computed tomography

The latest advance in CT relies on an array of parallel side-by-side detectors to further speed up data acquisition.

Computed tomography angiography (CTA)

Using the obtained CT information, computer display of contrast-filled vessels in a variety of three-dimensional views is possible.

Ultrasound (U/S)

Two-dimensional ultrasound

Using high-frequency sound to build up images of the interior of the body, the soft tissues and fluid collections are very well depicted.

Duplex Doppler ultrasound

Relying on the frequency alterations of reflected sound, flow patterns in vessels can be accurately determined.

Colour Doppler ultrasound

Superimposing a colour signal on the obtained velocity information allows rapid and easy detection of flow patterns.

Angiography

Angiography utilizes catheter-delivered intravascular bolus injections of iodinated contrast medium to view arterial and venous lumens and associated pathology.

Digital subtraction angiography (DSA)

Following the computer acquisition of images of intravascular contrast, a computerized subtraction technique allows the removal of distracting body structures from the angiogram.

Magnetic resonance imaging (MRI)

Spinning hydrogen protons present in the molecules of water of the body are subjected to a very strong magnetic field. Radio pulses are then used to disturb the proton spins, which in turn emit weak radio echoes. T1 and T2 echoes refer to the realignment and desynchronization of these proton spins respectively. These radio signals are mathematically used to create cross-sectional images of regions of the body in any plane. The technique is highly sensitive to soft-tissue structures and pathology, and can help determine the age of blood clot. Cortical bone and calcification are generally not well seen as they contain little water. The high-strength magnetic field does create problems in trauma patients, particularly regarding compatibility of life-support devices. A number of contraindications to MRI exist (see www.mrisafety.com).

Interventional radiology

This developing field makes use of image guidance to perform minimally invasive diagnostic and therapeutic procedures on patients.

Angiographic intervention

Embolization

Embolization is the deliberate occlusion of vessels by a range of catheter-delivered embolic agents. Gianturco coils (coiled spring wires) can be passed via a catheter lumen and packed into vessels, causing their occlusion. The vessel injury should ideally be at least 3 cm away from any vital parent vessel to permit safe embolization.

Particles

Embolic particles range in size from microns to millimetres in diameter. These would not be used in arteriovenous fistulae, as they could pass through the fistula into the pulmonary or systemic arteries. They may be temporary (such as gelatin sponge) or permanent (such as polyvinyl alcohol foam).

Other agents

These include the effective but dangerous liquid agents such as cyanoacrylate glue and ethanol.

Stents

These self-expanding or balloon-expandable tubular metal mesh devices have increasing application in trauma, largely as covered stents. Covered stents can be used to seal off and treat post-traumatic false aneurysms and arteriovenous fistulae. These devices are increasingly being used, but long-term follow up is still limited.

Drainages

Drainage catheters placed into collections or spaces using imaging guidance allow effective non-surgical treatment of collections.

Specific anatomical regions

Head

1 In a skull X-ray (SXR), evaluate for:
  - Vault fractures, especially those involving the sinuses or skull base
  - Basal fractures suggested by findings such as:
    - fluid levels in the sphenoid sinus
    - opacified middle-ear cavities
    - intracranial air
  - Depressed skull fractures
  - Intracranial air
  - Foreign bodies
  - Pineal shift (indicating midline shift)
  - The cranio-cervical junction, including the CO/1 relationship and the atlanto-dens interval

Additional notes. Slot fractures, such as those due to knife blade penetration, are often difficult to detect. It is important to remember with the patient supine for the lateral SXR using a horizontal X-ray beam technique, fluid levels appear vertical when viewing the SXR in the usual erect fashion. The fluid level may be easier to see by placing the lateral SXR in a nose-uppermost position.

Figure 9.1 CT brain demonstrating marked cerebral swelling with almost total obliteration of the CSF spaces, most notably the lateral (white arrow) and 3rd ventricles (black arrow)

Figure 9.2 CT brain demonstrating small amount of blood in the left lateral ventricle (black arrow), with extra-axial superficial collections of blood over the lateral fronto-parietal area (white arrow)

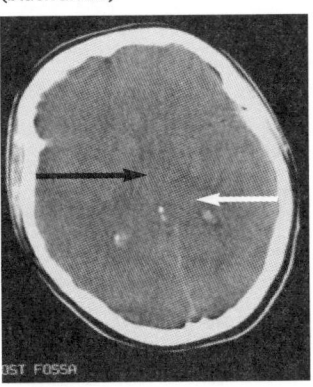
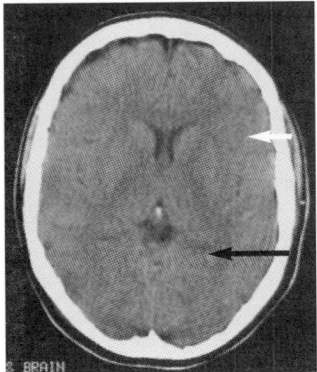

Table 9.1 Imaging recommendations for a CT scan of the head (Modified from reference 1)

Risks:	Low	Medium	High	Very High	Children
History	Minimal force	Inadequate history Stab head with loss of consciousness Penetrating eye injury Severe force fall of more than 60 cm or onto hard surface	Suspected FB or penetrating injury		Poor history
Consciousness	Fully oriented	Loss of consciousness	Depressed consciousness	Deteriorating consciousness	Loss of consciousness
Neurological defects	None, no amnesia	Neurological compromise Amnesia Headache Vomiting	Focal neurological features Disoriented Seizure	Confusion/coma	Neurological deficit
Examination	No serious laceration No haematoma	Scalp bruise Swelling Laceration over 5 cm in length or down to bone Inadequate examination	Sutural diastasis Skull fracture CSF from nose to ear Blood from ear Unstable Diagnosis uncertain	Open or penetrating injury Skull fracture Depressed or compound fracture Skull-base fracture	Tense fontanelle or sutural diastasis Possible NAI (non-accidental injury)
Action	Head injury observations	Head injury observations	CT head	Urgent CT head Urgent neuro-surgical/anaesthetist referral	CT head SXR and skeletal survey if NAI suspected

2   In a CT head, evaluate for:
   ● The presence of any midline shift.
   ● Symmetry between the two halves of the cerebral contents.
   ● Acute subdural and extradural haematomas. These are usually hyper-dense, but may rarely be isodense or hypodense, possibly due to anaemia and/or dilution by cerebrospinal fluid. Subacute subdural haematomas may become isodense with brain within a week and may therefore be more prone to being overlooked. Intravenous contrast is very useful in this circumstance, as it demonstrates the enhancing borders of subdural haematomas.

Facial region

The following table provides the appropriate radiological investigations required according to the nature of the facial injury.

Table 9.2 Imaging recommendations for the facial region (modified from reference 1)

Nose	Plain X-rays not helpful Other imaging only if requested by relevant specialist
Orbits	Facial X-rays
Blunt injury 'blow out' suspected clinically	Facial X-rays Low-dose axial and coronal CT/MRI an option
Penetrating injury **Radio-opaque foreign body** **Possible fracture orbital wall**	CT head Specialist referral. CT or U/S orbits if requested by ophthalmologist. MRI – beware intra-orbital metallic foreign bodies as these may move and damage the eye
Mid-face ● Tenderness over zygoma ● Mobile hard palate ● Infra-orbital sensory loss	Not urgent – delay facial X-rays if uncooperative CT if requested by maxillofacial specialist
Tenderness over mandible	AP X-ray, 2 obliques Orthopantomography Axial and coronal CT if requested by the relevant specialist

Foreign bodies

The following table provides the radiological investigations that may be useful in detecting foreign bodies.

Table 9.3 Imaging recommendations (modified from reference 1)

Type of foreign body	Recommended imaging	Further options
Metal/glass/painted wood	X-ray (remove dressings first), all glass is radio-opaque to some degree; some paint is also	U/S may be useful
Fish bone	Neck (lateral and frontal)	Endoscopy
Small, smooth foreign body	AP neck, CXR (to exclude presence in airways)	AXR if no passage after 6 days
Sharp or potentially poisonous foreign body (e.g. battery)	AXR	CXR if AXR negative
Large object	Inspect oropharynx visually Lateral neck (foreign body may impact at crico-pharyngeus), CXR	AXR if CXR negative (may need barium swallow or endoscopy)
Inhaled FB suspected	CXR/ expiratory view for air trapping	If CXR normal – bronchoscopy may still be needed

Cervical spine (C-spine)

Lateral cervical spine X-rays

- Routine evaluation of the cervical spine X-ray must include the alignment of the anterior and posterior borders of the vertebral bodies, the spinolaminar lines, the atlantodens-interval, the craniocervical relationships, the pre-cervical soft tissue, and the interspinous distances (see Figure 9.4).
- The atlanto-dens interval should not exceed 3 mm in adults and 5 mm in children up to five years of age.

Figure 9.3 Radio-opaque foreign body aspirated into right main bronchus, with distal right middle and lower lobe collapse/consolidation

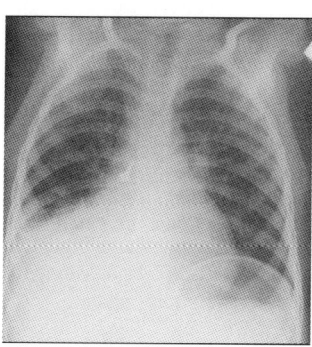

Figure 9.4 Lateral cervical spine X-ray demonstrating normal alignments; the anterior vertebral line (1), the posterior vertebral line (2), and the spinolaminar line (3)

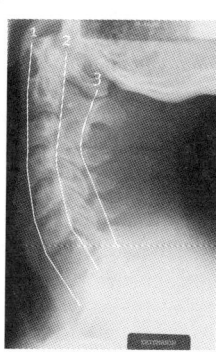

Table 9.4 Imaging recommendations for the cervical spine (modified from reference 1)

When there are:	
• No neck symptoms and the patient is alert and cooperative with no evidence of intoxication, and the neck is non-tender with no neurological signs	Imaging not required
Neck injury with pain, head injury or unconscious	NB Neck protection critical Cervical spine X-rays • Lateral • AP • Swimmer's or flying angel views including C7/T1 • Open mouth view of the peg
Neck injury with neurological deficit	Cervical spine X-rays as above, with • Urgent neurosurgical or orthopaedic referral, plus • MRI or CT myelogram if required by specialist

- On the lateral X-ray, above C3 the normal pre-cervical soft tissue measures up to a third of the width of the adjacent vertebral body; below C3 the same width as the vertebral bodies.
- The cranio-cervical junction relationship of CO/C1 must also be specifically evaluated (Figure 9.5).
- The bowtie sign of unilateral locked facets must be consciously sought, but the effects of rotation simulating this feature should also be known.

AP cervical spine X-rays
The alignment and spacing of the vertebral elements are important. The interspinous distances should be comparable to one another, and aligned on the AP view.

Open mouth odontoid peg views
Beware of the 'Mach' effect giving rise to pseudo-fractures of the peg. (This is a visual phenomenon caused by sudden changes in optical density, typically due to teeth or the occiput overlapping the odontoid peg.)

Figure 9.5 Lateral C-spine X-ray – the basion (inferior point of the clivus) should lie between 12 mm anterior and 4 mm posterior to the posterior axial line (a line drawn along the posterior body of C2). The line from the basion to the tip of the peg should not exceed 12 mm on the lateral C-spine X-ray.

Figure 9.6 Atlanto-occipital dislocation with a widened ADI

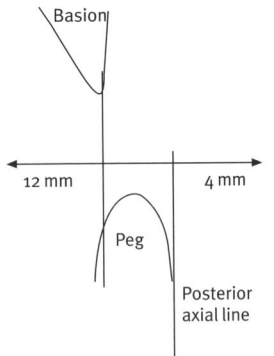

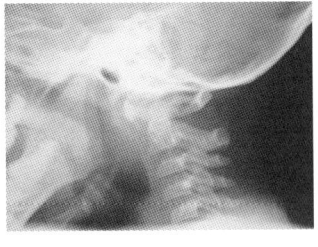

Thoracic and lumbar spine

Table 9.5 Imaging recommendations (modified from reference 1)

Clinical	Standard imaging	Specialized imaging
In a patient who is: • Awake, alert, asymptomatic, and examinable with no pain or neuro-logical deficit.	X-rays not required	
In a patient where: • There has been a significant fall, high-impact motor vehicle acci-dent, or other severe injury • Clinical evaluation is not possible • Local spinal pain is present • Neurological deficit is present	AP and lateral X-rays CT, MRI	

Flying angel or swimmer's view if C7/T1 junction is not seen
The C7/T1 junction must be seen to avoid missing injury.

Supervised erect flexion/extension views
These are indicated in patients with normal plain X-rays but:
• Persistent severe neck pain
• Suspected ligamentous injury
• Tenderness, especially with pre-vertebral soft tissue swelling

These flexion extension views may reveal soft tissue injuries by demonstrating widening of the interspinous distance and/or subluxation at the intervertebral spaces. These views should not be performed when any traumatic bony abnormality is present on the regular cervical spine X-rays, or in an unconscious patient.

CT cervical spine
CT scanning is very useful to further diagnose and characterize bony injuries, especially when cervical spine X-rays are equivocal, or with complex lesions.

MRI cervical spine
MRI very clearly shows soft tissue injuries such as disc herniation, ligamentous tears or epidural haematoma, as well as spinal cord oedema, contusion, or haematoma. MRI is especially useful when neurological damage is present.

Abdomen

Blunt abdominal trauma in adults is generally treated conservatively provided the patient is haemodynamically stable and there is no evidence of peritonism. For unstable patients, surgical exploration is appropriate.

Erect CXR

This is a sensitive means of detecting free subphrenic air where relevant. A right side up decubitus view is also a very sensitive way to detect free air – it is important that the patient be kept in this position for 5–10 minutes to allow the free air to percolate upwards over the lateral surface of the right liver.

CT abdomen

- Performs well in the detection of bony injury, pneumoperitoneum, and solid organ injuries, especially occult splenic or pancreatic trauma.
- The sensitivity of CT scan for detecting bowel perforations remains low, even with the addition of contrast.
- Free fluid in the peritoneal cavity, in the absence of any solid organ injury, should alert one to the possibility of a bowel perforation.

Table 9.6 Imaging recommendations

Blunt injury or stab abdomen	• Erect CXR + supine AXR	• CT for liver, spleen, pancreas, and kidneys as indicated • Role of U/S limited
GSW abdomen	• Erect CXR + supine AXR	• CT if conservative management considered
Major trauma	Stabilize first Protect C-spine • Minimal initial X-rays required in the polytrauma patient consist of C-spine, CXR, and pelvis	• CT head

Urological

Table 9.7 Imaging recommendations

Penetrating injury	• Microscopic haematuria	CT (or IVP)
Blunt injury	• Microscopic haematuria only	No specific urinary tract imaging required
Blunt injury	• Macroscopic haematuria	CT or IVP

Figure 9.7 CT scan of the abdomen demonstrating a major injury to the left kidney

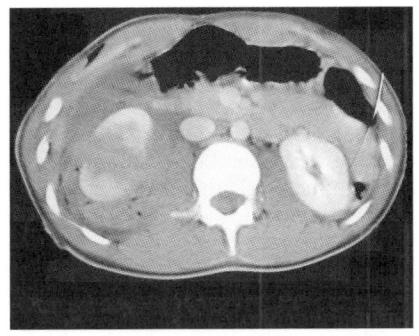

Pelvis

Table 9.8 Imaging recommendations

• A history of a motor vehicle accident or other significant injury	Pelvic X-rays
• The patient is not able to walk • Pain on compression of the pelvis • Rectal or vaginal bleeding • Severe multi-injury	CT

Pitfalls

- Develop a routine and stick to a consistent method of viewing X-rays, e.g. verify the patient name, date, and left/right markers on the image, evaluate the soft tissues, bones, and viscera successively.
- Use the 'bright light' to look at areas of concern.
- Do not stop searching for pathology once you have encountered one abnormality – the psychological phenomenon of 'satisfaction of search' is your enemy! Be doubly suspicious! This also applies to combined injuries such as aortic arch rupture, together with diaphragm rupture, head injury, and pelvic fractures, or associations between calcaneal and spinal injuries.
- Always ensure that the cervical spine is visualized down to T1.
- Find a good atlas of normal X-ray variants and keep it in the trauma unit.
- Don't forget to consider pre-existing pathology, with the increased risk of pathological viscera to trauma.

Reference

Radiation protection 118, Referral guidelines for imaging; UK Royal College of Radiologists and European Commission Directorate-General for the Environment. Luxembourg: Office for Official Publications of the European Communities (http://europa.eu.int/comm/environment/radprot/118/rp-118-en.pdf), 2000.

Antibiotics in trauma

Stephen Oliver

General principles

Consider the organisms likely to have been introduced as a result of the trauma: Was an area with significant normal flora involved? What was the likelihood of environmental contamination? Choose an antibiotic appropriate for those organisms.

Common organisms and their appropriate treatment

Staphylococcus aureus:	Cloxacillin for treatment of established infection; cefazolin most often used for prophylaxis
Streptococci:	Pencillin/Ampicillin; cloxacillin will also cover
Enterobacteria:	Aminoglycosides; cephalosporins; beta-lactam/betalactamase inhibitor combinations (co-amoxyclav); piperacillin/tazobactam
Anaerobes:	Metronidazole
Clostridia:	Penicillin or metronidazole

Additional points:
- Co-amoxyclav will cover *cloxacillin-sensitive* staphylococci, streptococci, many enterobacteria, and has the anaerobic cover equivalent to that of metronidazole.
- Most cephalosporins will cover *cloxacillin-sensitive* staphylococci and penicillin-sensitive streptococci.
- Combinations of short- and long-acting penicillins (e.g. Penilente Forte®) are more appropriate in certain 'early treatment' situations than benzathine penicillin. The latter gives sustained, but relatively low levels of penicillin.
- In patients with a history of allergy to penicillins:
  Clindamycin will cover both staphylococci and streptococci (and many anaerobes).
  Cephalosporins can be used (with caution) if the history is not one of anaphylaxis, bronchospasm, or other life-threatening reaction.
- When using aminoglycosides, it is essential to give an adequate first dose, irrespective of renal function (6 mg/kg for gentamicin, 15 mg/kg for amikacin).

True prophylaxis vs early treatment

True prophylaxis is the use of an antibiotic during a procedure in order to prevent infection. In this situation the antibiotic should be given before, and as close to the event as possible, and a single dose is all that is required. Most situations in trauma medicine involve early treatment (after the event) where there is a high probability of infection. Short courses of antibiotics are appropriate in these situations.

Prophylaxis/Early treatment recommendations for specific situations

Penetrating abdominal injury

- Penicillin, gentamicin, and metronidazole; or IV co-amoxyclav may be used (NB: IV co-amoxyclav is unstable and must be administered within three hours of being reconstituted).
- The first dose should be given pre-laparotomy – no need for subsequent doses if the gastro-intestinal tract is not penetrated.
- In cases where there has been soiling of the peritoneum, 48 hours of therapy is generally sufficient (recent studies have revealed no difference between 24 hours and five days of therapy).

Penetrating cranio-cerebral and spinal cord injury

- Cefuroxime 1.5 g, then 750 mg 8 hourly, plus metronidazole
- Five days of therapy are required.

Skull fractures

- *Base of skull:* Antibiotics have not been shown to decrease the incidence of meningitis – no prophylaxis recommended.
- *Compound depressed:* Cefuroxime 1.5 g, then 750 mg 8 hourly, plus metronidazole for five days of therapy.

Gunshot wounds

- *Abdominal injury:* As above for penetrating abdominal injury.
- *CNS injury:* As above for penetrating cranio-cerebral injury.
- *Soft tissue injury only:* 'Triple penicillin' (e.g. Penilente Forte®)1.2 mu. Consider broader cover, e.g. penicillin or cloxacillin, plus gentamicin and metronidazole if there is considerable tissue damage and especially in chest injuries that may have involved the oesophagus.

Intercostal drain insertion for traumatic haemopneumothorax

Antibiotic prophylaxis is not usually required. 'Triple penicillin' or broader cover may be used in situations where there is extensive soft tissue injury.

Bites

There is no clear evidence of the benefit for antibiotic prophylaxis in minor animal bites.

- Moderate to severe animal bites, all bites to the hand and all human bites should receive co-amoxiclav 625 mg (or 375 mg plus 250 mg amoxycillin) 8 hourly for five days (tetracycline or clindamycin are alternatives for penicillin-allergic patients).
- Patients presenting after 24 hours who do not have infected wounds probably do not need antibiotics.

Orthopaedics

Compound fracture. If the fracture appears clean, then penicillin G IV for 48 hours (this is for the prevention of clostridial infection); metronidazole should be used in penicillin-allergic patients. Any injury with significant contamination and large wounds with significant tissue destruction – cloxacillin, gentamicin, and metronidazole for 48 hours (this may need to be prolonged in some cases).

Open reduction and internal fixation of closed fractures. Cefazolin 1 g at induction, and then 500 mg 8 hourly for 24 hours.

Needle-stick injury or exposure to blood/body fluids

- Determine the type of body fluid involved (urine, faeces, saliva, and vomitus do not warrant prophylaxis.
- Determine the type of exposure – intact/non-intact skin, mucous membrane, penetrating injury.
- Determine the HIV status of the source patient and the injured person – consent required.
- See Table 10.1 for recommendations.
- *Two-drug regimen:* lamivudine 150 mg plus zidovudine 300 mg, both given 12 hourly – available in a fixed combination Combivir®.
- *Three-drug regimen:* As above, plus indinavir 800 mg 8 hourly (on an empty stomach).

Table 10.1 Recommendations for post-exposure prophylaxis (PEP) after exposure to infectious material (includes blood, CSF, semen, vaginal secretions, and synovial/pleural/pericardial/peritoneal/amniotic fluid) from HIV seropositive patients

Exposure	HIV status of source Unknown	Positive	High Risk*
Intact skin	No PEP	No PEP	No PEP
Mucosal splash/ Non-intact skin	Consider 2 drugs	Recommend 2 drugs	Recommend 2 drugs
Percutaneous (sharps)	Recommend 2 drugs	Recommend 2 drugs	Consider 3 drugs
Percutaneous (needle in vessels or deep injury)	Recommend 2 drugs	Recommend 3 drugs	Recommend 3 drugs

High risk * includes terminal Aids, seroconversion illness, or known to have a high viral load.

Treatment of some conditions that might be encountered in a trauma ward

Urinary tract infections

In catheterized patients with asymptomatic bacteriuria – remove or change the catheter and repeat the culture. If therapy is required:

- Single-dose therapy is never appropriate in catheterized patients.
- Co-amoxyclav, gentamicin, or cefuroxime are all suitable empiric choices – individual situations may dictate the choice.
- If the infection is hospital-acquired and more resistant organisms are prevalent, amikacin or a quinolone may be indicated.
- Therapy should be for a minimum of five days, 10–14 days if there are signs of upper tract infection (shorter courses can be employed with quinolones; three and seven days respectively).

Wound infection

Most wound infections are staphylococcal, and cloxacillin IV or oral flu-cloxacillin remain the best empiric choice.

- Wounds in areas where gram negatives and anaerobes may be more common should be treated with oral co-amoxyclav or IV cloxacillin, plus gentamicin and metronidazole if oral therapy is not appropriate.
- Clindamycin is a suitable choice for penicillin-allergic patients and in those who fail to respond to cloxacillin.

Nosocomial pneumonia

The treatment of nosocomial pneumonia will vary from hospital to hospital depending on the sensitivity patterns of local organisms.

- Generally a choice of a third or fourth generation cephalosporin (ceftriaxone, cefotaxime, or cefepime), or ampicillin plus amikacin would be appropriate.
- Patients who have been ventilated may be at risk of exposure to more resistant organisms in many units, and agents such as piperacillin/tazobactam, quinolones, or carbapenems may be required.

Meningitis

The organisms causing meningitis after trauma do not differ from those causing meningitis under other conditions except that *S. aureus* infections are more common.

- Ceftriaxone 2 g daily or cefotaxime 2 g 8 hourly are both effective for all these organisms and should be commenced empirically.
- Therapy should be adjusted once the sensitivity of the causative organism is known.
- Metronidazole should be added if the trauma involves the sinuses.

Brain abscess

Brain abscesses unrelated to trauma can usually be treated with penicillin and metronidazole if they are in the frontal area. Abscesses in the temporal area (otogenic) more often involve gram-negative aerobes and require ceftriaxone or cefotaxime in doses as for meningitis but with the addition of metronidazole for anaerobes.

Abscesses secondary to trauma may involve staphylococci, and cloxacillin 3 g 6 hourly (plus metronidazole) should be used if no gram-negative cover is required. Ceftriaxone or cefotaxime (plus metronidazole) as above should be given in cases where gram-negative organisms are likely.

Empyema

Organisms involved in empyemas include streptococci, staphylococci, anaerobes, and increasingly, gram-negative bacilli.

Antibiotic therapy should be guided by culture results but should empirically include cover for the range of possible pathogens.

Co-amoxyclav or a combination of cloxacillin, gentamicin, and metronidazole provide the required spectrum of action.

Septicaemia

The choice of antibiotic in a septicaemic patient must be governed by the likely origin of the sepsis. Penicillin, gentamicin, and metronidazole, a cephalosporin and metronidazole, or co-amoxyclav (IV) are appropriate for sepsis of abdominal origin and provide broad cover for cases of unknown aetiology.

Candida infections

If yeasts are cultured from a catheter urine specimen the catheter should be removed or changed and the culture repeated.

- Persistent presence of yeasts in a patient with signs of infection should be treated with amphotericin bladder washouts or oral fluconazole.
- Systemic candida (or other yeast) infection should be considered in patients with ongoing signs of sepsis despite adequate antibiotic therapy and in those where three days of amphotericin bladder washouts failed to eradicate the yeast.
- Isolation of yeasts from several local sites is an additional risk factor that may prompt commencement of antifungal therapy.
- The isolation of yeasts from a blood culture should always be taken seriously and treated with a minimum of two weeks of antifungal therapy.
- Amphotericin B or an azole (fluconazole) are currently the effective therapies available for these infections.

Pitfalls

- Urinary tract infections are the most common infections in trauma patients – remove the catheter as soon as possible.
- Think of joint penetration in animal bites that occur close to joints.
- If a patient is on a cephalosporin, it is not necessary to add cloxacillin for staphylococcal cover in most cases.
- If a patient is receiving co-amoxyclav, neither cloxacillin nor metronidazole are required as the co-amoxyclav provides both staphylococcal and anaerobic cover.

Recommended reading

Mandal A.K., Thadepalli H., Chettipalli U. 1997. Post-traumatic empyema thoracis: A 24-year experience at a major trauma centre. *Trauma*, Nov, 43(5):764–771.

Mandell, Gerald L., Bennett, John E., Dolin, Raphael 2000. *Principles and practice of infectious diseases.* Fifth edition. Edinburgh: Churchill Livingstone.

Smith P.F., Meadowcroft A.M., May D.B. 2000. Treating mammalian bite wounds. *J of Clin Pharmacy and Therapeutics*, 25:85–99.

Use of antibiotics in penetrating craniocerebral injuries. (Review) Working Party of British Society for Antimicrobial Chemotherapy. *The Lancet*, Vol 355, May 20, 2000.

11 Damage control surgery

Ken D Boffard, Elias Degiannis,
and Jonty Karpelowsky

The concept of damage control has gained increasing support among trauma surgeons as a valuable adjunct in the surgical care of the severely injured patient. Damage control is defined as preserving an incompletely repaired, but survivable anatomical form, in order to prevent the patient from progressing to an unsalvageable metabolic state of hypothermia, acidosis, and coagulopathy.

The usual endpoint of a surgical procedure is the restoration of disrupted anatomy. Technically, impressive repairs are often accomplished after hours of surgery. All too often, however, persistent operative efforts result in the exacerbation of underlying hypothermia, coagulopathy, and acidosis (the 'triad of death'), for which Moore coined the phrase 'the bloody vicious cycle'. The cost of metabolic failure is sepsis, multi-organ failure, and death. Never before has the surgeon been asked to operate to restore physiology.

Damage control (damage limitation surgery), therefore, is the technique where operative time and intervention are minimized in the grossly unstable patient. Rapid control of surgical haemorrhage and contamination, followed by transfer to the intensive care unit for physiological resuscitation and stabilization, and then return to theatre for the definitive procedure, can be life saving.

Damage control can be applied to all organ systems. It is divided into three phases:

1 Initial exploration
2 Secondary resuscitation
3 Definitive operation

Pathophysiology

Metabolic acidosis

With prolonged shock there is inadequate oxygen delivery to cells, which leads to metabolic acidosis, producing the by-product lactic acid. The accumulation of lactic acid results in metabolic acidosis (low pH on the blood gas analysis, a large negative base excess, and low bicarbonate values), which is mostly, in trauma patients, a direct result of tissue hypoperfusion.

All measures must be aimed at correcting the underlying hypoperfusion, by aggressive resuscitation. Simple correction of the pH by the administration of bicarbonate fails to address the underlying problem. A rise in the serum lactate is one of the most significant prognostic indicators of hypoperfusion (reflecting anaerobic metabolism). Although the lactate level should be regarded as the 'gold standard', the pH and base excess can be used as a guide to cell perfusion, worsening with ongoing shock, and improving as the patient is resuscitated.

A normal serum lactate level is < 2.5 mmol/litre.

Hypothermia

Hypothermia is an inevitable consequence of severe injury and subsequent resuscitation:

- Prior to arrival in hospital, heat losses occur as the patient lies exposed.
- During resuscitation the clothes are removed, cold fluids are commonly given, and the patient is exposed as procedures are performed.
- As body cavities are opened during surgery, the patient lies surrounded by wet drapes, leading to rapid evaporation and heat loss.
- The injured shocked patient has also been shown to have impaired thermogenesis.

Hypothermia has several consequences:

- It is in itself a very strong predictor of mortality.
- Myocardial function becomes depressed, further worsening perfusion.
- Clotting becomes severely deranged, leading to life-threatening coagulopathy.

Coagulopathy

Every aspect of normal physiological clotting is affected in the cold, acidotic, exsanguinating patient.

Platelets

Endothelial disruption leads to platelet plug formation, and activation of clotting factors.

Platelet function is affected by hypothermia and acidosis, possibly by affecting cyclo-oxygenase, leading to abnormal production ratios of prostaglandin.

Abnormalities have also been demonstrated in pathways responsible for the activation of proteins involved in platelet adherence.

Clotting factors

Clotting factors are a group of enzymes, which become activated via the external and internal pathways, ultimately resulting in fibrin clot formation and haemostasis. Enzymes are only able to function effectively within certain narrow temperature and pH limits. With progressive acidosis and hypothermia there is a steady decline in their function, with consequent coagulopathy and bleeding.

Fibrinolysis

The excessive breakdown of clot has not been clearly linked to disseminated intravascular coagulation and is usually related more to specific injury complexes, e.g. severe brain injury.

Dilutional coagulopathy

Massive transfusion has been clearly demonstrated as an independent risk factor and results from a decrease in both platelets and clotting factors. More recently, it has also been demonstrated that hypothermia and dilutional effects have an independent and exponentially additive effect on coagulopathy.

Figure 11.1 Pathophysiology of the 'bloody vicious cycle'

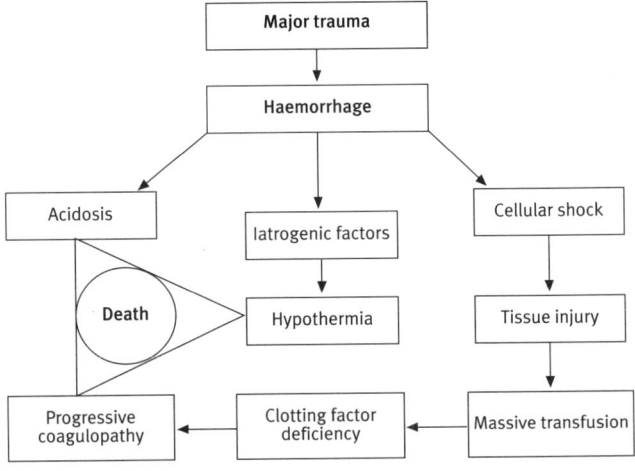

Figure 11.2 Overview of the damage control process

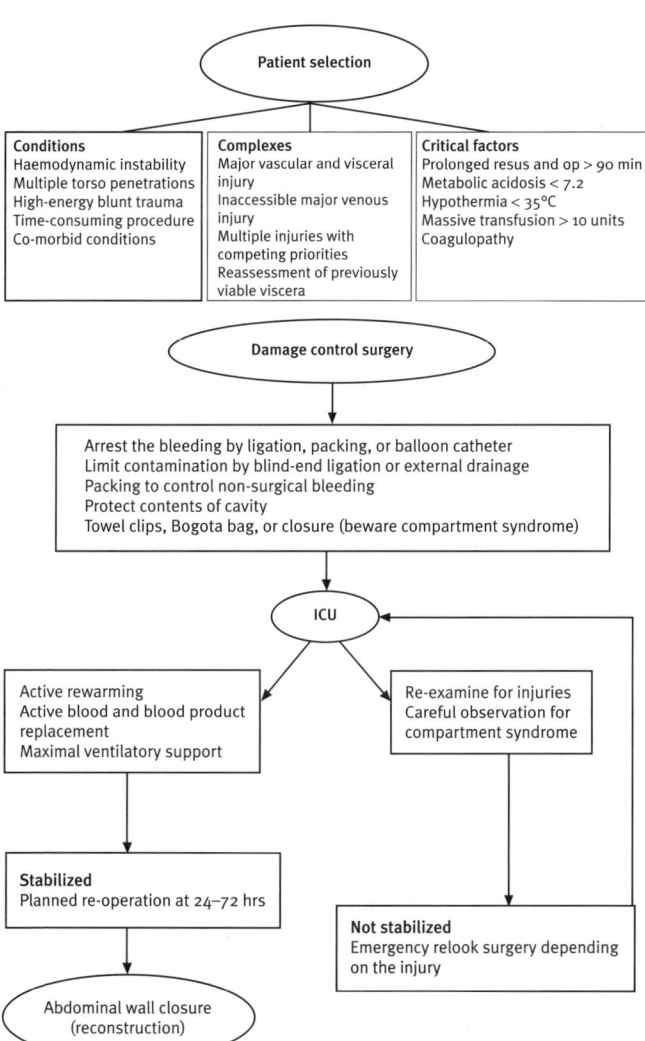

Damage control process

The main objective of damage control is to accomplish definitive operative management in a calculated, stepwise fashion based on the patient's physiological tolerance. There are five critical decision points in this process:

1 Patient selection
2 Initial surgery
3 Ongoing resuscitation and stabilization in the ICU
4 Re-operation planned as definitive surgery
5 Abdominal wall closure or reconstruction

Phase I: Patient selection

The success of damage control depends almost entirely on judicious patient selection and the timing of its implementation. Previously damage control was limited to patients with extensive liver damage but now it is based on a combination of the injury complex and the physiological parameters of the patient. Selection of patients is based on the following:

- Conditions
- Complexes
- Critical factors

Conditions

Condition on arrival should already alert the surgeon to the possibility of damage control. The following patients will probably require damage control, despite vigorous resuscitation:

- High-energy torso trauma
- Multiple torso penetration
- Co-morbidity (e.g. age, diabetes)
- Prolonged hypotension (Systolic BP < 75 mmHg)
- Profound haemodynamic instability
- Massive transfusion (> 10 unit blood requirement)

Complexes

The group of injuries found at the time of operation may suggest that the patient should undergo damage control surgery:

- Patients in whom there is inability to achieve haemostasis due to diffuse bleeding (e.g. in the liver) or inaccessible major venous injury (e.g. to the retrohepatic vena cava)
- Major vascular and visceral injury, e.g. bowel, duodenum, and inferior vena cava injuries
- Inaccessible major venous injury such as retrohepatic inferior vena cava or deep pelvic vessels
- Multiple injuries with competing priorities

- A time-consuming procedure is required in the presence of a rapid decline of physiological reserve, e.g. a Whipple's procedure
- Other injuries require non-operative control (e.g. severely fractured pelvis)
- Re-assessment of abdominal structures are required (planned relook)

Critical factors

Successful damage control is dependent on appropriate patient selection based on the following pre- and intra-operative findings:

- Prolonged resuscitation and operative time: total exceeding 90 min
- Inotrope requirements
- Systolic BP < 90 mm for more than 60 minutes
- Metabolic acidosis pH < 7.20
- Lactate > 5 mmol/litre
- Hypothermia < 35 °C
- Massive transfusion exceeding the patient's total blood volume (10 units)
- Coagulopathy as indicated by diffuse bleeding from all surfaces

While the above are only guidelines, irrespective of the setting, coagulopathy is the single most important reason for aborting a planned procedure or curtailing definitive surgery. It is important to abort surgery before coagulopathy becomes obvious.

Phase II: Initial exploration and damage control surgery

Once the decision to perform damage control surgery is made, an initial operative exploration is done, in order to:

- Arrest the bleeding
- Pack non-surgical bleeding
- Control contamination
- Protect the visceral contents

The technical aspects are dictated by the injury complex and the body cavity involved, but the principles and order of priorities are universal.

- The abdomen is opened through a long midline incision, and any clot or debris is removed.
- If exsanguinating haemorrhage is encountered, it must be controlled, either directly or by packing. The packing is then removed sequentially and all surgical haemorrhage within a particular quadrant is controlled before proceeding.

Arrest the bleeding

- Differentiate active surgical bleeding from the diffuse bleeding of coagulopathy and from venous beds.
- All active bleeding needs to be specifically controlled and will not stop by non-directed packing in the area.
- Initial control of vascular injuries is established using vascular clamps and suture ligatures.
- Simple lateral vessel wall repairs can be performed expeditiously.
- The procedures for haemorrhage control include ligation of accessible blood vessels, selective arterial inflow occlusion including intravascular balloons and vascular clamps. Penrose drains or Foley catheters with the balloon inflated provide excellent haemostasis along wound tracts, which might otherwise be inaccessible.
- Many venous injuries, including lacerations of the iliac veins and inferior vena cava can, as a last resort, be effectively controlled by ligation or packing.
- Even the 'difficult' retrohepatic vena cava is a low-pressure system and can be packed to arrest haemorrhage.
- Major arterial injuries usually require repair. Complex reconstruction in the physiologically unstable patient should be avoided. Temporary arterial stenting is an alternative with arterial reconstruction at re-operation.
- Complex repairs of bleeding solid organ injury should be avoided. Splenic and renal injuries should be managed by rapid resection. Hepatic injuries may require a variety of temporizing measures such as Pringle's manoeuvre, manual pressure, packing, and plunging (using Gelfoam® and thrombin or balloon catheter tamponade). Fibrin tissue sealants may have a place.
- Non-surgical bleeding, in itself a reason to institute damage control, is best controlled by packing.
- Surgical attempts to control such non-mechanical bleeding, especially from dissected surfaces, the liver, and retroperitoneum are usually unsuccessful.

Pack non-surgical bleeding

- A key principle in hepatic packing is that pressure applied by the packs should re-approximate the disrupted tissue planes. In order to achieve this, the affected liver lobe must be rapidly mobilized and the disrupted portions approximated by being sandwiched with orderly placed packs (above and below or in front of and behind the injured liver).
- Over-packing and under-packing, or packing in a wound cavity should where possible be avoided.

- Retrohepatic caval compression by the packs can result in sudden haemodynamic deterioration or undue tension observed during abdominal closure.
- Over-packing may result in an abdominal compartment syndrome.
- Under-packing results in failure of bleeding control. Packs rapidly become soaked with blood and haemorrhage continues underneath or around them. They should be immediately removed and properly re-applied.
- Packing is usually not effective in arresting haemorrhage from major arterial bleeders.
- Bleeding from the depth of an intrahepatic tract is normally dealt with by tractotomy to lay open the bleeding cavity for direct control of the bleeder. This procedure, as well as other complex procedures, such as complex resectional debridement, lengthy finger fracture techniques, and mesh hepatorrhaphy, should be avoided.
- Bleeding from a deep through-and-through penetration of the liver can be controlled by insertion of a Sengstaken-Blakemore tube into the tract. The gastric balloon is inflated outside (behind) the liver and serves as an anchor to preserve dislodgement of the catheter. The oesophageal balloon is then inflated inside the bleeding tract until haemostasis is achieved. The catheter is brought out through the skin and may be removed when coagulation is normalized without re-operation, simply by deflating both balloons and pulling them out. A similar technique using either a Sengstaken-Blakemore tube or large Foley catheter can be used in deep bullet tracts inside the pelvis.
- Interventional radiology for complex hepatic, pelvic, and muscle bleeding is of paramount importance and should follow the abbreviated surgical procedure when required.

Control contamination

- Following control of bleeding, attention is directed at containment of any enteric spillage.
- Contamination can be limited by either ligation of leaking ends, or external drainage, depending on the organ involved.
- Any violations of the GI tract should be treated with suture closure, or obstruction of the lumen with umbilical tapes, or staplers.
- No attempt to repair or formally resect the offending organ should be undertaken at this stage. Anastomosis and stoma formation should be deferred until later for definitive reconstruction. Any closed end of the bowel should be returned to the abdomen.
- Bile duct or ureteric injuries are temporized by ligation, stenting, 'tube ostomies', or simple drainage.
- Wide, closed suction drainage of pancreatic injuries is critical.

Protect visceral contents

Often primary abdominal fascial closure is not possible, secondary to oedematous bowel or haemodynamic instability.

Alternative methods of closing the abdomen include skin closure via towel clips or running suture, 'Bogota bag' placement (a three-litre sterile urologic irrigation bag sutured to the skin edges), prosthetic mesh insertion, or the 'sandwich technique' ('Vac-Pac'), using swabs and a plastic self-adhesive drape.

Phase III: Secondary resuscitation in the intensive care unit

The second phase in the damage control approach focuses on secondary resuscitation to restore the global physiological status of the patient, by correcting hypothermia, coagulopathy, and acidosis. This takes place in the intensive care unit where the patient undergoes invasive monitoring, complete ventilatory support, and aggressive fluid, blood, and blood product resuscitation. This is the key to resolution of the metabolic acidosis. The subsequent clearing of accumulated lactic acid is an indication of restoration of adequate tissue perfusion.

Haemodynamic status

- Patients are usually shocked on presentation to the unit, secondary to a combination of factors including fluid loss, ongoing bleeding, fluid extravasation into the body tissues, and myocardial depression.
- Patients require a combination of fluid and inotropes in order to achieve adequate tissue perfusion. The assessment of how much fluid and inotropes to give can be a difficult decision even in experienced hands, but fluid losses tend to be underestimated.
- Ongoing fluid resuscitation with blood and blood products is required to restore perfusion and correct coagulopathy.
- General oedema may represent endothelial dysfunction and extravasation of fluid into the tissue, whilst the intravascular compartment remains depleted.
- Response to resuscitation is detected clinically by observing heart rate, blood pressure, central venous pressure, improving urine output to greater than 0.5 ml/kg/hr, arterial pH, and base excess. A falling serum lactate is the most accurate assessment tool.
- Failure of the patient to respond to resuscitation indicates uncontrolled ongoing bleeding, underestimation of fluid requirements, or the onset of an abdominal compartment syndrome (see below).

Coagulation

- Coagulopathy is a multifactorial. Aggressive replacement of coagulation factors, fresh frozen plasma, and platelets is required. This contributes to fluid replacement and helps to stem ongoing blood loss by correcting the coagulopathy.

- Active rewarming of the patient is as important as coagulation factor replacement. Failure to achieve normothermia will result in persistent coagulopathy and ongoing bleeding.
- An INR of 1.5 and PTT < 1.5 × normal, with platelets greater than 80 000/mm^3 would be acceptable endpoints for correction of coagulopathy.

Acidosis

- The acidosis itself need not be addressed but during resuscitation it should improve, reflecting an improvement in tissue perfusion as resuscitation progresses and the hypothermia and coagulopathy resolve.
- Ideally, the base excess should be less than –5, the pH > 7.3, and the blood lactate < 2.5 mmol/litre within 12 hours.

Ventilation

- Goals are to maintain adequate oxygen saturation of greater than 92% or PaO$_2$ > 9.0 Kpa. This is often difficult in the presence of lung contusion, Acute Respiratory Distress Syndrome (ARDS), and fluid-filled lungs.
- High positive end expiratory pressure (PEEP) and inspired oxygen concentrations are often required. Evidence suggests that lower tidal volumes of 6–8 ml/kg should be used.
- No specific attempt should be made to control PCO$_2$ provided it does not lead to a marked respiratory acidosis.
- In addition to the primary pulmonary and intra-thoracic pathophysiology, high intra-abdominal pressures due to visceral oedema and packs cause further pulmonary compromise.

Temperature

- Normothermia is one of the most important priorities.
- Immediate and aggressive core rewarming not only improves perfusion, but it also helps reverse coagulopathy.
- Rewarming is initiated by elevating the room temperature, and using conductive and convective warming blankets and heated ventilation circuits.
- Space blankets in the hypothermic patient tend to be ineffective as there is little heat to reflect back.
- All intravenous fluids, blood, or blood products need to be prewarmed. As the body temperature normalizes, coagulopathy improves, but rapid infusion of clotting factors (fresh frozen plasma, cryoprecipitate, and platelets) is still required.

Table 11.1 Physiological endpoints within 12 hours

Haemodynamics	Urine > 0.5 ml/kg/hr, adequate CVP, BP, and pulse rate
Ventilation	$PaO_2 > 9.0$ Kpa
Coagulation	INR < 1.5 and PTT < 1.5 times normal, and platelets $> 80\,000$
Temperature	$> 36\,°C$
Acidosis	BE < -5, pH > 7.3, and lactate < 2.5

- An attempt must be made to maintain the patient in dry surroundings.
- Should hypothermia be persistent, invasive warming can be employed but this is not routinely recommended.

Physiological endpoints

It is important to attempt to reach physiologic normality as soon as possible, and preferably within a few hours.

Abdominal compartment syndrome (ACS)

- A potentially lethal complication that may occur during secondary resuscitation is the abdominal compartment syndrome (ACS). This is due to intra-abdominal hypertension (IAH), and is a complication of abbreviated laparotomy in up to 20% of patients.
- It results from ongoing haemorrhage into the abdomen or alternatively the development of oedematous bowel, both of which result in an elevated pressure in a fixed space. The result is compression of the kidneys, IVC, diaphragm, and mesenteric vessels, with associated poor bowel perfusion.
- Clinically, the most conspicuous signs of ACS are abdominal distension, progressive oliguria, and worsening hypoxaemia with elevated airway pressures. This is followed by cardiovascular collapse as a result of decreased venous return and myocardial dysfunction.
- The full clinical syndrome is easy to detect but ideally the diagnosis should be made early.
- Diagnosis is made by measurement of intra-vesical pressure (normal is less than 25 cm H_2O). This is done by simply infusing 50–100 ml saline into the bladder while clamping the catheter distal to the infusion point. The pressure in the bladder is then read as one would read central venous pressure (with a 3-way tap water manometer set) but using the catheter and the pubic symphysis as a zero point.
- Prompt operative re-exploration is mandatory. If surgical bleeding is found to be the cause, it should be controlled and the abdomen closed. If the cause of the compartment syndrome is oedema of the abdominal

Table 11.2 Recommendations for management of abdominal compartment syndrome

Grade	Bladder pressure cm H_2O	Recommendation
1	10–15	Maintain normovolaemia
2	16–25	Hypervolaemic resuscitation/decompress
3	26–35	Decompression
4	> 35	Decompression and revaluation for bleeding

contents, the abdomen should be closed using a 'Bogota bag' to reduce intra-abdominal pressure.

A simple guide has been put forward by Moore et al. (1998) in the presence of the clinically evolving syndrome (as shown in the table above).

Phase IV: Definitive operation

This operation usually takes place 48–72 hours following the initial operation and consists of re-exploration and definitive repair of the injuries. The decision to re-operate can be either planned or unplanned.

Planned surgery

Once the patient has been stabilized and the endpoints of resuscitation have been met, a return to the operating room is planned to complete the surgery in a stepwise and calculated manner. This is done at 24–72 hours depending on the type of damage control performed at the initial surgery. Blind bowel loops or obstructed vascular shunts mandate an earlier return, while isolated packed solid organs may be dealt with within 72 hours.

- Missed injuries are identified and reconstruction of bowel and vascular structures is performed, paying particular attention to avoiding high-risk anastomoses in an already hostile environment.
- Unpacking is carried out last, because if bleeding resumes, the operation will need to be aborted without reconstruction having taken place. After removal of packs, haemostasis is assessed and if required, packs can be replaced.
- All complex injuries are repaired with precedence being given to those involving the vasculature. Conservative principles are applied.
- Risky GI anastomoses or complex GI reconstructions should be avoided.
- If the abdomen can be safely closed without tension, then this is done. If not, it should be left open and contents protected by one of the methods mentioned elsewhere in this chapter.

Unplanned surgery

The unplanned decision to operate usually carries a high mortality, and is a decision forced upon the surgeon and patient. Unplanned surgery occurs as a result of:

- The presence of ongoing bleeding, despite normothermia and correction of coagulopathy, or the inability to keep up with transfusion requirements. This decision is best made by the operating surgeon and no fixed value can be given.
- The presence of abdominal compartment syndrome, causing haemodynamic, renal, and respiratory embarrassment.

Temporary abdominal closure

When closing the abdomen one needs to be aware of the significant danger of abdominal compartment syndrome (ACS). Should the abdominal volume indicate that the risk of ACS is high, a temporary low tension closure should be done.

- A plastic covering, e.g. 'Bogota bag' (a sterile 3-litre irrigation bag opened on three sides) is sutured to the skin edges.
- Alternatively, a sandwich ('Vac-Pac') technique can be used. An abdominal swab, covered on one side with an Opsite® drape, is placed, plastic side down, over the bowel and under the sheath. Above this two suction drainage tubes or large-caliber nasogastric tubes are placed and attached to suction. Finally the entire wound would be covered by a second large plastic drape.
- There are many techniques although none have been proven superior, but whichever technique is used, ensure protection of the intra-abdominal viscera, allow for expansion of the abdominal space, and ideally have a system for removal of fluid to prevent the patient remaining wet.

Final closure

The final phase of the treatment process would be the closure of the body cavity involved. Most work and problems have centred on closure of the abdomen. Closure can sometimes be achieved after a few days once visceral oedema has settled. Alternatively, a combination of granulation, with or without the aid of synthetic materials, with delayed skin grafts are used, and with correction of the ventral hernia several months later.

Damage control of specific organ systems

While the principles of damage control apply to all organ systems, the abdomen is the most common system involved in damage control surgery and there are a few specific issues worth mentioning.

Liver

Severe hepatic injury and resultant haemorrhage can be one of the most challenging problems facing the surgeon and often a reason for embarking on damage control surgery. Traditional techniques of partial liver resection, selective vascular ligation, or rapid regional debridement will carry a high mortality in the cold, acidotic, and coagulopathic patient. Other techniques for haemostasis are recommended.

Perihepatic packing can be used with large abdominal swabs placed above and below the liver in a manner to approximate disrupted segments and provide tamponade of bleeding. The packs can then be removed at second operation 48–72 hours later once the metabolic failure has been corrected. The value of this technique cannot be underestimated and provides a viable means of haemostasis even in the most devastating of injuries.

Should a small amount of debridement be required, the Pringle manoeuvre (atraumatic temporary occlusion of the portal triad) followed by the application of a large vascular clamp beneath a lateral segment of avulsed tissue, followed by ligating the tissue *en bloc* with 0 absorbable suture ties. Alternatively, horizontal mattress sutures using an atraumatic needle and 0 absorbable suture with omental plugs may be an option.

Damage control techniques in which tamponade rather than suture control is used include balloon tamponade, absorbable mesh tamponade, or perihepatic packing. Balloon tamponade using a Foley catheter or inflated Penrose drain is useful in controlling haemorrhage in a deep inaccessible missile tract.

Absorbable mesh is used to approximate disrupted liver segments under some pressure. The technique involves liver mobilization and circumferential wrapping of the liver with the mesh sewn to itself at various locations. The advantage of this technique is that the mesh need not be removed.

Spleen

For high-grade injuries the easiest method is still splenectomy. In very minor lacerations, direct suture may be a quicker alternative but in the presence of coagulopathy this is rarely a viable option.

Kidney

Injury to the kidney or adjacent renal vessels should be dealt with by nephrectomy should there be a normal contra-lateral kidney.

Abdominal veins

Ligation is the treatment of choice with severe injuries. The infra-renal IVC, internal, external, common iliac, or even the superior mesenteric and portal veins can be ligated in a shocked patient.

Pancreas

The shocked patient requiring re-operation will require very little aside from packing done at the initial operation. At re-operation drainage of non-ductal lesions can be done. Ductal injuries to the left of the mesenteric vessels are treated with distal pancreatectomy, and ductal lesions to the head of the pancreas can be assessed for a Whipple procedure in the stable patient.

Gastro-intestinal tract

Spillage control can be achieved by stapling off of bowel loops or ligation with umbilical tape. Colostomies and anastomoses should not be done in an already hostile field but rather left for the re-operation.

Thorax

Damage control in the chest has evolved in a slightly different manner. It originated with the emergency room thoracotomy in an attempt to restore physiology to the patient in extremis. While the principles remain the same, the focus in the chest has been on simpler and quicker but definitive procedures. The chest, unlike the abdomen where the midline incision is adequate for all injuries, requires different approaches depending on the site of injury.

- One of the best options is an anterolateral thoracotomy that can be extended across the midline, thus only leaving the posterior superior mediastinal structures fairly inaccessible.
- Pulmonary injuries can be rapidly dealt with by hilar cross-clamping or non-anatomic wedge resections using stapler guns. Pulmonary tractotomy with ligation of visible bleeders and air leaks may be performed after hilar control and often avoids formal resection.
- Cardiac injuries can be dealt with by a running Prolene® suture, a skin staple gun, or a balloon Foley catheter.
- The oesophagus is best dealt with by drainage and diversion with reconstruction at a later stage.
- Vascular injuries and non-surgical bleeding can be dealt with in the same way as in the abdomen.

The pelvis

The pelvis poses an extremely difficult problem with its rich blood supply and inaccessible anatomy. It requires a multi-disciplinary approach involving the radiologist, surgeon, and orthopaedic surgeon.

Any method that stabilizes the ring and diminishes intra-pelvic volume will stem the bleeding to a point. There-in lies one of the few uses of the MAST suit. A blanket or sheet placed around the pelvis and tied tightly, to minimize the pelvic volume, will tamponade bleeding, which is usually venous in origin.

Definitive stabilization has been advocated using early external fixation. Exploration of pelvic haematomas should be avoided as this may lead to fatal uncontrolled haemorrhage.

Problems and controversies

The logistics of damage control are not to be underestimated. It commits the medical team to a long and arduous task with immense consumption of resources in a group of patients who have up to 50% mortality. To be truly successful all staff members need to understand the rationale for treatment (including blood banks and laboratory staff).

The problem of patient selection and timing determines damage control techniques. Performing it on patients who are too ill and will die regardless, is a waste of resources. Performing it too early commits the patient to a long and unnecessarily arduous course.

There have been voices of concern that we have moved into a new paradigm of treatment without any firm scientific evidence. At present no level 1 evidence in the form of prospective randomized trials for patients of similar TRISS scores exists, the logistics of such a study are in itself problematic.

There are no hard and fast rules or recipe books for damage control surgery. Its success depends on the creativity and foresight of the surgeon and a dedicated postoperative ICU team. It is extremely demanding and often a demoralizing form of treatment, but is the only option for a patient who is spiralling into the inevitable 'Triad of Death'.

Pitfalls

- Waiting too long before embarking on damage control surgery.
- Packing liver without approximation of disrupted tissue planes.
- Leaving inadequately packed (bleeding) areas undisturbed in the false hope that the patient's coagulation mechanism and intra-abdominal pressure will effect haemostasis.

- Regarding raised intra-abdominal pressure as a useful adjunct for haemostasis.
- Failure to recognize in phase II that there has been failure of surgical control of haemostasis.
- Failure to diagnose abdominal compartment syndrome early.
- Failure to protect from hypothermia from the time of arrival in the emergency room.

Recommended reading

Feliciano, D., Moore, E. E., Mattox, K. L. 1996. *Trauma.* Third edition. East Norwalk: Appleton and Lange.

Hirshburg, A., Mattox, K. 1997. Damage control surgery. *The Surgical Clinics of North America*, Aug, Vol 77, No 4.

Moore, E., Burch, J. M., et al. 1998. Staged physiological restoration and damage control surgery. *World Journal Surgery,* 22:1184.

PART 2

Definitive management of injuries

12 Head Injuries

Fred van der Merwe

In South Africa and other developing countries, healthcare systems are burdened with high levels of trauma, of which head injuries contribute significantly to morbidity and mortality.

Given the high-risk nature of head injury, optimal initial management is mandatory. This includes recognition of the lucid interval, starting treatment within the 'golden hour', maintaining and supporting vital functions, recognition of associated injuries, and minimizing secondary insults. Early communication with a trauma surgeon or neurosurgeon is advisable.

The rehabilitation of a head-injured patient requires a multidisciplinary team approach, aiming to ultimately achieve reintegration into family and community.

The classification of head injuries is shown in the box on page 141.

Neuro-anatomy

Scalp

- Five layers cover the bone: Skin, Connective tissue, Aponeurosis, Loose areolar tissue, Pericranium.
- Well vascularized: potential for significant soft tissue swelling and blood loss

Skull

- Cranial vault (calvarium): thin temporal bone (fracture and haematoma)
- Base of skull: anterior, middle, and posterior parts

Meninges
- Pia, arachnoid, and dura mater (from inside to outside)
- Subarachnoid space contains cerebrospinal fluid and traversing vessels and nerves
- Subdural space (potential space) – subdural haematoma
- Epidural space (dissected space) – extradural haematoma
- Venous sinuses drain venous blood

Classification of head injuries
Mechanism of injury

• Blunt	High velocity (vehicular collision)	
	Low velocity (fall/blow to the head)	
• Penetrating	Gunshot	
	Stabs and other penetrating wounds	

Severity
- Mild   GCS (Glasgow Coma Scale) 14–15
- Moderate   GCS 9–13
- Severe   GCS 3–8

Morphology

• *Skull fractures*	Vault:	Linear/stellate
		Depressed/non-depressed
		Open/closed
	Basilar	With/without CSF (cerebrospinal fluid) leak
		With/without CN (cranial nerve) palsy
• *Intracranial lesions*	Focal	Epidural haematoma
		Subdural haematoma
		Intracerebral haematoma
		Contusion
	Diffuse	Mild concussion
		Classic concussion
		Diffuse axonal injury

Arterial supply

- Meningeal arteries supply the dura. Temporal skull fracture with middle meningeal artery (MMA) injury may cause the classical extradural haematoma.
- Main vascular supply to the brain traverses the dura mater.
- Carotid arteries form middle and anterior cerebral arteries (anterior circulation).
- Vertebral arteries form basilar artery and posterior cerebral arteries (posterior circulation).
- Communicating arteries complete the circle of Willis.

Brain

Supratentorial compartment
- Cerebrum: hemispheres separated by falx cerebri and connected via corpus callosum
- Frontal lobe: emotions, motor function, speech
- Parietal lobe: sensory function/spatial orientation
- Temporal lobe: memory, speech
- Occipital lobe: vision
- Cranial nerves I and II

Infratentorial compartments
- Cerebellum: coordination and balance
- Brainstem: Midbrain (in tentorial hiatus)
            Pons
            Medulla

Brainstem

- Nuclei of cranial nerves III–XII
- Reticular activating system (RAS)
- Ascending and descending tracts to and from spinal cord
- Vital centres: cardiovascular and respiratory centres
- Foramen magnum: brainstem transition to spinal cord; cerebellar tonsils lie just above the foramen

Cerebrospinal fluid (CSF)

- Choroid plexus in ventricles produces CSF
- Absorption by arachnoid villi into superior sagital sinus in midline
- CSF leak (target sign on pillow) carries risk of meningitis
- Hydrocephalus: obstructive (intra-ventricular obstruction)
            communicating(extra-ventricular obstruction)

Neurophysiology

Monro-Kellie doctrine

- The cranium is a non-expansile box, an increase in volume of any of the contents (haematoma, oedema, hydrocephalus, pneumocephalus) will cause raised intracranial pressure (ICP). Normal ICP $\leq$ 15 mmHg (2 kPa/22 cm H_2O).
- Pressure/Volume curve is non-linear: ICP rises exponentially as volume increases.

- High ICP will reduce cerebral perfusion; if not compensated, this will lead to cell death or irreversible damage.

Compensatory mechanisms for raised ICP

- Displacement of CSF
- Cushing reflex: triad of hypertension, bradycardia, and abnormal breathing patterns occurs when the cerebral perfusion pressure (CPP) ≤ 50 mmHg
- CPP = MAP (mean arterial pressure) – ICP (normal CPP(≥ 70 mmHg)
- MAP = $^1/_3$(systolic + 2[diastolic]) blood pressure
- Autoregulation keeps MAP at 50–150 mmHg
- Dysautoregulation is common in head injuries
- Unless systemic blood pressure is maintained and haematomas are timeously evacuated, compensatory mechanisms will fail and ICP may increase rapidly, leading to significantly reduced CPP.

Pathophysiology

Skull fractures

- Skull vault fractures: linear or depressed, closed or compound, with or without dural penetration or cortical damage.
- Base of skull fractures: anterior-, middle- or posterior fossa skull base may be affected.

Anterior fossa

- Frontal air sinus
- Ethmoid air sinus: CSF rhinorrhoea, raccoon eyes, subconjunctival bleeding
- Sphenoid air sinus: CSF rhinorrhoea, CN I injury (olfactory nerve: loss of smell), CN II injury (optic nerve: loss of light reflex and vision)

Middle fossa

- Mastoid sinus: Battle sign, CSF otorrhoea, rhinorrhoea (via Eustachian tube)
- Sphenoid sinus
- Cavernous sinus: CSF fistula
- Bony floor:
  Transverse fractures: CN VII palsy, CN VIII palsy, haemotympanum, fracture-dislocation of middle ear bones
  Longitudinal fractures: CSF and blood in external ear canal

Posterior fossa
- Clivus: CN VI injury (false localizing sign), eye movements impaired (Lat. Rect.VI; Sup.Oblq. IV; others III)
- Occipital bone: CN IX, X, XI, XII affected, no CSF leak, neck pain, nausea and vomiting may be present
- Penetrating fractures: Stab wounds and gunshot wounds

Problems: retained blades, infection, and vascular injury.

Focal intracranial lesions

Haematomas
- Extradural (EDH): characteristic lucid interval, 'talk and die' patients; emergency burrholes indicated, discuss with neurosurgeon
- Subdural (SDH): acute, subacute, and chronic SDH
- Intracerebral (ICH): traumatic and atraumatic (spontaneous ICH)

Contusions/Contusional haematomas

Figure 12.1 Burr holes and drainage of acute extradural haematoma

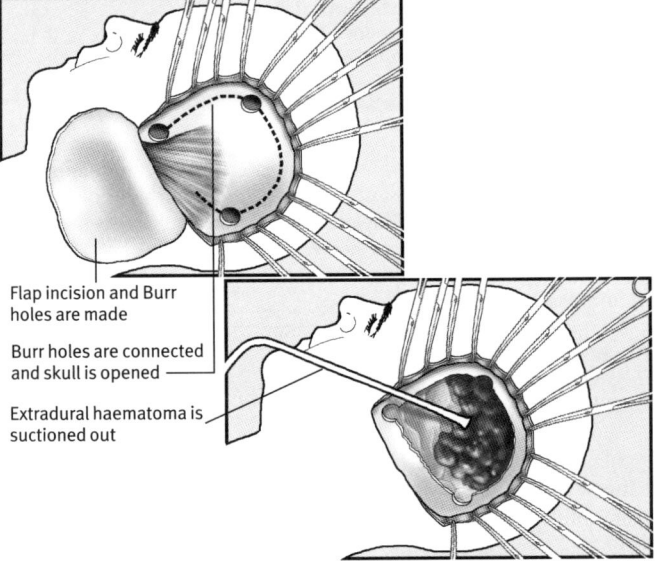

Flap incision and Burr holes are made

Burr holes are connected and skull is opened

Extradural haematoma is suctioned out

Diffuse brain injury

A spectrum of injury, caused by acceleration-deceleration type of injury with shearing of tissue. Findings on CT scan include punctate haemorrhages, coup-contracoup contusions, subdural haematomata, and burst lobe.

Mild concussion
- No loss of consciousness (LOC)
- Temporary neurological dysfunction
- Amnesia (retrograde or anterograde)

Classic concussion
- LOC < 6 hours
- Post-traumatic amnesia
- Post-concussion syndrome may follow

Diffuse brain injury (DBI)
- LOC > 6 hours
- Motor posturing
- Autonomic dysfunction

Herniation syndromes

Sub-falxine (cingulate gyrus) herniation
- L ⟷ R shift (requires pressure gradient between compartments)
- Vascular: anterior cerebral arteries and branches

Tentorial herniation
- Central herniation (brainstem)
- Up or downward herniation is possible, depending on whether pathology is above or below tentorium

Decreasing level of consciousness
- CNIII and CNVI deficit, cardiovascular, and respiratory effects

Lateral herniation (uncus)
- Ipsilateral dilated pupil (CNIII) with contralateral hemiplegia
- Long tract signs with depressed level of consciousness, or
- Kernohan-Woltman ipsilateral hemiplegia

Posterior herniation
- Posterior part of brainstem
- Parinaud phenomenon, ptosis

Foraminal (tonsilar) herniation

- Occurs late in the course of injury except in posterior fossa pathology
- Preterminal condition; characterized by apnoea
- Post-lumbar puncture: in the presence of raised ICP, always do CT scan before LP
- The only indication for an LP post-head injury is to exclude meningitis

Brain herniation

Through the wound, in cases of a compound depressed skull fracture with CSF and brain tissue leakage.

Primary vs secondary brain injury

Primary injury is the initial insult, including possible additional progressive damage over a period of six hours. Secondary injury is preventable in most cases by adhering to the ABC principles of trauma care.

Figure 12.2 Epidural haematoma and its consequences

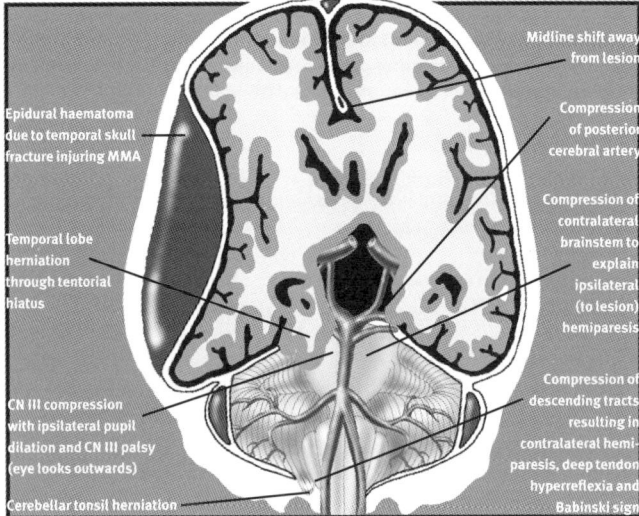

> The triad of depressed level of consciousness with an ipsilateral dilated pupil and contralateral (or ipsilateral) hemiparesis is a neurosurgical emergency.

Table 12.1 Causes of secondary brain injury

Systemic causes	Intracranial causes
Hypoxia	Haematomas
Arterial hypotension	Swelling/oedema
Hypercarbia	Raised ICP
Pyrexia	Herniation with brain shifts
Hypo/hypernatraemia	Infection
Anaemia	Seizures
Diffuse intravascular coagulopathy	
Hypo/hyperglycaemia	

Emergency management

Initially, the assessment and management of the head-injured patient should be done according to ATLS® principles, as for all seriously injured patients. During the primary survey, priority is given to the full ABC assessment and emergency management of life-threatening injuries, keeping in mind that head injuries are often associated with cervical spine and facial injuries. Pupils and level of consciousness are briefly assessed to determine whether the patient is Alert, responds to Verbal stimuli, or Pain, or is Unresponsive (AVPU). During the secondary survey, the level of consciousness is evaluated according to the Glasgow Coma Scale, together with cranial nerves, and extremity motor and sensory function.

Clinical assessment of the head-injured patient

The clinical assessment of the neurological status may be altered by concomitant injuries and insufficient cerebral oxygenation or perfusion.

GCS 14–15: Mild head injury
- Patient is awake and may be oriented.
- History is obtainable:
  Name, age, occupation
  Mechanism of injury

Table 12.2 Glascow Coma Scoring

Assessment area	Score
Eye opening (E)	
Spontaneous	4
To speech	3
To pain	2
None	1
Verbal response (V)	
Oriented	5
Confused conversation	4
Inappropriate words	3
Incomprehensible sounds	2
None	1
BEST motor response (M)	
Obeys commands	6
Localizes pain	5
Normal flexion (withdrawal)	4
Abnormal flexion (decorticate)	3
Extension (decerebrate)	2
None (flaccid)	1

Glascow Coma Score: (E+M+V); Best possible score = 15; Worst possible score = 3

> Time of injury
> Loss of consciousness: immediately post-injury, subsequent level of alertness.
> Amnesia: retrograde, antegrade
> Headaches: mild, moderate, severe
> Seizures

- Systemic injuries may be present, especially of the spine and facial bones.
- Limited neurological examination should be done.
- Cervical spine and other X-rays as indicated are required.
- Request blood alcohol level and urine toxicology screen.
- CT scan of the head is ideal in all patients, except completely asymptomatic and neurologically normal patients.

GCS 9–13: Moderate head injury
- Patient may be confused or somnolent, but is still able to follow simple commands.

- Initial examination is the same as for mild head injury, including baseline blood tests.
- CT scan of the head is obtained in all cases.
- The need for intubation should be considered if the patient is to be transported.

GCS 3–8: Severe head injury

The patient is unable to follow even simple commands because of impaired consciousness.

Assessment based on ABCDEs:

- Primary survey and resuscitation
- All patients require intubation
- Secondary survey and history
- Neurological re-evaluation:
  Eye opening
  Motor response
  Verbal response
  Pupillary light reaction
  Oculo-cephalic reflex (doll's eye movement) present/absent
  Oculo-vestibular reflex (cold caloric test) present/absent
- CT scan of the head is obtained in all cases.

Management of head injuries

Always assume cervical and other spinal injuries to be present, until excluded clinically and radiologically. Intoxication may mask head injury or an intracranial incident. If in doubt, admit to hospital for observation.

Management of mild head injury
Indications for admission

- No CT scanner available, or abnormal CT scan
- All penetrating head injuries
- History of loss of consciousness
- Deteriorating level of consciousness
- Moderate to severe headaches
- Significant alcohol/drug intoxication
- Skull fracture
- CSF rhinorrhoea or otorrhoea
- Significant associated injuries
- No reliable companion at home
- Unable to return to hospital promptly if necessary
- Amnesia

Discharge from Emergency Unit
- The patient does not meet any of the criteria for admission.
- Discuss need to return if any problems develop and issue an 'information sheet'.
- Schedule a follow-up visit, usually within one week.

Management of moderate head injury
Admit the patient for observation:
- Frequent neurological checks
- Follow-up CT scan if condition deteriorates or preferably before discharge

If the patient improves:
> Discharge when appropriate and follow up in clinic.

If the patient deteriorates:
> If the patient stops following simple commands, repeat CT scan and treat as for severe head injury.

Management of severe head injury
Aim to protect the brain, to create an optimum milieu for the recovery of the brain, and to prevent a secondary insult.

Initial assessment according to ATLS® principles
Airway
- Cuffed endotracheal intubation to maintain and protect airway
- Prevent aspiration
- Avoid hyperextension of C-spine during intubation

Breathing
- Normoventilate to a pCO_2 of 3.5–4.5 kPa
- Avoid aggressive hyperventilation
- Monitor blood gases, O_2 saturation
- PEEP of 5 is acceptable

Circulation
- Resuscitate with Ringer's lactate
- Adequate peripheral perfusion and urine output of 0.5–1 ml/min
- 0.9% saline solution for maintenance thereafter
- No glucose-containing solutions
- No hypotonic solutions
- Monitor intake and output (water and salt balance)
- Blood: urea, electrolytes, and glucose
  (Diabetes insipidus vs syndrome of inappropriate ADH secretion)

Useful drugs in head-injury management

Intubation

Midazolam (Dormicum®)

Anxiolytic, sedative, hypnotic, amnesic agent, subanaesthetic doses allow retention of pharyngeal reflex

Adult dose: 2.5–5 mg IV

Decrease dose in hypovolemic, hypothermic, or elderly patients

To prevent seizures

Phenytoin (Epanutin®)

Valproic acid (Epilim®)

Prophylactic anticonvulsants are optional to prevent early post-traumatic seizures (within the first week).

Prophylactic anticonvulsants are not recommended for preventing late post-traumatic seizures.

To control seizures if present

Diazepam (Valium®)

Adult: 10–20 mg IV

Child: 0.1–0.2 mg/kg IV

Followed by loading and maintenance dose of Epanutin® or Epilim®

To control raised ICP ('buying time')

Mild hyperventilation: $PaCO_2$ not less than 20 mmHg

Mannitol:

Starting dose 0.5–1 gram/kg over 30 min

Bolus administration is better than a constant infusion

Monitor hourly fluid balance and serum osmolality (< 320 mOsmol/l)

Furosemide: optional

Decadron: selected cases only (discuss with neurosurgeon)

To prevent vasospasm

Nimodipine (Nimotop®)

For traumatic SAH (discuss with neurosurgeon)

Antibiotics

Prophylactic versus therapeutic (discuss with neurosurgeon)

Nutritional support

Start early with enteral feeds if possible.

Deficits
- Monitor GCS, clinical trends, pupils, vital signs, O_2 saturation
- Invasive monitoring once in ICU

Environment
Maintain temperature during assessment and treatment of injuries.

Secondary survey
- Head-to-toe assessment for concomitant injuries
- Full neurological examination and documentation

Diagnostic tests (in descending order of preference)
- CT scan ideally for all patients with acute head injury
- Skull X-ray if CT scan is not available; normal skull X-ray does not exclude brain injury
- Cerebral angiogram in selected cases
- MRI (post-acute stage)

ICU preferable to ward admission
- Dedicated nursing care is essential
- The clinical trend is important
- Head positioning: flat to 15° head up in neutral position
- Monitoring:
  - BP, pulse, temp, O_2 saturation
  - PaO_2, $PaCO_2$, pH, urea and electrolytes, glucose
    ICP, CPP in selected cases

ICP monitoring indicated in severe head injuries
- Post-resuscitation GCS $< {}^9/_{15}$ with abnormal CT scan
- Normal CT scan with two or more of the following: age over 40 years; abnormal posturing; systolic BP $<$ 90 mmHg
- Selected patients with mass lesions

Management of specific problems
Stab wounds with slot fracture and/or retained knife blade
- Obtain a neurosurgical opinion
- X-rays (metallic vs non-radio opaque object), CT scan
- Don't pull it out (risk of major haemorrhage)
- May need angiogram prior to emergency procedure

Gunshot wounds. Prognosis depends upon:
- Missile ballistics
- Neurological condition on admission
- CT findings
- Intracranial complications

Brain death
- Definitive criteria to be followed
- Consult with neurosurgeon
- See chapter on Brain death and organ donation

Points of importance when referring a neurosurgical patient
- Age, mechanism of injury, associated neck injury
- Time of injury, presence of lucid interval
- Respiratory and cardio-vascular status
- Glasgow Coma Scale (GCS) score (eyes, verbal, motor response); pupillary reactions
- Other injuries
- Treatment given or planned
- Facilities and transport available
- Personal and past medical history

Surgical management

Wound care
- Tetanus toxoid, shave hair, adequate cleaning and debridement of wounds
- Suturing of skin only
- Pressure bandage
- Refer for neurosurgical opinion

Indications for surgery

Mass lesions
- Raised ICP with shift effect
- Herniation
- Decision based on clinical findings, radiology and ICP recording

Depressed fractures
- Debridement and dural repair required
- Need for cosmetic cranioplasty

CSF leak (persistent or complicated)
Anterior or middle fossa dural repair is required, as well as treatment of meningitis and its complications.

Penetrating injuries
- Presence of traumatic dissections, aneurysms, or arterio-venous malformations

- Traumatic carotid-cavernous fistula
- Abscess formation requires drainage
- Removal of foreign bodies

Sepsis
- Wound sepsis: superficial to galea aponeurotica, osteitis
- Intracranial infection: empyema, abscess formation
- Meningitis, ventriculitis may lead to hydrocephalus

Pitfalls

- Not identifying intra-cranial injury: alcohol and narcotic intoxication are commonly associated with head injuries and may erroneously be assumed to be the cause of altered levels of consciousness.
- Not recognizing retained knife blades which may not be clinically obvious; all penetrating head injuries should be X-rayed.
- Missed cervical spine fractures: C-spine immobilization is mandatory until adequate imaging excludes injuries. In the presence of cervical fracture, the entire spine should be reviewed.
- Omitting or delaying intubating the unconscious patient when indicated, will lead to aspiration pneumonia, as the unconscious patient cannot protect his/her airway (no cough reflex).
- Allowing the $PaCO_2$ values to drop below 3.5 kPa; do not over-ventilate the patient.
- Not identifying misplaced ET-tubes, which often occurs during emergency intubation or the subsequent period of transfer to trauma unit, scanner, or intensive care ward. Frequently re-verify the position of the ET-tube.
- Not recognizing metabolic disturbances: monitor fluid balance, sodium, electrolytes, and glucose levels regularly. Early enteral feeds are recommended.
- Not identifying intracranial complications early: regularly review vital signs and GCS, dedicated nursing care is imperative. Follow up CT scan if in doubt.
- Missing systemic injuries and other causes of pain: determine the cause of shock and/or restlessness. Ongoing bleeding, hypoxia, gastric dilatation, distended bladder, and pain from pressure ischaemia or undetected fractures may cause tachycardia or other abnormal parameters.
- Not referring to specialized facilities early: rehabilitation with a multi-disciplinary team approach yields the best results. Family support and integration into the community are important aspects of the recovery process.
- Not recognizing that hypotension is never due to blood loss from a head injury in an adult.

References and suggested reading

American College of Surgeons: Committee on Trauma. Advanced Trauma Life Support® 1997. *Student Manual.* Chicago: ACS.

Miller, J. Douglas. 1993. Neurological emergency: Head injury. *Journal of Neurology, Neurosurgery, and Psychiatry,* 56:440–447.

National Institute for Clinical Excellence (NHS). Head injury: Triage, assessment, investigation and early management of head injury in infants, children and adults. *Clinical Guideline,* 4 June 2003. www.nice.org.uk/pdf/cg4niceguideline.pdf

13   Spinal injuries

Pradeep Makan

The spine comprises the spinal column and the spinal cord. The spinal column is responsible for allowing trunk motion while at the same time affording protection to the spinal cord. When the spinal column fails, damage to the spinal cord may result in neurological compromise.

Mechanical forces involved in producing spinal injuries include hyperflexion, rotation, extension, vertical compression, and shear. These injuries arise from motor vehicle accidents, diving, falls from heights, and sporting accidents, e.g. rugby. Penetrating injuries (gunshot and stab wounds) may also result in cord damage, although the spinal column tends to be mechanically stable in these patients.

Spinal column injuries

Spinal injuries may be classified according to the mechanism of injury and are discussed below.

Flexion injuries

- *Flexion compression*, e.g. wedge compression and flexion teardrop fractures (see Figure 13.1)
- *Flexion distraction*, e.g. facet subluxation and dislocation, chance fracture (see Figure 13.2)
- *Flexion rotation*

Extension injuries

- *Extension distraction*, e.g. extension teardrop (see Figure 13.3)
- *Extension compression*, e.g. Hangman's fracture, which is fracture of the posterior elements of C2 and classified as an unstable fracture (see Figure 13.4)

Vertical compression

For example:
- Burst fracture
- Jefferson fracture (see Figures 13.5 and 13.6)
  - axial compression disruption of the C1 ring
  - usually a fourfold fracture of the anterior and posterior arches of C1

Figure 13.1 A typical hyperflexion injury C4 (arrow indicating the flexion teardrop). The large increase in the interspinous gap (indicated by the white line) suggests that this is a flexion injury rather than a vertical compression type injury

Figure 13.2 Chance fracture 1st lumbar vertebra, a horizontal fracture dividing the vertebral body into upper and lower halves. Also known as the 'lap belt' fracture. Commonly associated with intra-abdominal injuries

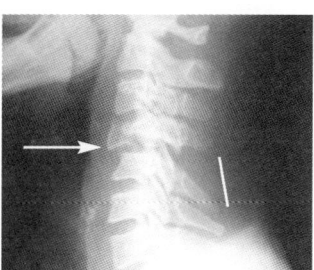

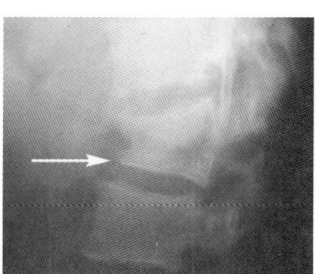

Figure 13.3 C2 extension teardrop; note the decrease in the interspinous gap

Figure 13.4 C2/3 fracture dislocation (Hangman's fracture); arrow indicates the site of the fracture through the pedicle of C2

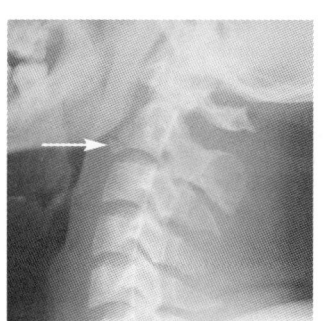

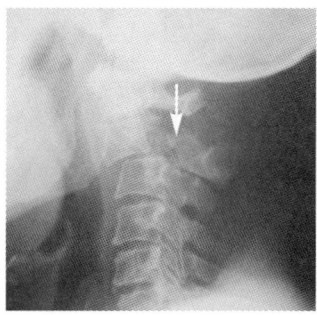

- the diagnostic crux is that the atlantic facets (usually both) overhang the axial facets
- classified as unstable

Shear

For example, bilateral facet dislocation (see Figure 13.7).

Additional spinal column injuries

Odontoid peg fractures

Three types are described:
Type 1 Fracture through tip of the peg (stable)
Type 2 Fracture through the base (unstable)(see Figure 13.8)
Type 3 Fracture through base and the vertebral body of C2 (unstable)

Rupture of the transverse ligament of the atlas (C1)

This rupture presents with a widened altanto-dens interval (ADI)(see Figure 13.9).

Spinal cord injuries

Spinal cord injuries may be complete or incomplete.

Complete spinal cord injury

Paralysis and loss of sensation occurs below the level of the cord injury. A level can usually be identified. Flaccid paralysis occurs below this level with absent tendon reflexes. Presence of the bulbocavernosus reflex in the absence of any motor or sensory sparing indicates a poor prognosis. The bulbocavernosus reflex is elicited by pulling on the urinary catheter with a finger placed in the anal canal. A positive reflex is when the anal sphincters are felt to contract when the urinary catheter is pulled. This is a primitive spinal reflex, which is usually absent when higher cortical control is present, but is present in complete spinal cord injuries when cortical control is absent. Priapism is common in high cord lesions and occurs secondary to paralytic vasodilatation.

Incomplete spinal cord injury

Incomplete spinal cord injury has a far better prognosis for recovering useful function and implies the presence of some motor and/or sensory

Figure 13.5 Jefferson fracture (arrow points to the fracture through the posterior arch of C1.) Note also the widened atlanto-dens interval. This should not exceed 3 mm in adults and 5 mm in children

Figure 13.6 Jefferson fracture on open mouth view. Note the overhang of C1 on the lateral mass of C2 and bony fragments

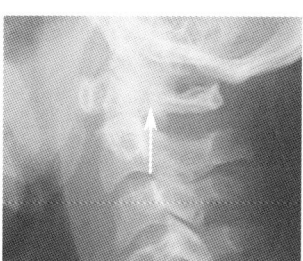

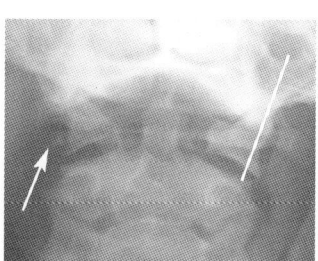

Figure 13.7 Bilateral facet dislocation C6 on C7 (Shear)

Figure 13.8 Type 2 odontoid peg fracture (note fracture through base of the dens)

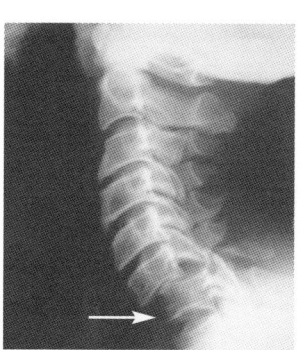

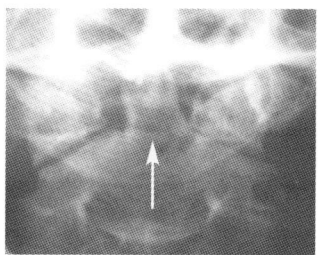

function below the level of the injury. Sparing of sensation ('sacral sparing') may be the only early sign of an incomplete cord lesion and it is important to determine if this is present.

Specific incomplete cord lesions are identifiable. They include:

Brown-Sequard syndrome. With this syndrome there is loss of power along with proprioception and impaired light touch on the same side as the lesion and loss of sensation to pain and temperature on the contra-lateral side.

Anterior cord syndrome. This is where there is severe motor loss, absent pain sensation with retention of vibration and position sense ('dorsal column sparing').

Central cord syndrome. This syndrome results in lower motor lesion of upper limbs and upper motor lesion of lower limbs.

Cauda equina syndrome. Saddle anaesthesia, loss of bladder and bowel control, and possible foot drop and foot intrinsic muscle weakness are indications of this syndrome.

Treatment of spinal injuries

- Treat life-threatening injuries.
- Typically with cord injuries, the patient will be in neurogenic shock due to a sudden cut-off of sympathetic tone and the resultant vasodilatation. The systolic blood pressure is often around the 90 mmHg level,

Figure 13.9 Rupture of the transverse ligament (ADI indicated by white line)

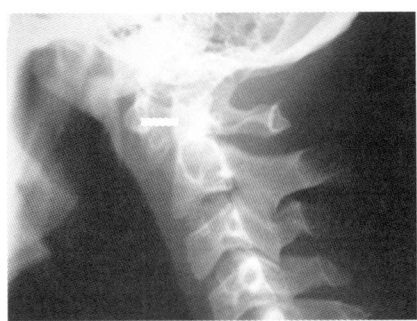

and this is sufficient provided there is adequate renal perfusion reflected by an adequate urine output. If there is concern over hypovolaemia, insert a CVP. Usually vasoconstrictors are not required.

- Maintain oxygenation saturation, i.e. airway ± ventilation.
- Restore spinal alignment with gentle manual traction – stop if patient resists.
- Apply cervical collar.
- Insert nasogastric tube.
- Insert a silastic urinary catheter.
- Administer steroids for incomplete blunt cord injuries presenting within 8 hours of injury. Recommended dosage is methylprednisolone 30 mg/kg stat followed by 5.4 mg/kg/hour over 23 hours. IV cimetidine should be administered concurrently to minimize the risk of gastrointestinal bleeding.
- Transfer patient to a suitable bed – at least six people are needed for a safe transfer.
- Administer pressure care, i.e. 3-hourly turning or lifting to prevent pressure sores.
- Initially treat all spinal injuries as unstable until adequate radiological assessment is obtained. If it is not possible to visualize injury on standard spinal radiographs, tomography, computer tomography +/- MRI is indicated. Determining whether a spinal injury is mechanically unstable may not be easy and requires assessment by an orthopaedic or spinal surgeon. Spinal instability implies that there is a risk of developing neurological compromise and/or a spinal deformity. If the spinal injury is stable, bedrest and analgesia are advised until the pain subsides. If the spinal injury is unstable, refer to spinal surgeon for possible surgical stabilization or continue bedrest until the injury stabilizes. Unstable cervical spinal injuries should be placed on neck traction, either by halter traction or by skull traction with callipers. Start with 2 kg and obtain a lateral spine radiograph to exclude vertical displacement as would occur with distraction injuries. Remove traction immediately if this occurs. Unstable thoracolumbar injuries should be placed on strict bedrest.
- Psychological support for patient and family must be provided.

Pitfalls

- There should be a high index of suspicion of a spinal injury in an unconscious patient in the presence of certain injury mechanisms, such as:
  - fall from a height
  - resuscitated drowning
  - traffic trauma

- head injury
- facial fractures
- paradoxical breathing
- hypotension resistant to resuscitation with warm peripheries
- bradycardia
- poor response to pain below a particular dermatome
- priapism
- lax anal sphincter tone
- urinary retention and overflow incontinence
- ileus

- Incomplete cervical spine X-rays and not visualizing the entire cervical spine down to T1.
- Missing abdominal injuries in cervical and high thoracic paraplegias.
- Mistaking a lower cervical lesion for an upper thoracic (T4) one, because the upper limb dermatomes have not been assessed. The supraclavicular nerves (C3–4) supply the upper anterior chest down to the 3–4th rib level.
- Low cervical and upper thoracic injuries are often difficult to visualize on standard radiographs. If suspicious of an injury at this level, request further investigations, i.e. tomography, computer tomography, ± MRI.
- Thoracolumbar injuries are often misdiagnosed as being mechanically stable. If unsure, consult an orthopaedic or spinal surgeon. It is important to repeat spinal radiographs following mobilization to assess whether a spinal deformity such as kyphosis is developing.

Recommended reading

Apley, A. G., Solomon, L. (eds.) 1993. *Apley's system of orthopaedics and fractures.* London: Butterworth Heinemann.

Bracken, M. B., Shephard, M. J., et al. 1990. A randomised, controlled trial of methylprednisolone or naloxone in the treatment of acute spinal cord injury. *NEJM*, 322:1405–1411.

Spinal Cord Injury Information Network. http://www.spinalcord.uab.edu/

14

Maxillo-facial trauma

Paul Bischoff

Trauma to the mid-face may be divided into soft- or hard-tissue injuries. Facial injuries are becoming increasingly common due to an increase in urban violence and warfare in South Africa, as well as sport-related injuries.

The soft tissues

The soft tissue manifestations may give an indication of the state of the underlying bony status. A subconjunctival haematoma may be indicative of a fracture of the orbit, thus necessitating more intensive investigations. However, isolated soft tissue injuries, in the absence of deep damage, should be treated in the same manner as injuries to the integument elsewhere, with particular emphasis on correct wound toilet, debridement, and accurate suturing to ensure optimal function and aesthetics post-operatively. As a general rule, soft tissue suturing should be left until all deeper structures have been attended to avoid unnecessary repetition of procedures.

Management

- Inspect to determine depth, extent, anatomical structures such as nerves or muscles involved, or the presence of debris, and palpate to identify inclusions.
- Determine the optimal timing of treatment, which can be delayed for some days if necessary.
- Ensure adequate haemostasis, and that physiologically appropriate dressings are placed.
- Choice of anaesthesia is dependent on the patient's cooperation and general state, i.e. severe injuries are best attended to in the operating room under general anaesthesia.
- Antibiotic regimen includes tetanus toxoid booster to patients previously immunized more than five years ago. Penicillin remains the antibiotic of choice.

Specialized structures

These include the ear, eye structures, facial (VII) nerve, and parotid duct. Special care should be taken to ensure that these are inspected and correct treatment instituted. Consultations with specialist services should be sought when doubts exist as to the extent of, or treatment indicated for such injuries.

The facial hard tissues

Fractures of the facial skeleton

These fractures are classified on an anatomical basis (see Figure 14.1).

Frontal sinus fractures

Diagnosis. This is confirmed on the basis of clinical signs, which include:

- Epistaxis and CSF (cerebrospinal fluid) rhinorrhoea
- Depression of the frontal (Glabella) region
- Peri-orbital emphysema and neurological deficits
- Pneumocephalus

Radiographs

Radiographs should include plain films to assess sinus air-fluid levels and asymmetries, as well as CT images to evaluate fractures, especially of the posterior walls.

Treatment

Following the administration of appropriate antibiotics (Penicillin G), displaced anterior wall fractures are elevated, usually via the laceration or coronal flaps. Displaced posterior wall fractures require neurosurgical intervention, via a coronal approach. Dural repair and sinus obliteration are used. Nasofrontal duct injuries are treated in various ways with complete removal of all mucous membrane and obliteration of the duct with fat graft being advocated by some workers.

Complications

Sinusitis, persistent CSF leaks, as well as mucocoeles, are reported.

Orbital fractures

Diagnosis. This is based on clinical signs such as:

- Ecchymosis, ptosis of the upper lid, deformity of the rim, as well as shift in the eye globe
- Paraesthesia of the supra-orbital or infra-orbital soft tissues
- Superior orbital fissure syndrome
- Restriction in upward gaze
- Enophthalmos
- Subconjunctival haematoma
- Diplopia

Visual tests including pupillary reflexes, acuity, and range of movement are essential aids to diagnosis.

Radiography
Radiography should include plane films supplemented by CT imaging (reconstructed views are ideal). (See Figure 14.2.)

Treatment
Direct visualization and rigid osteosynthesis with bone plates and screws is the treatment of choice. Treatment may be delayed for some days and tests repeated to ensure the injuries require surgical intervention to prevent complications such as:

- Blindness
- Infection
- Persistent ocular problems (diplopia, enophthalmos, and ectropion)
- Paraesthesias

Approach to the orbit is via subciliary, brow, or coronal incisions, this latter approach being useful in extensive injuries including orbital involvement.

Naso-orbital fractures
These injuries are often seen in association with other facial fractures such as frontal sinus – or Le Fort lll injuries. The nasal bones will be seen to be displaced.

Clinical features
- Peri-orbital swelling, oedema, or ecchymoses

Figure 14.1 Fractures of the mid-facial skeleton

Figure 14.2 Orbital fracture (inferior orbital rim)

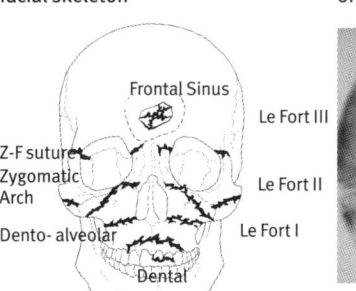

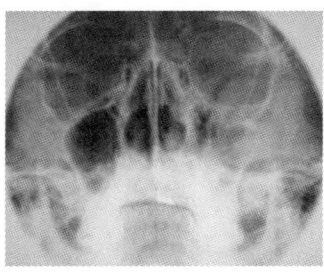

- Epistaxis
- CSF rhinorrhoea
- Pneumocephalus
- Telecanthus
- Obvious signs such as penetrating wounds, crepitations, and bony displacement

Radiographs
Radiographs should include lateral skull, Waters, and CT images to view deeper structures.

Treatment
Open reduction is the treatment of choice as the fractures can best be viewed and the stable periphery utilized to immobilize the loose fragments, using plates and screws, as well as direct wire osteosynthesis where indicated.

Bone grafts and implants are often needed to replace missing tissue, e.g. on the orbital floor (blow-out) and medial walls. Attention is also paid to the soft tissue structures, such as lacrimal apparatus and canthal ligaments. Canthopexy can be achieved using wire or screws. Soft tissue adaptation to the nasal bridge may require wire traction through the bridge of the nose.

Zygomatic fractures
The complex shape of the zygoma makes accurate interpretation of the fractures essential. Most fractures in this region are due to blunt trauma, the exposed position of the zygoma predisposing this site to depressed fractures. (See Figure 14.3.)

Diagnosis
- Orbital signs, e.g. ecchymoses, swelling, subconjunctival haemorrhage, restriction in motion, enophthalmos

Figure 14.3 Zygomatic fractures

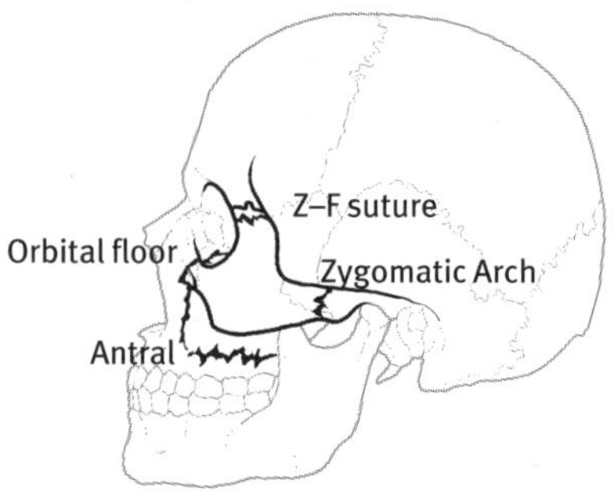

- Haemorrhages, e.g. epistaxis, oral bleeds
- Alteration in bony contours with palpable steps to the bone margins. Depression of the arch may impede mandibular movements
- Paraesthesias of the infra-orbital nerve

Radiographs

Waters and submento-vertex views are standard. The maxillary antra should be examined for step deformities as well as clouding, indicating haemorrhage into the sinuses. Axial and coronal CT views are a great help in visualizing important structures such as the orbit.

Treatment

Isolated arch fractures can be elevated via a Gilles temporal approach. Displaced fractures, especially those involving the orbital floor, are reduced and stabilized from an open approach, at the zygomatico-maxillary suture, and the infra-orbital as well as intra-oral regions, so as to visualize the floor of the orbit and facilitate direct osteosynthesis using light wires as well as bone plates.

Figure 14.4 Panorex of a dento-alveolar fracture (note the step in the occlusion)

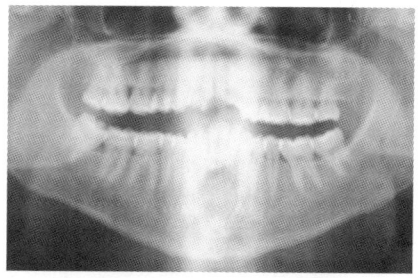

Figure 14.5 Le Fort II fracture; OM 30 degrees view

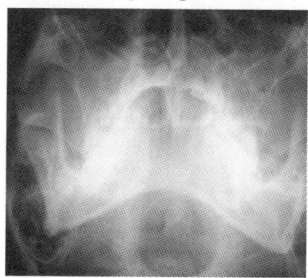

Maxillary fractures
Classification
1 Dento-alveolar
2 Le Fort I, II, III

Dento-alveolar fractures
Sections of the upper alveolus, including the roots of the teeth, may be fractured and are often best visualized on an orthopantomogram or indeed dental intra-oral views. (See Figure 14.4.) Teeth are attended to by the dentist, whilst alveolar fragments can often be stabilized using composite cements (dentist) or arch bars wired to adjacent teeth. The occlusion provides the template for ideal reduction as indeed it does in all jaw fracture treatment.

Le Fort fractures
Le Fort l: Low-level fractures above the roots of the upper teeth.
Le Fort ll: A pyramidal fracture which may be unilateral. Disjunction is detected at the infra-orbital region and there may be a mid-palatal fracture as well. (See Figure 14.5.)
Le Fort lll: Cranio-maxillary disjunction, with superior fractures running above the nose, involving the frontal sinus occasionally and leading to elongation of the face. The orbital extent of the fracture may vary enormously. Palatal fractures are seen.

Diagnosis
Clinically, there is:
- Massive facial oedema. Lacerations or abrasions are common
- Haemorrhage from nostrils, mouth, and skin. Bleeding may precipitate an airway obstruction
- CSF rhinorrhoea
- Mobility of the mid-face, with long-faced appearance and gross malocclusions
- Soft tissue swelling accompanied by emphysema
- Neurological deficits (Va and Vb)

Radiographic assessment
Films include P/A skull, lateral skull, and Waters views. The assistance of CT imaging is of great value in assessing the full extent of the injuries, and if neck trauma is suspected carotid angiography may be indicated.

Treatment
Mid-third facial fractures are treated relying upon the stable mandibular teeth to provide the template for reduction. Associated mandibular

fractures must first be attended to, after which the upper jaw is placed onto the lower counterpart. Interdental wires are used commonly, then the maxillary fractures are approached through skin and mucosal incisions to facilitate stable reduction.

The use of direct plate and screw osteosynthesis has meant that immediate post-surgical management and particularly nursing have been simplified as the jaws no longer need to be wired for any length of time.

The elongated face is reduced and suspensory wires placed, often in association with plates and screws. Care has to be exercised not to over-reduce, i.e. to shorten the face.

Antibiotics are mandatory and penicillin, in combination with a cephalosporin and metronidazole are indicated. A soft diet is also essential. Analgesia is routine, as these patients are often found to be relatively pain-free.

Figure 14.6 Mandibular fractures

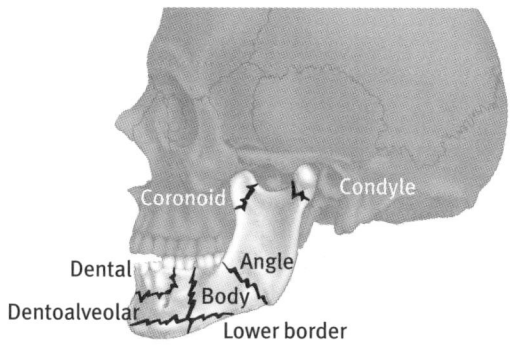

Figure 14.7 Bilateral mandible fractures

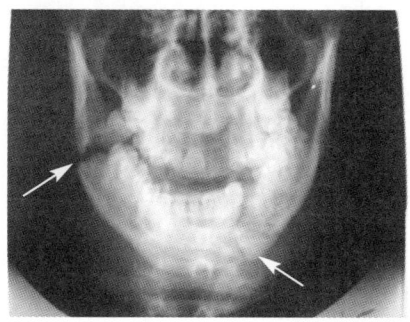

Mandibular fractures

These fractures are sub-divided into the various anatomical regions of the mandible (see Figure 14.6). General considerations are haemostasis, analgesia, and antibiotic regimes. Pain is usually not severe, and analgesia syrups may be adequate. For more severe pain, pethidine 75 mg IMI stat followed by post-operative analgesia syrups is indicated. Penicillin (2 million units pen G imi stat followed by oral penicillin VK 500 mg 6 hourly) as well as metronidazole 400 mg 8 hourly is the usual regime. Erythromycin or clindamycin are the drugs of choice in penicillin-sensitive individuals.

Patients actively bleeding should be nursed in the head-down position, with the head turned to one side to prevent aspiration. Temporary stabilization may be necessary to prevent excessive haemorrhage and this is best achieved by placing dental wires in situ.

Management

These common injuries are often compound into the oral region, as well as to the exterior, following blunt trauma to the lower face as in motor vehicle accidents or assaults, or as a result of sporting injuries. Associated dental injuries are always suspected, especially in cases of simple dento-alveolar trauma. Loose or avulsed teeth can be treated by the dental surgeon if the case can be seen in the first hour following the injury. However, the prognosis for re-implanted teeth falls rapidly if treatment is deferred beyond 90 minutes. Avulsed teeth can be transported either in the saliva in the buccal vestibule or in milk.

Diagnosis

- Pain at the site of the fracture, especially with mobility or attempts at chewing, as well as a degree of trismus
- Derangement of the dental occlusion. Check for gagging of the bite, i.e. premature contacts or gross step defects in the dental arches
- Paraesthesia in the distribution of the inferior alveolar nerve, i.e. at the chin region on the affected side if unilateral
- Sublingual haematoma due to tearing of the lingual periosteum
- Haemorrhage from the fracture site and associated soft tissues

Radiology

The orthopantomogram (Panelipse view) is the gold standard for mandibular fracture diagnosis. (See Figure 14.8.) Lateral oblique views combined with PA mandible are useful, as are CT images of the temporo-mandibular joints.

Treatment

Closed reduction. Reduction may be closed using simple eyelet wiring and intermaxillary wiring, or elastic traction utilizing stainless steel arch bars. This will, in most cases, satisfy all requirements of reduction and immobilization, the dental occlusion providing the template for ideal reduction. Immobilization is usually maintained for 5–6 weeks. An adequate dentition is required to facilitate the placement of wires.

The considerations of choice of technique, closed vs open, may be affected by:

- Site of fracture, i.e. teeth in vicinity, distal to the last tooth, health of adjacent teeth
- Degree of displacement of the fragments, i.e. large displacement generally indicates open treatment
- Type of fracture, i.e. condylar (closed generally) vs body or angle where displacement may be great
- Choice of anaesthesia and condition of the patient
- Concurrent injuries such as mid-facial trauma, or head injuries where nursing considerations must be met
- Comminuted fractures may preclude open reduction as stripping of periosteum may compromise the blood supply and thus the prognosis for the fragments

Open reduction. In cases involving simple (not multiple) comminution of the mandible, or where adequate reduction is not possible using the eyelets mentioned above, open techniques are indicated. The patient's nutritional requirements should also be borne in mind where intermaxillary fixation is contemplated. Open techniques are indicated where extensive mid-facial injuries exist, in order to maintain the vertical dimension of the face. Open reduction involves either external incisions (or the use of lacerations), as well as mucosal incisions within the oral soft tissues to approach the fracture sites, after which the bone fragments can be accurately aligned and fixated either with wire osteosynthesis, or direct bone fixation with plates and screws, lag screws, or wires. Often dental arch bars are required to stabilize the dental aspect.

In edentulous cases, plates and screws are of great importance in stability.

In children, care should be exercised if open techniques are envisaged, as the developing tooth buds are in danger of being damaged by drills and screws. Condylar fractures in children are usually treated by closed reduction, with elastic traction to train the dental occlusion, supplemented by gentle physiotherapy. Prolonged fixation in this group may lead to haematoma organization and ankylosis, so duration of fixation should not exceed 14 days.

Teeth in the fracture line, especially where demonstrable loosening has occurred, should be extracted to avoid post-operative sepsis. Impacted or unerupted teeth can be observed but should be removed at the first sign of infection developing.

Pitfalls

- Mandibular fractures are usually bilateral until proven otherwise. Look for a second fracture.
- A haematoma in the floor of the mouth is often suggestive of a fractured mandible.
- Exclude aspiration of avulsed teeth in dento-alveolar fractures by doing a CXR.
- A flame-shaped lateral subconjunctival bleed is often suggestive of a zygomaticofrontal or lateral orbital wall fracture.

Recommended reading

Journal of oral rehabilitation AST. Franks (ed.) Published on the Web by Blackwell Science Ltd.
http://www.blackwellpublishing.com/journal.asp?ref=0305–182x&site
Mathog, R.H. (ed.) 1992. *Atlas of craniofacial trauma.* Philadelphia: W B Saunders Co.

15

Ear and nasal injuries

Johannes Fagan

Ear injuries

Ear injuries should always be excluded in the presence of open or closed head trauma, or blast injuries. Apart from trauma to the external ear, ear trauma may manifest as dizziness, deafness, and bloody or cerebro-spinal fluid (CSF) otorrhoea.

Auricle

The auricle consists of a cartilage framework, covered by skin. Nutrition to the cartilage is derived from the perichondrium. Even minor deformities of the auricle can be disfiguring. Therefore great care should be taken to carefully repair auricular injuries, and to manage auricular trauma appropriately in order to avoid perichondritis and resorption of cartilage.

Auricular haematoma

This is caused by blunt trauma and results in a tensely swollen auricle. The haematoma between the perichondrium and cartilage causes resorption of cartilage and a cauliflower ear deformity.

Acute management

Complete evacuation of haematoma by aspiration or incision is required. Apply a pressure dressing on both sides of the auricle, secured by through-and-through nylon sutures, for seven days to prevent re-accumulation of haematoma.

Auricular laceration

The different types of laceration require different treatment:
- Simple laceration: Suture meticulously.
- Denuded cartilage: Perform a full-thickness post-auricular skin graft.
- Perichondrium intact: Requires an immediate graft.
- Perichondium denuded: Delay skin grafting until covered by granulation tissue.

Auricular avulsion

Partial
Small avulsions (< 2 cm): Perform a primary repair
Large avulsion (> 2 cm): Requires a local or regional flap, with or without a cartilage graft
Total
Place auricle in sterile plastic bag, and transport in iced water (not ice, to avoid freezing).
Re-implanatation will require a microvascular anastomosis.

Auricular bites
The management of auricular bites is as follows:
- Antibiotics
- < 12 hrs old: Primary repair
- > 12 hrs old: Allow to heal by secondary intention with dressings

Ear canal

The outer half of the canal has a cartilaginous wall. The medial half has a bony wall. The canal is lined by skin, which is very thin over the bony section. The principal objective is to avoid canal stenosis.

Haematoma, laceration of the canal
- Consider a temporal bone fracture.
- Drain the haematoma.
- Stent the canal with antibiotic/antiseptic-impregnated ribbon gauze.

Tympanic membrane
Most traumatic perforations heal spontaneously. Disruption of the ossicular chain may cause conductive or sensorineural deafness and vertigo.
- Small perforation: Advise the patient to keep ear dry, and consult otolaryngologist within a few days.
- Large perforation: Refer to otolaryngologist to attempt to approximate free edges of the perforation.
- Vertigo/imbalance/nystagmus: Refer to otolaryngologist for audiogram and complete assessment.

Nasal trauma

Nasal trauma manifests with external nasal deformity and nasal obstruction. In more severe midfacial trauma, an orbital haematoma, visual disturbance due to orbital fractures, or CSF rhinorrhoea may be present. A septal haematoma requires prompt drainage.

Nasal fracture

The nasal skeleton consists of the nasal bones, upper and lower nasal cartilages, and cartilaginous and bony nasal septum. Radiology is seldom required because the need for intervention is dictated by external nasal deformity.

Nasal deformity

Nasal deformity requires a closed reduction under local (LA) or general anaesthetic (GA) within a week.

Soft tissue swelling obscures nasal contour

- Reassess for nasal deformity at approximately five days.
- Closed reduction once swelling has subsided.

Epistaxis post trauma

- Use nasal decongestant and local anaesthetic.
- Locate the bleeding vessel and cauterize.
- If this fails: Use anterior nasal packing with an antiseptic-impregnated ribbon gauze.
- If this fails then: Reduce the nasal fracture, and pack the nose.
- Further failure to control the bleeding will require posterior and anterior packing of the nose.
- Failed control is an indication for either embolization or ligation of sphenopalatine and ethmoid vessels.

Nasal septal haematoma

Failure to recognize and treat a septal haematoma may result in a septal abscess, and in resorption of nasal septal cartilage, loss of dorsal nasal support, and nasal deformity. It presents with nasal blockage, and a submucosal swelling of the nasal septum.

Management
- Incise and drain under general anaesthesia.
- Transseptal quilting sutures.
- Pack the nose.
- Administer a broad-spectrum antibiotic.

Pitfalls

- Skull-base fracture into middle ear may present as CSF rhinorroea (drains along eustachian tube).
- Swollen face may obscure a nasal fracture – therefore reassess for nasal deformity after swelling has subsided.
- A meningitis following blunt trauma to the head implies a base of skull fracture is present.

Recommended reading

Cummings, C. 1996. *Otolaryngology head and neck surgery.* St Louis: Mosby.
Kerr, A. (ed.) 1997. *Scott-Brown's otolaryngology.* Sixth edition. London: Butterworth-Heinemann Medical.

16   The injured eye
Thomas Eshun-Wilson

Eye injuries are frequently associated with trauma to the head and cervical regions and this may result in a delay in diagnosis. It is important, however, that these injuries are detected early in the assessment of the injured patient and that the ophthalmologist is included as part of the management team.

History

Take a history from the patient:
- Document the time of the injury.
- Establish the mechanism of trauma:
    - *blunt* – fist, shoe, brick
    - *chemical* – acid/alkali
    - *penetrating* – knife, glass, foreign body.
- Establish previous ocular history.

Examination

Perform a primary survey and attend to the survival of the patient first.
As part of the secondary survey, make use of a bright light source, close to the eye; directly and from the side; examiner's eye close to the injured eye. Local anaesthetic drops (Minims Benoxinate HCl 0.4%®) should only be used for examination and the performance of minor procedures. They should not be used as treatment. Fluorescein drops are used to detect any corneal abrasions. In order to retract the eyelids use paper clips.

External examination of the eye

Note if any of the following are present:
- Any fractures – skull, maxilla, zygoma
- Wounds – clean/septic
- Involvement of the eyelids – margin, intact cannalicular system
- Orbital rim – palpate for fractures, emphysema
- Ocular movements

Ocular examination
Always compare the injured eye with the other eye.

- Check visual acuity:
  - ability to count fingers
  - ability to detect hand motions
  - perception of light
  - no perception of light (NPL)
- Pupillary reactions
- Conjunctiva – presence of haemorrhage or laceration
- Sclera – look for uveal prolapse (dark brown tissue)
- Cornea – any laceration, ulcer, uveal prolapse
- Anterior chamber: presence of pus (hypopyon), blood (hyphaema)
- Pupil – should be round – if peaked implies prolapsing iris
- Lens – any cataract
- Retina:
  - presence/absence of the red reflex
  - orange reflection indicates choroidal blood
  - inspect the optic disc and blood vessels

Do not dilate both eyes with tropicamide drops. Dilate only the involved eye if the injury is not obvious. Beware that small upper-lid lacerations are often associated with large posterior scleral lacerations. Lid margin wounds need to be sutured by a specialist because incorrect apposition of the wound will result in a lid notch, which will constantly abrade the cornea.

Investigations

The following needs to be done:
Blowout fractures: X-ray (Waters view) or CT scan
Foreign body: X-ray looking straight, up, down, or CT scan
Stabbed eye: CT scan of the brain and orbits (objective evidence of globe disruption, and a significant number of patients will have intracranial penetration)

Management of specific injuries

Anterior segment

- *Arc eye:* double pad; Chloromycetin®ointment; analgesia (expect pain for 48 hours)
- *Chemical injury:* immediate irrigation with 2–3 litre Ringer's lactate or water; apply local anaesthetic drops; refer after $^1/_2$ hour of washing, including sweeping under the eyelids
- *Corneal abrasion:* Chloromycetin®ointment; apply an eye pad; refer next morning

- *Corneal ulcer:* Refer
- *Corneal foreign body:* Apply local anaesthetic drops; attempt removal with a cotton bud; Chloromycetin® plus eye pad; if unsuccessful refer within 24 hours
- *Hyphaema:* Refer for assessment and treatment of raised intra-ocular pressure, which can be blinding
- *Mydriasis:* If vision is normal, steroid drops and refer in two days

Blunt trauma

- *Decreased vision* from uveitis/retinal oedema – refer within 24 hours
- *Blowout fracture* (depressed fracture orbital floor with incarcerated tissue) – refer within 48 hours
- *Orbital haemorrhage* – acute proptosis – refer immediately

Penetrating trauma

- *Lid laceration.* Suture and administer tetanus toxoid; if involving margin/cannalicular system refer within 48 hours
- *Eyeball penetration.* (Corneoscleral incised wounds) – do not remove the knife/nail if in situ; keep nil by mouth; perform a CT scan of the brain and orbits and refer for removal.

Pitfalls

- Missed subtarsal (under the upper lid) foreign body.
- Missed intra-ocular foreign body (history of hitting metal onto metal).
- Missed corneal ulcer (stains green with fluorescein drops under blue light).
- Missed large posterior scleral laceration because lid injury is small.
- Inadequate wash-out for chemicals.
- Pupil reactions not tested.

Recommended reading

Chua, C. N., Salluotio, B., Frackiewicz, S. Eye casualty. Oxford Eye Hospital website on common ocular emergencies and referrals. http:/www.eye-casualty.co.uk.
Kanski, J. J. 1999. *Clinical ophthalmology.* London: Butterworth-Heinemann.

17 Penetrating neck injuries

Jenny Edge

Penetrating neck injuries are commonly seen in South Africa. Many are minor injuries of no significance but they can be deceptive in appearance. The platysma covers (and hides) many structures in the neck. Accurate assessment of whether the injury has penetrated the platysma is mandatory. If it has, the injury should be regarded as potentially serious.

This chapter provides a logical approach to the accurate assessment and management of injuries to the neck.

Classification of penetrating neck injuries

A penetrating neck injury is one that has penetrated platysma. To assess this, the wound may need to be infiltrated with local anaesthetic, cleaned and carefully examined without precipitation of bleeding. If the platysma has not been penetrated, then simple wound management is sufficient.

Injuries penetrating the platysma should be classified as:
- Posterior triangle (behind the posterior border of the sternocleidomastoid muscle)
- Anterior triangle (in front of the posterior border of the sternocleidomastoid muscle)
- The anterior triangle is subdivided into Zone I, Zone II, and Zone III. Zone I is below the cricoid cartilage, Zone III above the angle of the mandible, and Zone II lies in between.

Figure 17.1 Zones of the anterior triangle of the neck

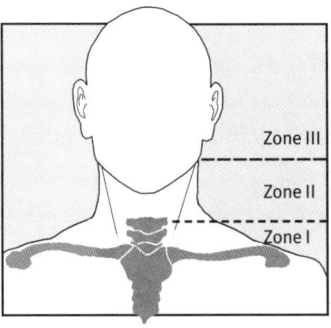

The anatomical structures potentially injured fall into six groups:

1 Blood vessels
2 Nervous system
3 Respiratory system
4 Digestive tract
5 Lymphatic system
6 Glands

Although the position of the entry wound does not rule out injury to other anatomical areas, it is useful to consider the structures lying in the areas of subdivision.

Posterior triangle

- Generally these injuries are less likely to injure the major structures.
- The spinal cord, brachial plexus, and vertebral arteries may be at risk.
- If the injury is very low, the subclavian vessels or the lung apex could be involved.
- Suspected vertebral artery injury should be managed with arteriography and embolization whenever possible.

Anterior triangle

Zone I

- Blood vessels: aortic arch, subclavian, and innominate vessels
- Nerves: brachial plexus, left recurrent laryngeal nerve, spinal cord, sympathetic trunks
- Respiratory: trachea, apex of the lung
- Digestive: oesophagus
- Lymphatic: thoracic duct on the left

Zone II

- Blood vessels: carotid vessels, internal jugular vein
- Nerves: vagus, recurrent laryngeal, phrenic nerve
- Respiratory: trachea, larynx
- Digestive: oesophagus
- Thyroid gland

Zone III

- Blood vessels: carotid vessels, internal jugular vein
- Nerves: cranial nerves VII–XII
- Respiratory/digestive: pharynx
- Parotid gland

Primary survey

The assessment and management of penetrating neck injuries must follow the ATLS® primary survey principles.

Airway

- Airway compromise may be directly due to the injury, or secondary, e.g. oedema secondary to haematoma, or vocal cord paralysis secondary to injury to the recurrent laryngeal nerve.
- If the airway is compromised, oral intubation should be attempted whenever possible, but facilities to perform an emergency surgical airway procedure must be present.
- If there is an obvious open injury to the airway, it is better to consider tracheostomy as soon as possible.

Breathing

The apex of the lung may extend into the neck, or the wound may penetrate into the chest. Always do a chest X-ray to check for a haemo-/pneumothorax.

Circulation

- Vascular injuries may present as neurological complications, e.g. neurological fall-out in the distribution of the middle cerebral artery may be secondary to a carotid artery injury.
- Obvious bleeding should be managed by direct pressure. A high-flow intravenous line should be set up.

Disability

Neurological deficit may be secondary to vascular injury, cranial nerve, or spinal cord damage.

Exposure/environment

Look for other injuries – keep in mind that additional injuries may also be present.

If bleeding is uncontrolled, the patient should go directly to the operating theatre; if it is controllable, proceed to the secondary survey.

Secondary survey

History

Establish the mechanism of injury, note voice change, ask about chest pain, dysphagia, haemoptysis, weakness, paresthaesia, or numbness in the arms.

Examination

Assess for the presence of:

- Local bleeding, pulsation, bruit, absent pulses, expanding haematoma
- Air in soft tissues, distended neck veins
- Fluid leaking from the wound (saliva, CSF, lymph)
- Cranial nerve deficit, particularly CNVII–XII, Horner's syndrome
- Loss of sensation, pulses, and power in the upper limbs
- Loss of sensation and power in the lower limbs
- Pneumo-/haemothorax, abnormal breathing pattern (e.g. diaphragmatic breathing)
- Frequent reassessment of the airway is mandatory to check for impending obstruction due to oedema.

> Does the patient require operative management? If yes, the patient should go straight to theatre. If there is no urgent indication for surgery, the wound should be classified according to zone, and further investigations should be done.

Investigations

In the stable patient who has no immediate indication for surgery, the blood vessels, respiratory, and digestive systems should be investigated to rule out injury. This may be done primarily by surgical exploration, or by utilizing special investigations which may obviate the need for surgery. Zone II injuries are readily exposed and accessed, and are therefore often surgically explored without pre-operative investigations. The structures in Zone I or III are more difficult to visualize intra-operatively and need more pre-operative planning and preparation.

Chest X-ray

Do not sit patient up if there is an open wound; it may cause a fatal air embolism.

Cervical spine X-ray

Look for the presence of fractures, foreign bodies, or air in soft tissues.

Arteriography

Zone I: Consider if there is any indication of a vascular injury: blood pressure difference of more than 10 mmHg in either arm, widened mediastinum on chest X-ray, bruit or haematoma.

Zone III: Consider if there are stigmata of vessel injury (bruit, neurological deficit, or haematoma).

Spiral CT scan

A spiral CT scan may be considered if an aortic injury is suspected.

Endoscopy

An endoscopy may show oesophageal injury: the success of utilizing either rigid or flexible endoscopy depends on the skill and experience of the endoscopist.

Gastrografin® swallow

The Gastrogafin® swallow is not sensitive for Zone III injuries, but is sensitive for lower injuries.

Laryngoscopy

Laryngoscopy may be used diagnostically and therapeutically: blood clots may be removed.

Management

- If all the investigations are normal, the patient may be observed overnight and discharged home if there is no deterioration.
- A haemothorax should be managed accordingly.
- If the investigations are abnormal, the patient should be referred to a surgeon.

Operative management

Aim

- To ascertain the extent of the injuries
- To restore vascular continuity where indicated and stop haemorrhage

Figure 17.2 Management of penetrating neck injury

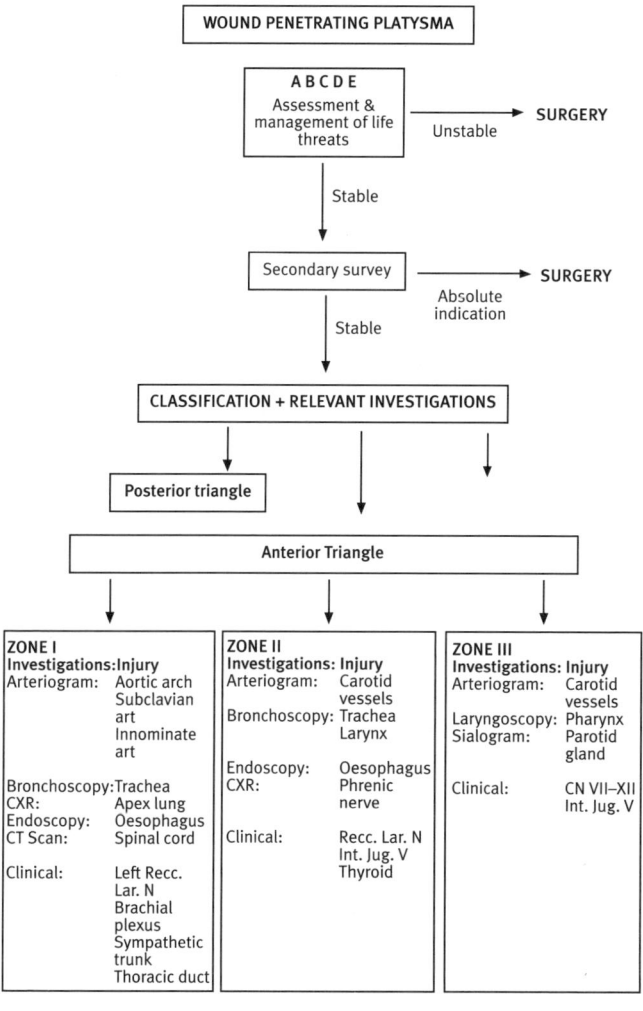

- To repair any structural damage
- To drain when indicated

Position and anaesthetic
- General anaesthetic with a definitive airway
- Patient supine with the table flat
- Place head on head ring with the face turned away from the side of injury provided that no injury to C-spine exists
- Clean skin to xiphisternum to allow for extension of incision

Incision
Anterior to and parallel with sternocleidomastoid: this allows extension superiorly for Zone III injury or inferiorly for Zone I injury as indicated.

Exposure and control
- Mobilize sternomastoid muscle and retract the muscle laterally to expose the internal jugular vein (IJV).
- Lateral retraction of vessels allows access to the midline structures.
- Medial retraction of the vessels allows exploration of the prevertebral fascia and vertebral arteries.
- Explore tract of injury.
- If haematoma is encountered, then aim to achieve vascular control above and below the suspected area of injury before exploring the haematoma.

Figure 17.3 Anterior sternocleidomastoid incision

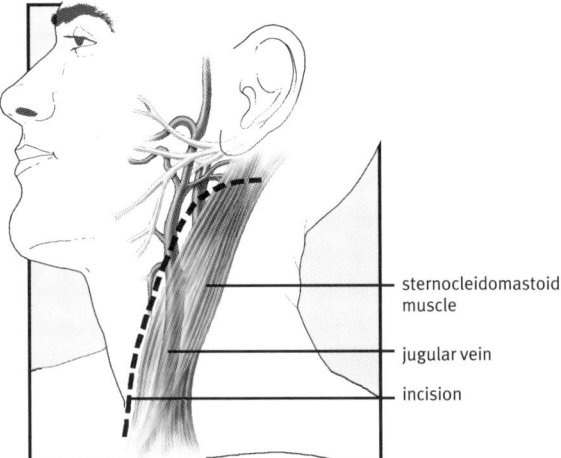

sternocleidomastoid muscle

jugular vein

incision

Vascular injuries

- The carotid artery is crossed anteriorly by the middle thyroid and facial veins, which may both be divided.
- The vagus nerve lies posteriorly and the hypoglossal nerve anteriorly: both of these should be preserved.
- To explore the carotid more distally, the posterior belly of the digastric may be divided and the sternocleidomastoid divided near its origin from the mastoid bone (*Note:* The glossopharyngeal, facial, and accessory nerves are at risk).
- Whenever possible, aim to repair the carotid artery. A direct repair may be possible if there is a stab wound. In the case of blunt injury or gunshot wound, ensure that all damaged vessel walls are resected. The area of adventitial bruising may be greater than the area of direct damage.
- Venous injuries should be treated by ligation of the vessel. The IJV is extremely thin walled, and susceptible to damage during mobilization.
- When a vascular injury in Zone I is suspected, an elective sternotomy (or occasionally a 'trap door' extension) should be considered.

Oesophageal injuries

- The oesophagus is a thin-walled, poorly vascularized structure, and must be explored delicately and carefully for an injury.
- It may be repaired directly using a monofilament or multifilament absorbable suture.
- Identification may be aided by passing a nasogastric tube.
- Always drain the area with a soft drain.

Figure 17.4 Exposure of the oesophagus and left recurrent laryngeal nerve

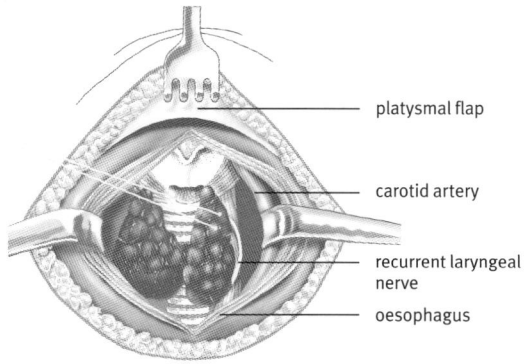

platysmal flap

carotid artery

recurrent laryngeal nerve

oesophagus

Tracheal injuries
Repair tracheal injuries directly with an absorbable suture.

Thyroid injuries
- The main aim is to prevent any bleeding.
- Rarely a thyroid lobectomy may be performed but care must be taken to avoid damage to the recurrent laryngeal nerve. The left nerve lies in the tracheo-oesophageal groove but on the right, it runs from infero-lateral to supero-medial.

Root of the neck
- The incision may be extended laterally to expose the structures at the root of the neck.

Figure 17.5 Exposure of the proximal subclavian vessels

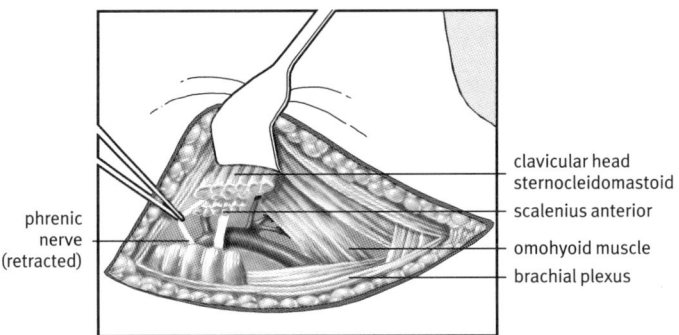

phrenic nerve (retracted)

clavicular head sternocleidomastoid
scalenius anterior
omohyoid muscle
brachial plexus

Figure 17.6 Exposure of the proximal vertebral artery

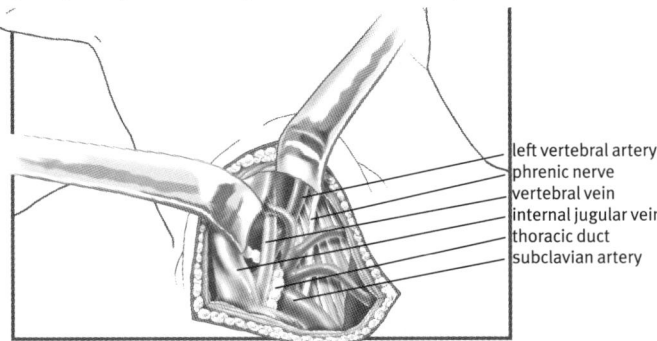

left vertebral artery
phrenic nerve
vertebral vein
internal jugular vein
thoracic duct
subclavian artery

Figure 17.7 Exposure of the distal vertebral artery

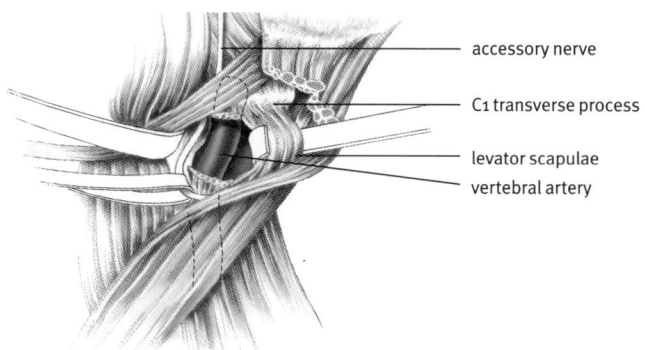

— accessory nerve

— C1 transverse process

— levator scapulae
— vertebral artery

- The scalenus anterior may be divided to expose the subclavian artery (note that the thoracic duct lies nearby).

Vertebral artery
- Exposure of this vessel is difficult and any suspected injuries are best treated by selective embolization by the radiologist where possible.
- If not, exposure can be gained by retracting the IJV medially and the carotid artery laterally. The sympathetic chain lies anterior to it.

Closure
- Close in layers with absorbable sutures.
- Leave a drain if there is any suspicion of an oesophageal injury or any haematoma.

Pitfalls
- Not adhering to ABCDE for the initial management of the patient.
- Not recognizing airway problems that may not be due to the initial injury and may develop over time. Always frequently reassess the airway.
- Not doing a thorough assessment of platysmal penetration. The wound should *never* be probed as bleeding is sure to be precipitated.
- Penetrating neck injuries may involve the lung or mediastinal structures. The chest should always be assessed.
- Vascular injuries may cause neurological manifestations.

- During operative procedures, always aim to get control of a vessel above and below the area of injury: arterial injuries may be more extensive than initially seen and veins must be adequately mobilized prior to attempted ligation.
- Always drain a suspected oesophageal injury.

References and recommended reading

Ballantyne, J., Harrison, D. F. 1986. *Rob and Smith's Operative Surgery.* Fourth edition. London: Arnold.

Ellis, B. W., Paterson-Brown, S., Bailey, Hamilton. 1995. *Hamilton Bailey's emergency surgery.* Twelfth Edition. London: Butter Hein Med.

Madiba, T. E., Muckart, D. J. 2003. Penetrating injuries to the cervical oesophagus: Is routine exploration mandatory? *Annals of the Royal College of Surgeons of England,* May, 85(3):162–6.

Wilmore, D. W., et al. (eds.) 2002. *ACS surgery: Principles and practice.* New York: WebMD Corporation.

Cardiac injuries

Andrew Nicol

Penetrating cardiac injuries

The prehospital mortality rate for penetrating cardiac injuries is 86%. Of the fatal penetrating chest injuries, 50% are a direct result of a cardiac injury. In view of the high mortality, it is essential to diagnose and treat appropriately the potential survivors who arrive in the emergency department.

Clinical presentation

Always be suspicious of a penetrating cardiac injury in the presence of a stab wound in the precordium or epigastrium and where the bullet tract has passed close to the heart.

The four major presentations are:

1. Hypovolaemic cardiac arrest
2. Exsanguinating thoracic haemorrhage
3. Cardiac tamponade
4. Stable haemopericardium

The majority of patients present in the first three categories.

- Exsanguinating haemorrhage implies bleeding into the thoracic cavity through the pericardial laceration and this is usually detected after insertion of an intercostal drain.
- Cardiac tamponade occurs when the wound in the pericardial sac has sealed and the collected blood in the pericardial sac results in a diminished left ventricular end-diastolic volume from the pressure effect.
- Beck's triad (the classical presentation of cardiac tamponade, which is present in 75% of cases) consists of:
  1. Hypotension
  2. Raised JVP
  3. Muffled heart sounds
- Pulsus paradoxus (weakening of the pulse on inspiration – increased venous return on inspiration results in less space for the left ventricle to fill) is found in 11% of patients with cardiac tamponade.
- The stable haemopericardium may be a diagnostic challenge and the patient may be remarkably stable. Warning signs are a period of unexplained hypotension in the prehospital phase and a tachycardia. Always

listen for cardiac murmurs, which may indicate a traumatic septal defect, and a pericardial rub.

Diagnosis of cardiac injuries

- The vast majority of cardiac injuries are fairly easily diagnosed – a precordial injury presenting with hypovolaemic shock or features of cardiac tamponade.
- A further subset will be diagnosed at surgery where, particularly for thoraco-abdominal gunshot injuries, a subxyphoid window should be performed prior to laparotomy if the bullet tract is close to the heart so as to exclude a cardiac injury. A positive subxyphoid window will be an indication to perform a median sternotomy. If the patient is sufficiently stable and mobile ultrasound is available, this can be performed prior to surgery instead of the subxyphoid window.
- The usual diagnostic work-up for a suspected cardiac injury is as shown in the diagram below.

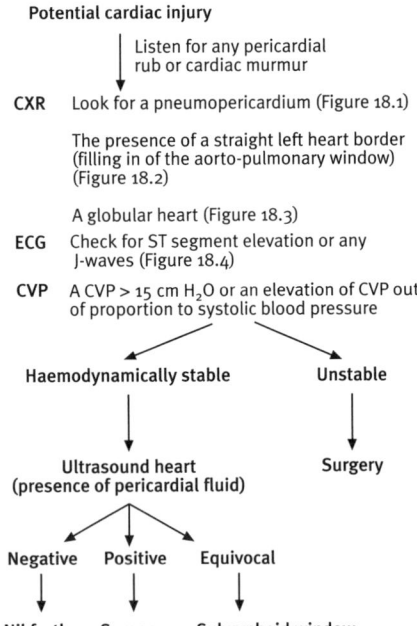

Potential cardiac injury

Listen for any pericardial
rub or cardiac murmur

CXR   Look for a pneumopericardium (Figure 18.1)

The presence of a straight left heart border
(filling in of the aorto-pulmonary window)
(Figure 18.2)

A globular heart (Figure 18.3)

ECG   Check for ST segment elevation or any
J-waves (Figure 18.4)

CVP   A CVP > 15 cm H_2O or an elevation of CVP out
of proportion to systolic blood pressure

Haemodynamically stable   **Unstable**

Ultrasound heart
(presence of pericardial fluid)   **Surgery**

Negative   **Positive**   **Equivocal**

Nil further   **Surgery**   **Subxyphoid window**

Figure 18.1 CXR following a stab to the left chest with a pneumoperi-cardium. The major differentiating feature between a pneumopericardium and a medial pneumothorax is that in the former, the attachment of the pericardium stops at the level of the aortic arch. A medial pneumothorax will continue above this level.

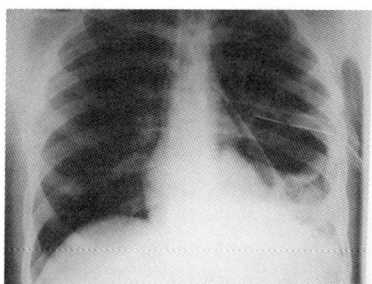

Figure 18.2 CXR with a straight left heart border indicating a haemopericardium

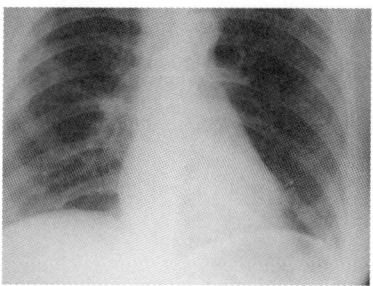

Figure 18.3 Globular heart in a patient presenting one month after a precordial stab

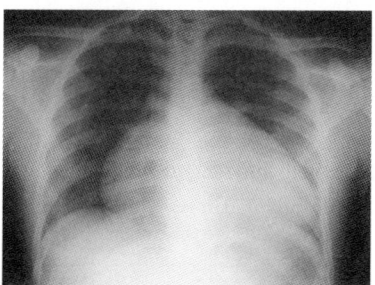

Figure 18.4 J-waves on an ECG

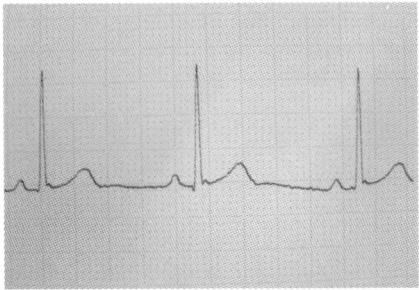

- Any suspicious feature on the CXR, ECG, or CVP requires an ultrasound of the heart to be performed.
- If the patient is haemodynamically unstable, the surgical options consist of: an emergency department thoracotomy, a subxyphoid window in theatre to confirm the diagnosis, or a median sternotomy/thoracotomy. No unstable patient should leave the resuscitation room for investigations.
- Diagnostic needle pericardiocentesis is not indicated as it is unreliable as a diagnostic tool – false-negative rate 10–80%, false-positive rate 10%.
- The sensitivity of ultrasound in detecting pericardial fluid varies and a left-sided haemothorax may make visualization difficult. Any equivocal studies should have a diagnostic subxyphoid window performed in theatre.
- An elevated CVP may also be due to:
  - tension pneumothorax
  - overzealous fluid resuscitation
  - straining
  - pain
- A subxyphoid pericardial window remains the gold standard for the diagnosis of cardiac injuries.

Surgical management of penetrating cardiac injuries

Emergency department thoracotomy (EDT)

An EDT is currently only indicated in penetrating trauma. It is imperative that the patient, who will not survive the transfer to the operating theatre and the subsequent delay in management, is identified and an EDT performed. The survival rate is higher for patients with penetrating cardiac injuries operated on in the operating theatre (86% survival in theatre vs 38% survival for EDT). The left antero-lateral thoracotomy allows the quickest access for an EDT. The indications for an EDT are:

- Asystole with signs of life in the preceding five minutes
- Pulseless electrical activity on an ECG monitor with cardiac arrest
- Hypovolaemic cardiac arrest in hospital
- A hypotensive patient with a precordial injury, who has a systolic blood pressure of less than 70 mmHg, is not responding to fluid resuscitation, and will not survive the 10-minute delay to transfer into theatre.

Median sternotomy vs thoracotomy

- As a general rule, if a penetrating injury is medial to the mid-clavicular line, then a median sternotomy should be performed. This allows better access to the heart and the intra-thoracic great vessels.
- Penetrating injuries lateral to the mid-clavicular line should have a thoracotomy performed. This allows easier access to the lung.
- The rare patients presenting with a second cardiac injury with an old sternotomy scar, should be entered through a thoracotomy.
- A cardiac injury with a penetrating injury on the right side of the chest should undergo a right antero-lateral thoracotomy.

Subxyphoid window

- A positive subxyphoid window for a haemopericardium remains an indication for sternotomy and definitive repair of any cardiac injury.
- Pericardial drainage alone in patients with a stable haemopericardium, who are not actively bleeding at surgery, and where the injury is >24 hours old, may be an option but further studies are required.

Intracardiac fistula and valvular injuries

- If these are found intra-operatively and the patient is haemodynamically stable, then the chest is closed and a cardiac catheterization is performed at six weeks. A significant proportion of these fistulae will close spontaneously.
- Any patient with a cardiac murmur should have echocardiography performed, provided they are haemodynamically stable.

Intracardiac missiles

- The risk of potential complications of the missile (missile embolism/endocarditis/thrombo-embolism) must be weighed up against the safety of its removal. Generally missiles that do not move on sequential X-rays can be well tolerated.

Coronary artery injuries

- Major proximal injuries tend not to survive.
- Distal injuries may be ligated. If the heart goes into ventricular fibrillation, then the suture should be removed and coronary artery bypass grafting is required. This may be performed on cardiac bypass or on the beating heart.

Blunt cardiac injury (BCI)

The true incidence of BCI is unknown but is estimated to vary between 15 – 75% of patients after blunt-chest trauma. BCI was formerly known as a myocardial contusion. The current management strategy for BCI is outlined in the diagram below.

- Inotropes/anti-arrhythmics should be administered as required.
- Cardiac troponin and CK–MB fractions do not appear to be useful.
- For patients with confirmed BCI requiring surgery, invasive pulmonary artery monitoring should be used.

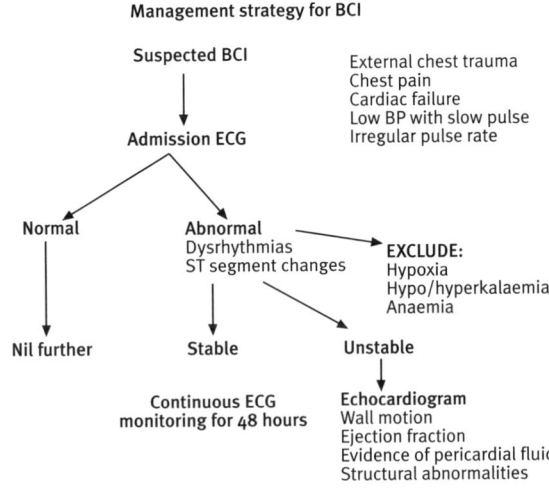

Management strategy for BCI

Suspected BCI
- External chest trauma
- Chest pain
- Cardiac failure
- Low BP with slow pulse
- Irregular pulse rate

↓

Admission ECG

Normal → Nil further

Abnormal
Dysrhythmias
ST segment changes

EXCLUDE:
Hypoxia
Hypo/hyperkalaemia
Anaemia

Stable → Continuous ECG monitoring for 48 hours

Unstable → Echocardiogram
Wall motion
Ejection fraction
Evidence of pericardial fluid
Structural abnormalities

Operative technique for cardiac injuries

Front room thoracotomy

Preparation
- Intubate and ventilate.
- Administer morphine 10 mg and midazolam 10 mg IVI.

Incision
- Extend from the costal margin on the left to mid-axillary line in 5th intercostal space. Avoid injuring the internal mammary artery.
- If the entrance wound is on right side of chest, consider a right antero-lateral thoracotomy (better access to right side of the heart).
- Incise the skin, subcutaneous tissue, pectoralis major, and the inter-costals down to the pleura.
- Incise the pleura and use a Mayo scissors to divide the remaining muscle and pleura – avoid injury to the underlying lung.
- Insert a large Finochietto retractor.
- Note: It is not necessary to divide to costal cartilages as this usually results in injury to the internal mammary artery.

Surgical procedure
- Apply an Allis clamp to the pericardial sac to elevate it away from the heart.
- Incise the tented up portion of the pericardium.
- Incise the pericardium towards the right shoulder so as to avoid injuring the phrenic nerve (if a left thoracotomy is performed).
- Remove the clot from the pericardial sac.
- Site of the injury will be evident from the colour of the blood – dark, unoxygenated blood will indicate a right-sided lesion.
- Apply digital pressure to the wound.
- In larger lacerations of the atria, a Satinsky clamp can be applied (do not use this on the ventricles).
- For larger wounds, a Foley catheter can be inserted through the injury, the balloon inflated and pulled back against the heart to tamponade any bleeding – a clamp should be placed across the Foley catheter to stop blood pouring out of the catheter.
- For right-sided injuries, total inflow occlusion can be achieved by cross-clamping the superior and inferior vena cava; this may be used for only 2–3 minutes before the heart stops beating.
- Injuries to the heart should be sutured with a 2–0 polypropylene (Prolene®) suture either interrupted or as a mattress suture.
- Gentle approximation of the edges of the wound is required. Pledgets (Teflon®) may be used to prevent the suture tearing out.

- Wounds close to the coronary arteries require a mattress suture that must be placed beneath the vessel and then tied so as to avoid ligating the artery.
- Skin staples have also been described for use in closing cardiac wounds.
- Once the laceration has been repaired, inspect the posterior surface of the heart for a through-through injury – this manoeuvre will dramatically decrease cardiac output and any injury must be dealt with rapidly. If the hole is in the posterior atrio-ventricular groove then cardiac bypass may be required.
- Once haemostasis has been achieved, the patient is taken to theatre where the chest is washed out and a pericardial and two intercostal drains are inserted.
- Closure of the pericardial sac is controversial; if it is performed then a small space should be left open at the inferior aspect. The pericardial sac should be drained.
- The internal mammary artery is inspected for any damage and then the chest is closed in layers.

Subxyphoid window

This procedure is best performed under general anaesthetic although it has been described under local. It remains the gold standard for the diagnosis of a cardiac injury.
- Incise the skin for 6 cm over the xyphisternum.
- Incise through the rectus sheath but do not enter the peritoneal cavity.
- Dissect bluntly (swab on a stick) up over the top of the diaphragm.
- Place a Langenbeck retractor under the xyphisternum.
- Wipe the pre-pericardial fat away to visualize the pericardial sac.
- Elevate the pericardial sac with an Allis clamp and incise next to the tented up portion.
- Insert a Metzenbaum scissors and make a 5 cm incision into the pericardium.
- A positive pericardial window for blood in the acute trauma setting will indicate a median sternotomy is required.
- For negative pericardial windows, a soft pericardial drain is inserted and the wound is closed in layers.

Pitfalls

- Waiting too long until attempting an emergency department thoracotomy.
- Using external chest compression in penetrating hypovolaemic cardiac arrest when internal cardiac massage is required.

- Infusing large volumes of fluid into the patient presenting with cardiac tamponade pre-operatively.
- Not being scrubbed and gowned before the induction of the anaesthetic for a cardiac injury as the patient may suddenly decompensate.
- Missing the gradual enlargement of the heart on CXR in a patient with a penetrating chest injury.

Recommended reading

Asensio, J., Montgomery Stewart, B., Murray, J., et al. 1996. Penetrating cardiac injuries. *Surgical Clinics of North America,* 76:685–724.

Duncan, A. O., Scalea, T. M., Salvatore, J. A., et al. 1989. Evaluation of occult cardiac injuries using subxyphoid pericardial window. *Journal of Trauma,* 29:955–960.

Knudson, M. 1992. Emergency department thoracotomy for trauma: A reappraisal. *Advances in Trauma and Critical Care,* Vol 7:133–157.

Nagy, K. K., Krosner, S. M., Roberts, R. R., et al. 2001. Determining which patients require evaluation for blunt cardiac injury following blunt chest trauma. *World Journal Surgery,* 25:108–111.

Von Oppell, U. O., Bautz, P., De Groot, M. 2000. Penetrating thoracic injuries: What we have learnt. *Thoracic Cardiovascular Surgery,* 48:55–61.

19 Blunt chest injuries

Douglas M G Bowley, Elias Degiannis,
Martin D Smith

The majority of significant blunt chest injuries occur during motor-vehicle accidents. Speed is a critical factor; a 10% increase in impact speed translates into a 40% rise in the case fatality risk for both restrained and unrestrained occupants.

The mechanism of injury relates to rapid deceleration at the moment of impact and the interaction of the occupant (or pedestrian) with the mass of the vehicle.

Chest injuries are often life threatening, either in their own right or in combination with other system injuries.

The initial priorities for patients with chest trauma are to ensure patency of the airway, adequate ventilation, and restoration of an effective circulation.

Pulmonary contusion

Pulmonary contusion is a result of bleeding into the pulmonary parenchyma.

- It usually occurs beneath fractured ribs or a flail segment in adults. It may be present in children in the absence of fractured ribs (due to the elasticity of their rib cage).
- It is the most commonly diagnosed intrathoracic injury in victims of blunt trauma and is an independent risk factor for pneumonia and acute respiratory distress syndrome (ARDS).
- Significant contusions are often not diagnosed until 24 hours after admission as the CXR signs are typically delayed and often underestimate the degree of the pulmonary injury.
- Respiratory dysfunction arises due to a combination of:
  - Lack of pulmonary function in the contused segment
  - Remote lung injury mediated by cytokines released by the trauma to the lung parenchyma

Treatment

Treatment relies on recognition of the pulmonary contusion, adequate analgesia, good physiotherapy, and supplemental oxygen. In patients with pulmonary contusion, avoidance of overtransfusion with intravenous fluids is sensible, but restriction of fluid as a treatment is not advised.

Rib fractures

Fractured ribs are a clinical and not a radiological diagnosis.
- Palpation over the chest wall must be performed to elicit any tenderness or crepitations to suggest an underlying rib fracture.
- Associated injuries are:

Fractures ribs 1–3	Subclavian artery/brachial plexus
Fractures ribs 3–7	Haemo-/pneumothorax
	Pulmonary contusion
Fractures 8–12	Diaphragm
	Intra-abdominal trauma (liver/spleen)

Management

Patients with fractures of only one or two ribs can usually be discharged home provided that there is no underlying pulmonary pathology (chronic obstructive pulmonary disease), the CXR is normal, and the patient is able to cough adequately with analgesia.

Fractures of three or more ribs require admission for adequate analgesia. The patient must be able to cough so as to prevent atelectasis and a subsequent pneumonia from developing.

Flail chest

Flail chest is defined as a fracture of two or more ribs in two or more places with resultant paradoxical movement of a segment of the chest wall. This paradoxical movement (recession of the chest wall on inspiration) may be apparent only after 24 hours.
- The blunt force required to disrupt the integrity of the thoracic cage typically produces an underlying pulmonary contusion.

Figure 19.1 CXR demonstrating a pulmonary contusion after blunt trauma

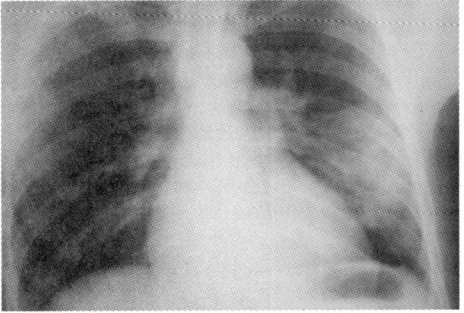

- Traditional treatment has been the use of positive pressure ventilation (IPPV) to 'internally splint' the chest until fibrous union of the broken ribs occurred. Ventilation is still often required, especially in patients with multiple injuries.
- Continuous positive airway pressure (CPAP) via a tight-fitting face-mask is effective management of a flail chest and may avoid intubation and ventilation, and the complications associated with this, including hospital-acquired pneumonia. Hospital stay may also be reduced. Close monitoring of the patient's respiratory rate and $PaCO_2$ levels are required.

Treatment
As with all pulmonary injuries, the cornerstones of treatment include effective use of analgesia and aggressive physiotherapy.

Analgesia in blunt chest trauma

Fractured ribs are extremely painful and inhibit the patient from taking deep breaths and coughing; leading to respiratory dysfunction due to atelectasis, retention of secretions, and pneumonia.

All patients should receive oral paracetamol and a non-steroidal anti-inflammatory medication, in the absence of contraindications.

A **pleural block** may be used if the patient has an intercostal drain in situ and the patient is carefully monitored in a high-care environment.

A mixture of 10 ml of 0.5% bupivacaine and 40 ml of sterile water is introduced into the chest using the intercostal drain, which is then clamped for five minutes and the patient encouraged to change position to distribute the mixture around the pleural space. The duration of effective analgesia is approximately four hours. This technique is not appropriate if the chest drain is bubbling, as a tension pneumothorax can occur in the presence of an active air leak. Bilateral pleural blocks should not be used.

Intercostal nerve blocks can provide highly effective analgesia for patients with an isolated fractured rib:
The fractured rib, plus the rib below and the rib above are blocked by injection of 3 to 5 ml of local anaesthetic (0.5% bupivacaine and 1% lignocaine mixture) at the lower edge of each rib approximately 2.5 cm from the midline posteriorly. It is necessary to inject the rib above and below because of the crossover of innervation between ribs. Aspiration is performed before infiltration to avoid inadvertent intravascular injection and care must be taken to stay within the maximum dosage of local anaesthetic.

The single injection technique provides analgesia, which lasts for 6 to 10 hours and may not need to be repeated.

Intravenous morphine (20 mg morphine in 200 ml of normal saline – 1 mg per 10 ml) used as a continuous infusion provides excellent analgesia. Start at 2 mg per hour and increase (up to 4 mg per hour) until the patient is able to cough effectively.

A high thoracic epidural should be considered early in the patient with extensive rib fractures. This should only be performed when the patient can be monitored in an intensive care unit but it is extremely effective and if used early may avoid the problem of respiratory failure and ventilation.

Aortic injuries

Traumatic aortic injuries (TAI) cause or contribute to 15% of fatalities due to MVA. Most patients with TAI die before they reach hospital, and the vast majority will have major co-existing thoracic and extra-thoracic injuries. The mechanism of injury is major deceleration trauma, most often during MVA, but also after falls from a height or crush injuries to the torso. Three mechanisms are thought to contribute to aortic rupture:

- Shearing stress generated by differential movement between a fixed portion of the aorta and a relatively more mobile portion.
- A very high peak of intraluminal pressure occurring during the moment of the accident.
- Crushing of the aorta between the chest wall and the spinal column (so-called osseous pinch).

The majority of blunt TAIs occur at the aortic isthmus, defined as the proximal descending aorta within one centimetre of the origin of the left subclavian artery. This is where the aorta is fixed by the ligamentum arteriosum.

Figure 19.2 Supine CXR showing a widened mediastinum associated with traumatic aortic injury (TAI)

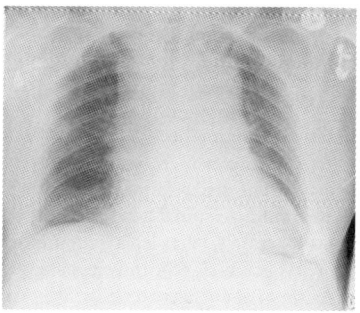

Figure 19.3 Angiogram with fusiform enlargement of the aorta due to a TAI

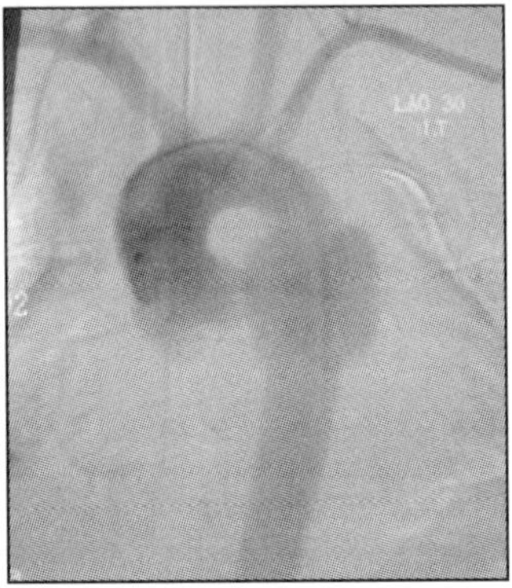

Diagnostic modalities

TAI is suspected in patients with a suitable mechanism of injury and suspicious features on initial CXR. The most sensitive CXR findings of aortic injury are widening of the mediastinum (> 8 cm at the arch in a supine film) and an abnormal or indistinct aortic contour. The initial chest X-ray may be reported as normal and a high index of suspicion is required by emergency room personnel in order to diagnose TAI.

Aortography is still the 'gold standard' diagnostic tool for TAI, with sensitivity of almost 100% and specificity of 98%.

Helical CT scanners with intravenous contrast have the advantage of being non-invasive and are able to demonstrate injuries other than TAI. There is some concern about the ability of CT to diagnose aortic branch injury and the effectiveness of CT depends greatly on the available expertise.

Transoesophageal echocardiography (TEE) has also been used to evaluate TAI. This is highly operator dependent and certain anatomical regions (the arch and supra-aortic branches) are difficult to visualize.

Operative techniques

The traditional operative repair has been called 'clamp and sew'. A clamp is placed proximal to the rupture, usually between the left common carotid and left subclavian artery. The distal clamp is placed as high as possible on the thoracic aorta, to minimize spinal cord ischaemia and reduce back-bleeding from intercostal vessels. Paraplegia is an important complication of operative repair of TAI and is significantly less likely if cardiac bypass is used. The involved segment of aorta is excised and a primary anastomosis or a graft is performed.

The increasing sophistication of endovascular techniques has led to attempts to treat TAI using vascular stents, thus avoiding the considerable morbidity of open repair. This approach holds great promise for the future.

Blunt tracheobronchial injuries

Blunt tracheobronchial injuries constitute a small fraction of admissions to trauma centres, as many patients die before they reach hospital.

The *mechanism of rupture* is thought to be due to a combination of shearing forces between the two relatively fixed areas of the tracheobronchial tree (the cricoid and the carina) and a sudden increase in intraluminal pressure caused by reflex closure of the glottis, together with compression of the thorax.

The location of the lesions appears to be constant with 80% occurring within 2.5 cm of the carina, 15% are tracheal, and 5% are distal bronchial lesions.

Subcutaneous emphysema and severe dyspnoea are the most common initial signs. CXR may reveal pneumothorax, pneumomediastinum, and the 'fallen lung sign' where the apex of the lung is seen at the level of the carina, which is diagnostic of main bronchial rupture.

Treatment

This is primarily surgical, although if the transection is less than one third of the circumference of the airway and the lung is fully expanded, conservative treatment may be applied successfully.

The optimum procedure is debridement of the ends of the damaged airway and primary anastomosis. Good results are likely in 90% of cases.

Diaphragmatic injuries

Reported incidence of diaphragmatic rupture is between 0.8% and 1.6% of patients admitted to hospital with blunt trauma.

- Left-sided injuries predominate. Under-diagnosis of right-sided injuries, hepatic protection of the right hemi-diaphragm, and weakness of the left side at points of embryological fusion have all been proposed to explain the preponderance of left-sided injuries.
- The diagnosis of ruptured diaphragm is frequently missed in the acute phase. Always suspect in the patient with respiratory distress and a flail chest.
- There is no single investigation that provides a reliable diagnosis of diaphragmatic rupture at presentation. Between 33% and 70% will be diagnosed on initial CXR. Elevation of the hemi-diaphragm on plain CXR may represent diaphragmatic rupture, visceral herniation, or

phrenic nerve paralysis. Diaphragmatic rupture can only be diagnosed on radiographs if herniated stomach or bowel is constricted (the 'collar sign') as it transits the torn diaphragm or if the tip of the nasogastric tube resides above the diaphragm.

- The reported sensitivity of CT for diaphragmatic tears is low and varies between 14% and 61%. Sensitivity is improved if there is herniation of intra-abdominal contents into the chest.
- A combined barium meal and enema may be performed to confirm the diagnosis of acute diaphragmatic herniation.
- Suspected diaphragmatic injury can also be accurately evaluated by video-assisted thoracoscopy (VATS) or laparoscopy.

Figure 19.4 A CXR after blunt trauma showing colon, stomach, and small bowel in the chest

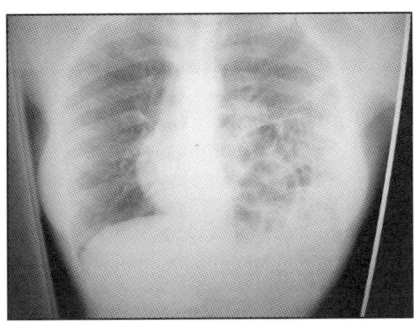

Figure 19.5 A barium swallow confirming the presence of an acute diaphragmatic hernia with stomach in the chest

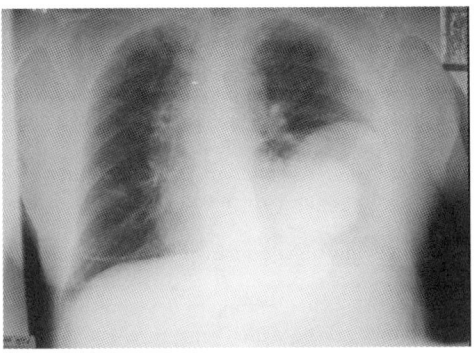

Treatment

Acute diaphragmatic injuries are best approached through the abdomen, as approximately 90% will have an associated intra-abdominal injury. During a laparotomy for blunt trauma, the surgeon must make a point of assessing both domes of the diaphragm for injuries.

Oesophageal rupture

Rupture of the oesophagus from blunt chest trauma is very rare.

Clinical signs, such as mediastinal air, are often subtle and overshadowed by serious injuries to other organs. Associated tracheobronchial rupture may occur. Delay in diagnosis is associated with significant morbidity.

Pitfalls

- Underestimating the degree of lung injury at first assessment. Close observation and frequent re-evaluation of patients after severe blunt chest injury are mandatory.
- Inadequate analgesia after chest injury. This leads to hypoventilation, retention of secretions, and pneumonia. Good analgesia facilitates physiotherapy, which together reduces pulmonary morbidity.
- Failing to recognize significant intrathoracic injury. A high index of suspicion is required to diagnose aortic, bronchial, and diaphragmatic rupture, with liberal use of diagnostic studies.
- Assuming that lack of evidence of chest wall trauma in children means there is no intrathoracic injury.

Recommended reading

Mattox, K. L., Feliciano, D. V., and Moore, E. E. 2000. *Trauma*. Fourth edition. New York: McGraw-Hill.

20

Penetrating chest injuries

Douglas M G Bowley, Elias Degiannis,
Martin D Smith

In modern-day civilian practice, thoracic injury accounts for 20% of deaths due to trauma. Eighty-five per cent of thoracic trauma may be managed without operative intervention. The mainstays of management are the provision of an adequate airway, oxygenation, tube thoracostomy, analgesia, and physiotherapy.

Initial assessment

Resuscitate patients according to the ATLS® protocols.

Primary survey

Airway and cervical spine protection

Exclude airway obstruction from vomitus, blood, or an expanding haematoma. Secure a definitive airway (cuffed tube in the trachea) if there is any doubt about airway patency. Ensure adequate cervical spine protection until cleared on clinical and radiological findings.

Breathing

Listen for air entry bilaterally. Exclude a tension pneumothorax clinically. This is suggested by an external wound with an elevated jugular venous pressure (JVP), hypotension, decreased breath sounds on the affected side, and tracheal shift to the contra-lateral side. An intercostal drain (ICD) should be placed immediately if the patient is hypoxic and clinical signs suggest a pneumo/haemothorax – do not wait for a chest X–ray (a needle thoracocentesis may be used initially while the equipment is set up). Avoid covering sucking wounds without inserting a chest drain.

Circulation

Look for signs of cardiac tamponade (hypotension with an elevated JVP may also be due to a tension pneumo/haemothorax).

Exposure and preventing hypothermia

Undress the patient. Perform a careful examination of the front and back for other injuries – it is surprisingly easy to miss a small penetrating injury to the torso. The patient should be log-rolled until the cervical spine is cleared.

Adjuncts to primary survey

- Perform a cervical spine X-ray – always exclude an injury unless the patient is fully conscious, complains of no neck pain, and is not drunk.
- Look on chest X-ray (CXR) for any pneumo/haemothorax, pneumo-mediastinum, pneumopericardium, enlarged heart, pulmonary contusion, or air under the diaphragm on erect films. A widened mediastinum is a sign of an intra-thoracic great vessel injury and in a stable patient will require an angiogram.
- Look for blood in the nasogastric tube, which may indicate an oesophageal or stomach injury.
- Observe the cardiac leads for any ST segment elevation, which may suggest a cardiac or pericardial injury.

Secondary survey

It is important to determine the tract of any gunshot injury so that an appropriate assessment is made – determine through which anatomical structures the bullet may have passed. Entrance and exit wounds must be identified, as well as any retained bullets (retained missiles require a lateral X-ray of the area to ascertain the position).

- All patients with injuries below the nipples anteriorly or below the tip of the scapula posteriorly, must have an abdominal injury excluded.
- All penetrating neck injuries must be considered to have a thoracic injury until proven otherwise.

Specific injuries

Oesophageal injuries

The overall mortality for oesophageal injuries is 40%. It is vital to determine if the oesophagus is injured early as the morbidity and mortality increase with a delay in diagnosis.

Clinical features

Pain on swallowing (odynophagia) is the most common symptom of oesophageal injury but the symptoms and signs may be very non-specific. Other clinical features suggestive of oesophageal trauma consist of:

- Dysphagia
- Blood in the NGT
- Haematemesis and haemoptysis
- Leak of saliva from neck

- Leak of gastro-intestinal contents into the chest drain
- Subcutaneous emphysema
- Mediastinitis – late presentation of a missed thoracic oesophageal injury
- Transmediastinal penetrating trauma

Special investigations

The radiological features will consist of:

- Pneumomediastinum on CXR (see Figure 20.1)
- Pre-vertebral air (air in the soft tissue) on lateral C-spine X-ray (see Figure 20.2)

Any clinical suspicion of an oesophageal injury will warrant further investigations.

Figure 20.1 CXR with air in the mediastinum

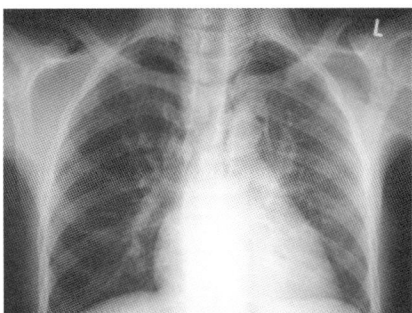

Figure 20.2 Lateral neck X-ray with pre-vertebral air

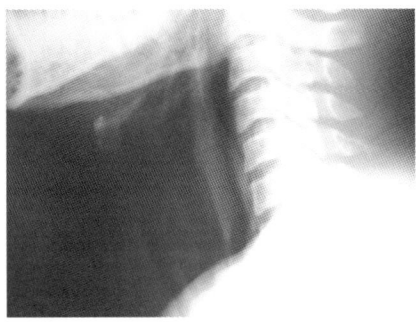

Figure 20.3 Algorithm for the management of a suspected thoracic oesophageal injury

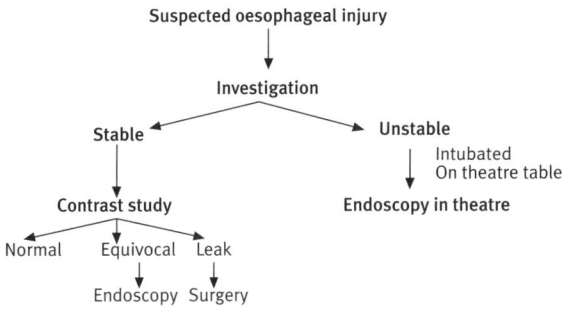

Figure 20.4 A contrast study of a stab to the thoracic oesophagus with a leak as indicated by the arrow

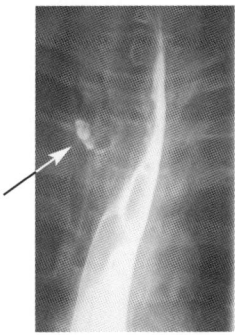

Contrast study

For the stable, co-operative patient a simple contrast swallow study is recommended. Avoid gastrograffin if there are signs of a traumatic tracheo-oesophageal fistula as gastrograffin is toxic to the lung parenchyma.

Endoscopy

Patients requiring emergency surgery for the commonly associated major airway or vascular injuries should be endoscoped on the theatre table. Rigid or flexible oesophagoscopy should be used depending on the available expertise. If endoscopy is not available and the patient has been intubated, the NGT may be pulled back into the pharynx and the contrast may be inserted via the NGT.

Surgery

- Perform a primary repair in a single layer with wide drainage and a NGT passed through the repair for feeding. Even after delayed diagnosis this is the preferred management as it maintains a functional oesophagus and prevents the need for successive operations. For combined oesophageal and tracheal injuries, a muscle flap must be interposed.
- Diverting procedures or oesophagectomies are only undertaken as a last resort and usually in a patient who is septic and requires ligation of the oesophagus with a gastrostomy and feeding jejunostomy. When the patient is more stable, an oesophagectomy and finally a gastric pull-up will be required.

Tracheo-bronchial injuries

The presentation of thoracic tracheo-bronchial injury depends on whether the injury is confined to the mediastinum or communicates with the pleural spaces. Injuries confined to the mediastinum will present with a pneumomediastinum. An injury that communicates with the pleural space usually presents with a pneumothorax, which persists despite adequate placement of chest drains, and a bronchopleural fistula (continuous bubbling into the underwater drain).

- Bronchoscopy is the most reliable means of diagnosis.
- Rigid bronchoscopy requires a general anaesthetic and should be avoided in a patient with a cervical spine injury.
- Flexible bronchoscopy also allows for evaluation of the larynx and controlled insertion of an endotracheal tube if required.

Management

The majority of tracheo-bronchial injuries may be handled non-operatively. The indications for surgery are:

- Massive subcutaneous emphysema with airway obstruction (rare)
- Massive air leak
- Persistent air leak into the intercostal drain >10 days

Figure 20.5 Algorithm for the management of a suspected tracheal injury

Suspected tracheo-bronchial Injury

Clinical: Massive subcutaneous
emphysema
Large air leak with
collapsed lung despite
two chest drains on
suction

Bronchoscopy

Transmediastinal gunshot injuries

These injuries carry a high mortalitity. The management decisions will depend on the haemodynamic stability of the patient and on determining the tract of the bullet and the potential structures that may have been damaged.

- An angiogram and a contrast study of the oesophagus are the minimum investigations required in the stable patient.
- A spiral CT scan may be used to determine the tract of the bullet and aid in whether the tract has passed close to the aorta or oesophagus and help decide on whether the other investigations are required.

Figure 20.6 Management strategy for a transmediastinal GSW

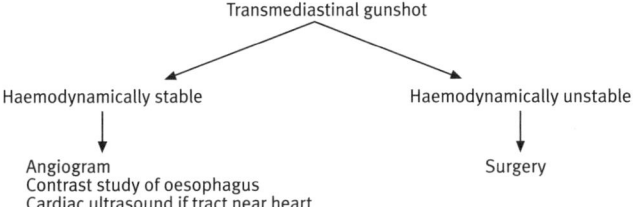

Transmediastinal gunshot

Haemodynamically stable   Haemodynamically unstable

Angiogram
Contrast study of oesophagus
Cardiac ultrasound if tract near heart

Surgery

Pneumothorax

A pneumothorax implies the presence of air in the pleural space between the parietal and visceral pleura resulting in partial or complete collapse of the lung. It may be caused by blunt or penetrating trauma or may arise spontaneously in a patient on a ventilator or with underlying lung disease.

Classification

A pneumothorax is classified as:

- Open – air derived from the exterior
- Closed – air from damage to the lung parenchyma or airway

Figure 20.7 A CXR showing a right-sided pneumothorax

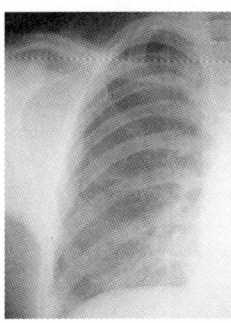

Management
Large pneumothorax
A large pneumothorax is more than 1.5 cm in size with the measurement taken from the inside of the 3rd rib to the margin of the lung. A minimum 28 FG intercostal drain should be inserted in the adult, a 32 FG if there is an associated haemothorax.

Small pneumothorax
A small pneumothorax < 1.5 cm in size measured from the inside of the 3rd rib to the margin of the lung, may be treated without an intercostal drain provided:
- It is unilateral
- The patient is not on a ventilator (positive pressure can exacerbate the pneumothorax)
- No air travel is planned
- The patient does not require a general anaesthetic

The patient should be kept in hospital and have a follow-up X-ray in 12 hours. If there is no increase in size of the pneumothorax, the patient may be discharged home. If the pneumothorax has increased in size, then a drain should be placed.

Figure 20.8 Algorithm for management of a pneumothorax

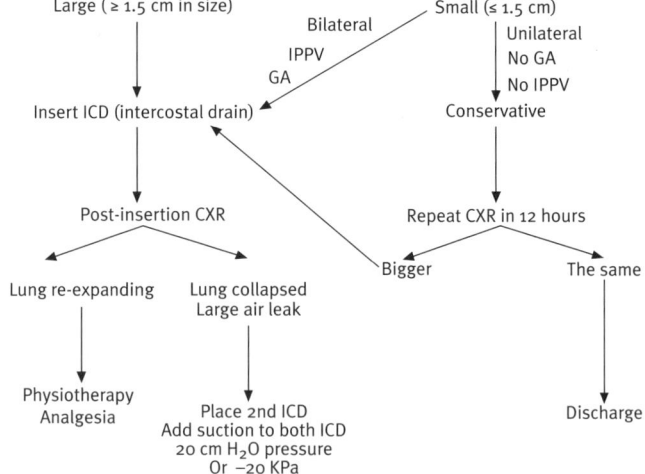

Tension pneumothorax

Chest wounds can act as one-way valves – allowing air to enter during inspiration but not allowing air to escape – this results in an increase in pressure in the pleural cavity and will result in mediastinal shift with a reduction in cardiac output.

Clinical presentation

- Hypoxia
- Anxiety
- Severe dyspnoea
- Elevated JVP
- Trachea shifted to opposite side

Management

Tension pneumothorax is a clinical diagnosis, there is no time for X-rays. Treatment is insertion of a large-bore needle into the 2nd intercostal space mid-clavicular line to decompress the pneumothorax, followed by insertion of a chest drain.

Open pneumothorax

With larger penetrating wounds, air may preferentially enter the pleural cavity via the wound rather than through the trachea. If an open wound exceeds 2/3rd of the cross-sectional area of the trachea in a patient breathing spontaneously, effective ventilation may cease.

Management

Complete occlusion of the wound will lead to a tension pneumothorax. Appropriate management is to place a plastic dressing over the wound and to tape it on three sides, so as to allow air to escape but not to enter the pleural cavity. Once the patient is in hospital, a chest drain should be inserted and the wound debrided and closed.

The addition of suction to an intercostal drain

Low-pressure, low-volume suction should be used via a Drager pump. This should not exceed 20 cm H_2O or −20 KPa.

- Watch for the development of a 'Tidal Steal' phenomenon – where in large air leaks the patient may lose his/her entire tidal volume through the intercostal drain. After the placement of suction the patient will become hypoxic.
- Keep the suction on until the lung has re-expanded completely for at least 24 hours.

Figure 20.9 How suction is applied to an intercostal drain bottle

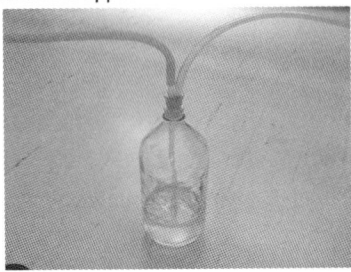

Problem cases with a pneumothorax

- The lung has not re-expanded after the insertion of an intercostal drain. Place the intercostal drain on suction. If the lung remains collapsed then insert a 2nd intercostal drain and place both drains on suction.
- There is continuous bubbling from the intercostal drain.
  Check to see that there is no air leak from the system – all tubing is sealed and tight – if there is no leak from the system, this implies a bronchopleural fistula – the majority of which will seal spontaneously with intercostal drainage. If this does not seal after 10 days, surgery will be required.

Haemothorax

A haemothorax is the presence of blood in the pleural cavity. Large haemothoraces may produce a tension haemothorax with a shift in the mediastinum.

The clinical features are those of a pleural effusion, namely:

- Dullness to percussion
- Decreased air entry

Radiological signs

The radiological signs of a haemothorax will vary, depending on whether the X-ray is supine or erect, and the amount of blood present in the chest. There are four different patterns of haemothorax on CXR that may be encountered:

1 Supine haemothorax (supine CXR)
2 Classical crescent shape (erect CXR)
3 Haemo-pneumothorax (erect CXR)
4 Subpulmonic haemothorax (erect CXR)

Figure 20.10 The classical crescent shape of a haemothorax on an erect CXR

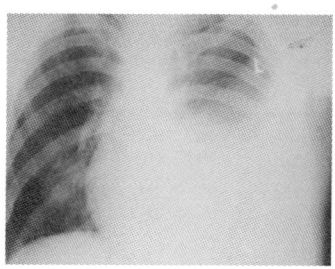

Figure 20.11 The haemo-pneumothorax with an air-fluid level (outline of the collapsed lung indicated with arrows)

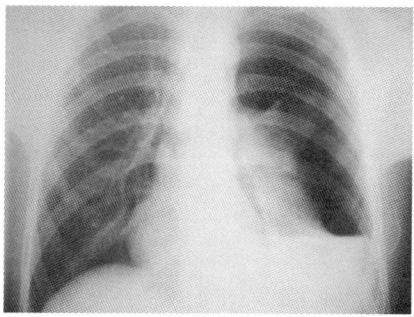

Figure 20.12 (a) A sub-pulmonic left-sided haemothorax on an erect CXR

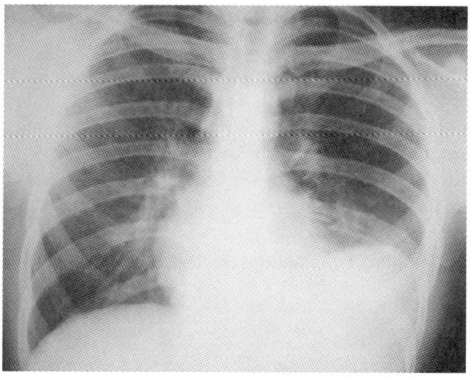

Figure 20.12 (b) A left lateral decubitus X-ray of the same patient in 12 (a) Note the run-off of blood as indicated – this is probably in the region of 400 ml. All the features of a sub-pulmonic haemothorax are well represented in Figure 12 (a). An ICD is indicated for this patient.

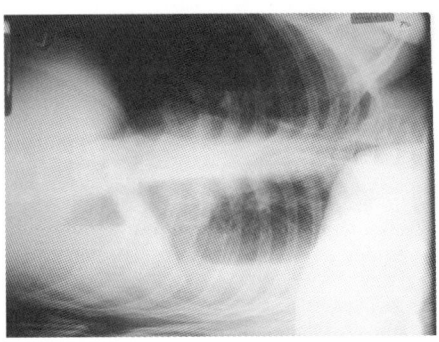

- When a CXR is performed in the supine position and a haemothorax is present, the X-ray findings will range from a complete white-out of the affected side (if there is a large amount of blood) to an increased opacification of the affected side when compared to the opposite side (if there is a small amount of blood).
- The classical crescent shape of the haemothorax is seen on an erect CXR. A combined pneumothorax with an air-fluid level indicates a haemo-pneumothorax.
- A subpulmonic haemothorax implies that there is blood above the diaphragm but sitting below the lung – this collection may be significant – features on X-ray that are suggestive are:
  - elevated hemi-diaphragm
  - a lateral hump to the shape of the diaphragm
  - fluid in the costo-phrenic recess.
- The diagnosis of a subpulmonic haemothorax is made by performing a lateral decubitus X-ray, with the 'sick side' facing downwards, and one should then check for any run-off. If the run-off is thicker that 1.5 cm, an intercostal drain should be placed.
- An intercostal drain should be inserted if one expects to get at least 200 ml of blood from the pleural cavity.

Massive haemothorax

A massive haemothorax (> 1.5 litre of blood) causes a shift of the mediastinum, compression of the lung on that side, with reduction in breath

sounds and features of hypovolaemic shock. Immediate drainage of
> 1.5 litre of blood into an intercostal drain is an indication for an urgent
thoracotomy and operative haemostasis.

Management of an intercostal drain

- Perform a post-insertion CXR to check the position of the drain.
- Ensure adequate analgesia.
- Refer for physiotherapy.
- It is preferable that the patient be placed in a chair.
- Monitor amount of blood drained (> 200 ml blood drained per hour is
  an indication for thoracotomy).
- Watch Hb and temperature.

Criteria for removal of an intercostal drain
The lung must be fully expanded on CXR, there must be < 50 ml drained
over the last 12 hours and there should be no bubbling when the patient is
asked to cough.

Technique of removal of an intercostal drain
- Explain removal to the patient.
- Ask the patient to valsalva (continuously blow out against the back of
  his/her hand).
- Whilst the patient is performing the valsalva, cut the securing suture
  and tie the purse-string suture securely.
- Place a dry dressing at the site.

Further follow-up post-removal of intercostal drain
All patients should have a follow-up CXR performed within three days
after discharge. A chest injury form should accompany the patient detail-
ing the symptoms that would indicate that the patient should return
immediately to hospital namely:
- Severe chest or abdominal pain
- Sudden shortness of breath
- Coughing up of blood
- Painful swallowing or difficulty in swallowing
- Bleeding or discharge from the drain site
- Fever and a temperature
- Abdominal cramps

Common complications post-intercostal drain insertion
Clotted haemothorax
Confirm that the blood has clotted by performing a lateral decubitus X-ray
and checking for run-off; if there is run-off, insert an intercostal drain if

> 200 ml of blood is expected to drain. On CXR it is extremely difficult to distinguish between pneumonic consolidation and clotted haemothorax, and a CT scan is often required to make that differentiation. If the patient is symptomatic or if > $^1/_4$ of the extent of the pleural cavity is involved with a clotted haemothorax, surgery is required.

Empyema

The presence of a temperature, dyspnoea, and decreased breath sounds should alert one to the possibility of an empyema (pus in the pleural cavity).

- Intravenous antibiotics with *S. aureus* cover should be started and the site of the collection identified and drained with an intercostal drain.
- An AP and lateral CXR usually indicate the position of the collection but an ultrasound is more accurate to determine the exact site.
- A thoracotomy must be performed for patients not responding to antibiotics and chest drainage.

Thoracic duct injuries

The presence of chylous material in the chest drain after penetrating trauma heralds an injury to the thoracic duct. The features of chyle are:

- Milky appearance (colourless in patients kept nil by mouth)
- Separation into a creamy upper layer on standing
- Fluid becomes clear when mixed with ether
- Relative density 1 012–1 015
- Triglyceride level > plasma triglyceride level
- Cholesterol: triglyceride ratio < 1
- Protein content of 20–30 g/l

Management

Initial conservative management for a period of 7–14 days provided nutritional and metabolic status is not compromised.

- Keep patient nil by mouth.
- Give medium chain triglycerides (MCTs) via a NGT (these do not pass through the lymphatic system).
- Monitor chyle output.

Indications for surgery

- Chyle leak > 1 litre per day for > 5 days
- Failure of conservative management with persistent leak
- Nutritional complications from chyle loss

Surgical management

- 5 g of cream orally four hours before operation.

- Ligation of thoracic duct in Poirier's triangle if the leak is in the upper thorax or neck. Poirier's triangle is the region between the internal carotid artery, arch of the aorta, and the vertebral column. Elective ligation may also be performed in the upper abdomen or lower thorax where the anatomy is more constant.

Penetrating diaphragm injuries

GSWs that have traversed the peritoneal cavity require a laparotomy because of the high incidence of associated visceral injuries (95%). In stab wounds to the lower left thorax, a diaphragm injury will occur in 22% of patients. Because the diaphragm normally rises to the level of the 5th rib with expiration, it is frequently penetrated by wounds to the anterior chest below the nipple line. As a result of the intermittent negative intrathoracic pressure, abdominal viscera can herniate through diaphragmatic defects. Subsequent vascular compromise of the incarcerated viscera can lead to strangulation.

Clinical features

Clinical evidence of a diaphragm injury following a lower *thoracic* stab wound consists of:
- Air under the diaphragm
- Omentum herniating through the wound
- Left upper quadrant tenderness
- Leakage of bowel contents

Special investigations

- U/S and CT have a low sensitivity in detecting isolated diaphragmatic injuries in the absence of bowel herniating into the chest.
- Laparoscopy/thoracoscopy are probably the most sensitive investigations. The isolated injury can also be repaired through the minimally invasive route.

Surgical repair

- *Acute diaphragmatic wounds* should be approached via a laparotomy due to the high frequency of associated injuries. The wounds should be accurately sutured with a non-absorbable suture material.
- *Chronic diaphragmatic injuries* with bowel herniation are best managed with a thoracotomy. A laparotomy may also be required to free all the adhesions.

Surgical guidelines

Indications for an immediate thoracotomy/sternotomy

- Cardiac tamponade
- Loss of thoracic wall
- Tracheo-bronchial injury
- Oesophageal injury
- Thoracic great vessel injury
- Drainage > 1.5 litre of blood on chest drain insertion
- Continued bleeding > 200 ml per hour into chest drain.

Immediate thoracotomy

Outcomes after surgical intervention are improved if the surgery is performed in the theatre rather than the emergency room.

- If the patient is critically unstable, an emergency department thoracotomy should be performed.
- With penetrating unstable thoraco-abdominal injuries, the blood loss into the intercostal drain may often be from the abdominal cavity.

Delayed thoracotomy

Delayed thoracotomy may be required for unrecognized or incompletely treated acute injuries.

Indications for a delayed thoracotomy

- Clotted haemothorax
- Empyema not responding to conservative management
- Persistent air leak
- Chylothorax not responding to conservative measures
- Diaphragmatic hernia

Video-assisted thoracoscopy

The most widespread application of video-assisted thoracoscopy is in the treatment of clotted haemothorax.

- A CT scan of the chest must be performed pre-operatively to define whether the opacification on the CXR is parenchymal (atelectasis or pneumonic) or represents a retained haemothorax.
- Best results are obtained if performed within 10 days of the injury otherwise adhesions may make the procedure difficult.
- If a decortication is required, this is best performed via a thoracotomy.

Pitfalls

- To wait for a CXR before treating a tension pneumothorax.
- Closing a sucking chest wound before inserting a chest drain.
- Failure to examine the oesophagus intra-operatively when performing a thoracotomy for penetrating trauma.
- Failure to investigate for an oesophageal or tracheo-bronchial injury in the presence of a pneumomediastinum on CXR.
- Assuming that a haemothorax or pneumothorax is not present because they were not seen on supine CXR.

Recommended reading

Boffard, Ken (ed.) 2003. *Manual of definitive surgical trauma care.* London: Edward Arnold.

Knottenbelt, J. D., Van der Spuy, J. W. 1990. Traumatic pneumothorax: A scheme for rapid patient turnover. *Injury,* 21:77–80.

Merrigan, B. A., De Winter, D. C, O'Sullivan, G. L. Chylothorax. (Review) *British Journal of Surgery*, 1997, 84:15–20.

Shaw, J. M., Navasaria, P . H., Nicol, A. J. 2003. Laparoscopy assisted repair of diaphragm injuries. *World J Surgery,* 27:671–674.

21

Abdominal injuries

Jacques Goosen, Jerome Loveland

Blunt and penetrating abdominal injuries are both common and potentially life threatening. Gunshot wounds are replacing stab wounds as the most frequent cause of penetrating (abdominal) injury. For example, over the past 17 years, the trauma unit of the Johannesburg Hospital noted a 13-fold increase in gunshot wounds requiring resuscitation (Khavandi, et al., 2002). The higher the velocity of the bullet, the greater the area of degenerative changes of tissue surrounding the tract of the bullet. Necrosis and delayed perforation may follow. The direction and depth of penetrating wounds cannot be accurately assessed from the appearances of the skin defect.

Because of the high rates of road traffic accidents, intra-abdominal injury due to rapid deceleration, shearing, or compression of viscera is common in the developing world.

Victims of interpersonal violence should be considered to be at risk for blunt abdominal injury. Very few victims can remember the exact details of the altercation.

There is a shift towards non-operative management of haemodynamically stable patients with blunt, solid visceral injury.

Triage

Triage aims to direct the patient to the closest appropriate facility. Physiological parameters, e.g. Trauma Scores, tend to under-assess the severity of injury. Injury characteristics, such as mechanism, type, and site of injury, deceleration rate and degree of deformation of the vehicle etc., provide an indication of energy transferred. 'Major' mechanisms of injury therefore mandate immediate callout of the best surgical teams at a facility that can provide the highest level of care available. Traditional assessment by staff of sequentially increasing levels of experience result in delayed decision-making and delayed definitive care.

Initial assessment

The Advanced Trauma Life Support (ATLS®) programme correctly ensures that the initial assessment of injured patients is protocol driven. During a crisis, there is very little opportunity for lateral thought or prolonged consideration of the alternatives.

Primary survey

The aim of the primary survey is to identify and manage the threats to life in order of their priority.

'A' Abdominal injury may cause airway compromise, when hemorrhagic shock is so severe as to cause loss of consciousness, usually at a systolic blood pressure below 70 mmHg.

'B' Every chest injury can potentially be associated with penetration of the abdominal cavity. Major injury to the lower chest is commonly associated with upper abdominal injury.

'C' For potential abdominal injuries, assessment of the circulation includes:

- Assessment of tissue perfusion and degree of shock
- Assessment of cardiac function
- Determining the source of bleeding (chest, abdomen, pelvis, limbs, or external)
- Stopping the bleeding
- Volume resuscitation

For hypotensive victims of penetrating truncal trauma, delay of aggressive pre-operative fluid resuscitation improves outcome, provided that surgery can be done soon (Bickell, et al., 1994). Aim to provide volume resuscitation to a systolic blood pressure of at least 90 mmHg. Limiting the time from injury to definitive therapy is a principal determinant of survival.

'D' Paraspinal penetrating injury may cause damage to the spinal cord, retroperitoneal and/or intraperitoneal structures. Spinal cord injury above the level of T6 may mask abdominal signs due to the loss of somatic sensation. Decreased levels of consciousness mask abdominal signs.

'E' Active re-warming during and after resuscitation is vital. A core temperature of less than 35 °C (hypothermia) equates with a mortality of 34%, and a core temperature of 32 °C or less equates with a mortality of close to 100% for severe trauma (Jurkovich, et al., 1987).

Resuscitation and monitoring

- Before the patient is X-rayed, all bullet wounds should be marked with radio-opaque markers (paper clips), to determine bullet tracts. This will prevent the embarrassment of missed visceral injury due to stray bullet tracts. Marked wounds and/or bullet fragments must correspond and be visualized on truncal X-rays.
- Any penetrating injury between nipples and knees may enter the abdominal cavity, and assessment should include X-rays of chest and abdomen.

- The abdomen should be watched for distension during resuscitation. A distending abdomen is indicative of massive haemorrhage (and imminent death) until proven otherwise.
- Non-responders to volume resuscitation require immediate control of haemorrhage. Temporary responders to volume resuscitation are in the same (sinking) boat.

Secondary survey

- The majority (70–80%) of patients requiring laparotomy for abdominal injury declare themselves on arrival with peritonism, evisceration, or shock in the presence of a distending abdomen. These clinical findings all mandate urgent laparotomy.
- Assessing abdominal injury is based on simple actions, i.e. inspection, palpation, percussion, and auscultation.
- Bowel sounds can still be present with significant visceral injury.
- Blood on rectal examination implies bowel perforation and laparotomy.
- Special investigations are indicated where diagnostic ability is decreased (doubtful clinical signs), level of consciousness is decreased (including intoxication), or sensation is decreased (high spinal cord injury).

Special investigations

The issue is to operate as soon as possible on those requiring definitive surgery, to avoid non-therapeutic/negative laparotomy (acute peri-operative morbidity of 53% with associated injuries, 22% in those without associated injuries), and to avoid (septic) complications induced by delayed laparotomy (Weigelt & Kingman, 1988).

- For abdominal injury, all commonly used special investigations may show free intra-peritoneal fluid (high sensitivity). None can consistently identify the organ injured (lower specificity).
- Diagnostic peritoneal lavage (DPL) is still the mainstay for assessing the doubtful abdomen, especially where radiological experience is limited. For penetrating injury, the cut-off point is more than 10 000 red cells/mm^3 and particularly a white cell count of more than 50 cells/mm^3. For blunt injury, the cut-off point is more than 100 000 red cells/mm^3, or more than 500 white cells/mm^3. Vegetable fibres are rarely identified in clinical practice.
- A negative DPL comfortably excludes the need for laparotomy for intra-peritoneal injury, but not retro-peritoneal injury. DPL is very sensitive in the diagnosis of haemoperitoneum, but has a poor specificity due to its inability to diagnose organ injury or the need for therapeutic laparotomy.

- Screening DPL, followed by abdominal CT if positive, is a safe, efficient method of evaluating adult blunt abdominal trauma. The combination reduces time to evaluate the abdomen, does not result in increased non-therapeutic laparotomies, results in fewer missed injuries, and reduces overall use of abdominal CT, when compared to either DPL or CT alone (Mele et al., 1999).

- Sonar of the abdomen for free fluid (Focused Abdominal Ultrasound, or FAST) is non-invasive, cheap, easily repeated, but highly operator dependent. In experienced hands, FAST is 93.4% sensitive and 98.7% specific in the detection of hemo-peritoneum (Rozycki & Shackford, 1996). For occasional operators, FAST is best repeated after four hours. It is the investigation of choice for children, pregnant patients, or patients with fractured pelvis because it is non-invasive.

- Despite its high specificity in studies from single centres (by experts), sonar has an unexpectedly low sensitivity for the detection of both free fluid and organ lesions. In clinically suspected (blunt) abdominal trauma, another assessment, e.g. helical computed tomography, must be performed regardless of the initial ultrasonographic findings (Stengel et al., 2001).

- To date, the criteria for clinical efficacy using sonar for blunt abdominal trauma have not been fulfilled in terms of technical capacity, diagnostic accuracy, diagnostic effect, therapeutic effect, or patient outcome. It is not (yet) the standard diagnostic test in the evaluation of blunt abdominal trauma (Pearl & Todd , 1996).

- For haemodynamically stable patients, a positive DPL or FAST may be followed by a contrast-enhanced CT scan (CE-CT). Haemodynamic stability can be defined as patients maintaining parameters of perfusion in the normal range after infusing a maximum of 2 000 ml crystalloid during resuscitation.

- The current trend towards non-operative management of blunt abdominal trauma decreases non-therapeutic laparotomy from 35% to 14% (Lukan et al., 2001), but is still in development. Level 1 evidence is not yet available. The indications for laparotomy increase with the presence of a vascular blush, grade (grade 4–5) of solid visceral injury, and number of solid organs injured (Omert et al., 2001). Clinical deterioration (evidence of ongoing bleeding) is the most important indicator for laparotomy. Hollow visceral perforation is indicated by free gas, free fluid in the absence of solid visceral injury shown on CT scan, increasing number of solid organs injured (> 3) and mandates laparotomy. Altered level of consciousness is not a contraindication to non-operative management of blunt abdominal trauma.

- Age > 55 years and female gender show a greater failure rate of non-operative management, longer stay in hospital, and greater mortality for non-operative management, at least for splenic injuries (Harbrecht et al., 2001).

- Laparoscopy can be performed under local anaesthetic and sedation, and will detect anterior, antero-lateral, and many lateral penetrations of the peritoneal cavity. It is not able to exclude GIT injuries, once penetration of the peritoneum has taken place (Bautz, 1994).
- Penetrating injuries of the back and flanks cause significant visceral injuries less commonly than anterior penetrating wounds, due to the protection afforded by the 10–15 cm thick lumbar muscles.
- Penetration of retroperitoneal structures is best assessed by triple contrast CT scan (contrast per mouth, per rectum, and intravenously – stable patients only) with an accuracy of 97.8% (Easter et al., 1991).
- In the absence of a CT-scanner, the second best option for penetrating injury to the back and flank is a combination of repeated clinical examination by the same surgeon, sonar of the abdomen looking for collections, water-soluble contrast enema, and laparotomy in case of unresolved doubt. Retroperitoneal sepsis due to a missed visceral perforation can turn into a catastrophe.
- Rectal injuries are easily missed, because of the soft tissue surrounding the pelvis, especially the buttocks, and inadequate perineal or rectal examination.
- Sigmoidoscopy is mandatory in suspected rectal injury, more so by identifying blood in the rectal canal, than by visualizing perforation. Contrast studies are rarely, if ever, required for suspected rectal injury. Colostomy is indicated for grade 3 (or more severe) anal injuries, or any penetrating rectal injury (Levy et al., 1995).
- Haematuria, whether macroscopic of microscopic, declares injury to the urinary tract, except ureteric injury, where 34% of injuries do not manifest haematuria. In addition, excretory urography is only 14% sensitive, suspicious in 42% for penetrating ureteric injury. Most ureteric injuries are due to penetrating injury, and are identified on exploration of haematomas in proximity (Azimuddin et al., 1998).
- Unstable patients demonstrating haematuria require emergency room or on-table excretory urography, if only to demonstrate the presence and function of the contra-lateral kidney.

Management: Laparotomy or not?

Selective conservatism in the management of stab-wounds of the abdomen is well established. The patient is reassessed for peritonism by the same surgeon at a specified interval – four hours later. Failure to improve implies laparotomy (Demetriades & Rabinowitz, 1987).

For gunshots, the standard is laparotomy. Selective conservatism for gunshot wounds of the abdomen allows avoidance of laparotomy in 38% of patients, a 14% rate of negative laparotomy, and 0% mortality due to missed injury. This policy is reserved for experienced surgeons (Velmahos et al., 2001).

For blunt abdominal injury, the trend is toward non-operative management in haemodynamically stable patients without evidence of hollow visceral perforation. Review of available guidelines did not show any level-1 evidence, but only level-2 evidence, to support this.

Any blood found on rectal examination implies visceral penetration or less commonly, ano-rectal injury, and mandates sigmoidoscopy to identify the source.

Our retrospective data indicates that the cost of managing generalized peritonitis due to the delayed diagnosis of visceral perforation, is 17 times that of a non-therapeutic laparotomy.

Pitfalls

- Failure to call out a trauma team for a patient suffering a 'major' mechanism of injury.
- Underestimating the impending disaster of a distending abdomen in a shocked patient.
- Exposing the patient to hypothermia.
- Failure to match bullet holes and/or bullets on X-rays.
- Diagnostic dalliance, instead of immediate surgery, for a 'non-responder' or 'temporary responder' to volume resuscitation.
- Failure to do a complete rectal and perineal examination on every victim of major trauma.
- Failure to personally re-examine a patient admitted for abdominal observation, irrespective of special investigations performed, or the lack of sleep.
- Delay to theatre, once the decision to operate is made.
- Ultimately, a negative laparotomy is better than a positive postmortem.

References and recommended reading

American College of Surgeons, Committee on Trauma. Advanced Trauma Life Support®; Program for Physicians. American College of Surgeons. 1997.

Azimuddin, K., Milanesa, D., Ivatury, R., et al. 1998. Penetrating ureteric injuries. *Injury*, 29(5):363–7.

Bautz, P. Laparoscopy in trauma. 1994. In *Trauma Yearbook '94*. Johannesburg: Helm Publishing. 18–20.

Bickell, W. H., Wall, M. J., Pepe, P. E., et al. 1994. Immediate versus delayed resuscitation for hypotensive patients with penetrating torso injuries. *New England Journal of Medicine,* Oct 27, 331(17):1153–4.

Demetriades, D., Rabinowitz, B. 1987. Indications for operation in abdominal stab wounds. A prospective study in 651 patients. *Annals of Surgery,* 205:129–131.

Easter, D. W., Shackford, S. R., Mattrey, R. F. 1991. A prospective, randomized comparison of computed tomography with conventional diagnostic methods in the evaluation of penetrating injuries to the back and flank. *Archives of Surgery,* 126:1115–1119.

Harbrecht, B. G., Peitzman, A. B., Rivera, L., et al. 2001. Contribution of age and gender to outcome of blunt splenic injury in adults: Multicenter study of the Eastern Association for the Surgery of Trauma. *Journal of Trauma,* 51:887–805.

Jurkovich, G. J., Greiser, W. B., Luterman, A., et al. 1987. Hypothermia in trauma victims: An ominous predictor of survival. *J. Trauma,* 27:1019.

Khavandi, A., Bowley, D. M. G., Boffard, K. D., et al. 2002. A seventeen-year review of the pattern of trauma at the Johannesburg Hospital: The malignant epidemic is worsening. *SAMJ,* 92:798-802.

Levy, R. D., Strauss, P., Aladgem, D., et al. 1995. Extraperitoneal rectal injuries. *J Trauma,* 38(2): 273–277.

Lukan, J. K., Carillo, E. H., Franklin, G. A., et al. 2001. Impact of recent trends of noninvasive trauma evaluation and nonoperative management in surgical resident education. *J Trauma,* 50:1015–1019.

Mele, T. S., Stewart, K., Marokus, B., et al. 1999. Evaluation of a diagnostic protocol using screening diagnostic peritoneal lavage with selective use of abdominal computed tomography in blunt abdominal trauma. *J Trauma,* 46(5):847–852.

Omert, L. A., Salyer, D., Dunham, M., et al. 2001. Implications of the 'contrast blush' on computed tomographic scan of the spleen in trauma. *J Trauma,* 51:272–278.

Pearl, W. S., Todd, K. H. 1996. Ultrasonography for the initial evaluation of blunt abdominal trauma: A review of prospective trials. *Ann Emerg Med,* 27(3):353–361.

Rozycki, G. S., Shackford, S. R. 1996. Trauma ultrasound for surgeons, in E. Staren, M. E. Arregui (eds.) *Ultrasound for the surgeon.* Philadelphia: J B Lippincott-Raven, 23–25.

Stengel, D., Bauwens, K., Sehouli, J., et al. 2001. Systematic review and meta-analysis of emergency ultrasonography for blunt abdominal trauma. *Br J Surg,* 88:901–912.

Velmahos, G. C., Demetriades, D. D., Toutouzas, K. G., et al. 2001. Selective nonoperative management of 1 856 patients with abdominal gunshot wounds: Should routine laparotomy still be the standard of care? *J Trauma,* 234:395–403.

Weigelt, J. A., Kingman, R. G. 1988. Complications of negative laparotomy for trauma. *American Journal of Surgery,* 156:544–547.

22

Practical trauma laparotomy

Sandie R Thomson

Definitive treatment of all injuries at the time of the initial surgery is the goal for the majority of trauma victims. This approach is suitable for stable patients and those patients who undergo an operation after a period of observation and investigation. It is also appropriate for those with single injuries causing haemodynamic instability.

In a small group of unstable patients with multiple injuries, damage control type procedures are recommended and primary anatomical reconstruction is not appropriate.

Preparation for laparotomy

Preparation of theatre

- Warm theatre, warm IV fluids, and prepare external warming devices such as hot air blankets and warming mattress.
- Anticipate the possibility of additional assistance, staff or instruments required, such as extra suction, sternotomy saw, or vascular instruments.

Positioning and incision

- For laparotomy the supine position is usually used.
- In patients with suspected or confirmed perineal or rectal injury, the Lloyd-Davis Trendelenburg position allows access to these areas.
- The shocked patient is prepped from nipple to groin.
- The possible need for sternotomy, thoracotomy, saphenous vein graft, or positioning of stomas and drains must be considered.
- A midline incision allows rapid entry and good access to all areas of the abdomen.

Early laparotomy

Securing haemostasis

- First stop the bleeding and then proceed to a systematic laparotomy.
- Note that massive blood loss can occur from single injuries.
- Identify the source of bleeding rapidly as the tamponade effect of the closed abdomen is immediately lost when the abdomen is opened.

- Blood is best removed by scooping with packs as suction as this stage is too slow.
- The spleen, small-bowel mesentery, liver, and retroperitoneum are the most likely sources of profuse haemorrhage and these organs should be inspected in that order or as dictated by site of injury.

The profusely bleeding spleen

Examination and mobilization

If the right upper quadrant is the origin of haemorrhage, the spleen is usually the source. Strong retraction of the lower costal margin, with good suction, allows inspection and palpation. If the spleen is bleeding briskly, it is brought up into the wound. The surgeon's left hand draws the posterior rim of the spleen medially, allowing division of the peritoneum and then the lienorenal ligament. In rapid bleeding and poor visualization these attachments can be broken with one's fingertips.

Opening the lesser sac

The greater curvature of the stomach is pulled superiorly and the transverse colon inferiorly. The gastrocolic omentum, now taut, is divided transversely in the relatively avascular plane below the gastro-epiploic arch. The tail of the pancreas and splenic hilum are now in view. The splenic artery can be occluded between the left thumb and index finger to obtain a degree of haemorrhage control and to review the extent of the injury. This is particularly useful in the child where splenic salvage is desirable.

Splenectomy

Hilar vascular injury and gross disruption of splenic substance require splenectomy. Division of the short gastric vessels and the gastrosplenic ligament allows exposure of the hilum and adjacent pancreas. The splenic pedicle can be mass ligated, or artery and vein tied individually. The former may result in damage to the tail of the pancreas. This is not desirable but is certainly not a disaster.

If there is any doubt about the integrity of the pancreatic tail a drain should be inserted. Once the spleen is out, it is important to check the stumps of the artery and vein, and the greater curvature of the stomach for serosal tears and bleeding.

Summary

- Identify the bleeding source; hilum or pulp.
- Bring into the wound by dividing the lienorenal ligament.
- Open the lesser sac to gain access to the splenic pedicle.

- Gain digital control of the pedicle.
- Reassess.
- Decide on splenectomy or preservation.
- Divide short gastric vessels.
- Ligate and divide the pedicle.

Bleeding from the stomach

The stomach is a highly vascular organ and direct injuries can result in brisk and continued bleeding. These injuries should be quickly closed with a running all layers suture.

Branches of the left gastric can bleed profusely and direct suture ligation is the quickest and safest solution.

Access to the posterior surface of the stomach is as for exposure of the splenic hilum.

Bleeding from the small bowel mesentery

The small bowel and its mesentery is delivered from the abdominal cavity and obvious haemorrhage is controlled by digital pressure, and then discreet clamping and suturing.

- This rarely causes significant ischaemia if not immediately adjacent to the bowel.
- If the superior mesenteric artery is injured in the base of the mesentery, one should use digital pressure, not clamps, and proceed as for a central haematoma.

Major bleeding from liver

Major liver injuries, particularly on the right, with retrohepatic caval venous bleeding are uncommon and usually associated with multiple injuries. This usually necessitates a damage control approach and liver packing (see chapters on Damage Control and on Liver Injuries).

- When there is brisk bleeding from an obvious capsular and parenchymatous rupture, apply Pringle's manoeuvre (digital compression of the hepatic artery and portal vein at the foramen of Winslow).
- An angled vascular clamp can be applied subsequently.
- To control arterial bleeding from the depths, finger fracture of the parenchyma with inflow control allows suture ligation of the identified bleeding points.
- The left lateral segments are easy to compress to control venous bleeding.

The systematic laparotomy

Once haemorrhage has been controlled, one should proceed to a systematic laparotomy.

The hollow viscera

Long-acting hydrolysable sutures are used for all bowel repairs. Whether a single or double layer, continuous or interrupted anastomosis is constructed, healing will usually occur, provided that well-vascularized tissue is meticulously sutured. Gentle inspection of the segment can be used to ensure that no leakage of luminal content takes place at the suture line.

The small bowel

The small bowel, the most frequently injured hollow viscus, is then thoroughly inspected, loop by loop, and placed on and covered by warm wet packs.

- All injuries must be identified and gross spillage controlled using soft bowel clamps or Babcocks.
- Single perforations are simply closed. If two perforations are nearby, the bridge of tissue is divided and the defect sutured transversely to avoid narrowing of the lumen.
- Some destructive injuries will require resection and anastomosis, as will areas rendered ischaemic by the injury or by control of mesenteric haemorrhage.

The stomach

The stomach is largely situated in the intrathoracic portion of the abdomen and is vulnerable to transdiaphragmatic injury.

- Injuries are likely to be missed at the gastro-oesophageal junction, the greater curve at the omental and splenic attachments, the lesser curve at the gastrohepatic ligament and the posterior wall of the stomach.
- The rich blood supply of the stomach ensures that gastric wounds heal well, provided they are detected and repaired.
- Control bleeding with bowel clamps, digital pressure or Babcocks, debride wound edges if required, and do a full-thickness running suture.

The colon

Inspection of the whole colon is now done.

- Overt colon perforations, particularly of the transverse and sigmoid portions, should be appropriately controlled until repaired.

- Any smell, staining, or haematoma at the flexures or in the paracolic gutters mandates mobilization to identify or exclude injuries.
- Division of the lateral peritoneal attachments allows complete circular inspection and identification of all injuries.
- In stable patients, irrespective of the mechanism of injury, intraperitoneal primary closure (including resection and anastomosis), performed with technical competence, is the repair of choice for all identified colon injuries.

The rectum

If digital examination, proctoscopy, or sigmoidoscopy reveal fresh blood in the bowel or mixed with the stool, a rectal injury must be assumed and treated.

- Patients with suspected rectal injury should be operated in the Lloyd-Davis position.
- Anaesthetic tubing is placed in the rectum pre-operatively, and held in place with a peri-anal purse string suture.
- The free end of the tubing is then placed in a large deep bucket (preferably covered) at the base of the theatre table.
- At laparotomy, anterior and lateral perforations in the upper third of the rectum should be primarily repaired.
- Loop colostomy with distal rectal washout should be performed. This defunctions the rectum and removes faecal matter to prevent the fuelling of sepsis in the pararectal tissues.
- The peritoneum, if intact, is left alone and the rectum is not extensively mobilized to look for holes in the lower two thirds.

Loop colostomy and washout

A loop colostomy can be created in order to perform distal rectal washout.

- A mobile segment of sigmoid colon is looped with a latex tube through a gap in the mesenteric border.
- A grid-iron incision is made in the left illiac fossa and the loop pulled through. Don't make this opening too big.
- The main abdominal wound is isolated with towels or packs and a 24-gauge Foley catheter inserted through a purse string into the exteriorized loop.
- Irrigation is commenced with normal saline till the effluent is seen to be clear. The catheter is then removed and the small hole closed with the purse string to prevent spillage whilst the abdomen is closed and dressed.
- The latex rubber tube is secured as a bridge to the skin and the stoma opened.

- At the end of the abdominal procedure the tube is removed from the anus and the rectum is then cleansed per anum with swabs on sticks soaked in chlorhexidine.
- Perineal, buttock, or sacral wounds should be debrided and drained or loosely packed with gauze. If there is no wound into the presacral space it is not opened up to place a drain.

The diaphragm

Diaphragmatic injuries are frequently associated with penetrating chest trauma below the nipple and with disruptive pelvic fractures due to blunt trauma. Associated liver spleen or colon injury is not uncommon.

- The diaphragm should always be routinely inspected to ensure that herniation through the diaphragmatic wound is detected.
- Enlarge the diaphragmatic wound as this simplifies the reduction of the contents; usually stomach, colon, or spleen.
- The thorax can then be thoroughly washed out, and an intercostal drain inserted prior to the diaphragmatic repair.
- Use a continuous non-absorbable suture.
- Once the first stitch is placed and tied, it can be used to pull the diaphragm inferiorly to make the remainder of the suturing simpler.

The retroperitoneum, duodenum, and pancreas

(See chapters on Pancreatic and duodenal injuries.)

The retroperitoneal area requires detailed inspection because it is easy to miss an important injury. Haematoma, oedema, crepitus, and/or bile staining along the lateral margin are indicative of an injury; usually of the duodenum but occasionally the colon.

The physiological functions of the duodenum make this segment of bowel unforgiving of any technical or judgemental errors in the wound management. Kocher's manoeuvre will expose the back of the duodenal loop and will allow adequate inspection of the kidneys and ureters.

- Simple repair after debridement of contused wound edges will be suitable for most injuries.
- A single layer inverting suture placed transversely or obliquely avoids lumenal narrowing.

Drainage procedures

- Some duodenal wounds are extensive with considerable tissue loss.
- Defects involving the 2nd part of the duodenum with the ampulla of Vater exposed, are covered with a mobilized Roux-en-Y loop anastomozed to the excised duodenal wound in an end-to-side fashion.

- It is important to drain the area adequately and gain distal jejunal access (jejunosomy feeding tube) for post-operative nutritional support should a controlled fistula occur.

Examination of the pancreas
- Exposure of the duodenum also reveals both surfaces of the head of the pancreas. The neck, body, and tail are accessed by opening the lesser sac, as described for access to the splenic hilum.
- Pancreatic ruptures vary from a superficial crack in the capsule, without any involvement of ducts, to a complete transection or disruption. Rupture of the pancreas may not immediately be identified due to the presence of haematoma.
- The capsule must be incised, and blood and clot sucked and mopped away, to allow a parenchymal injury to be identified.

Pancreatic injuries
- Simple drainage is effective in the majority of minor and moderate injuries with parenchymal damage.
- For isolated transection of the neck or proximal body of the pancreas the alternatives lie between distal pancreatectomy or pancreatico-enteric anastomosis without resection.
- This technique avoids a tedious dissection of the pancreas to free it from the tributaries of the splenic vein and thus reduces the risk of concomitant splenectomy with its attendant risks. (See section Pancreatic and Duodenal injuries.)
- More severe injuries are discussed in the section on Damage control surgery.

Retroperitoneal haematomas

Central retroperitoneal haematomas
Central haematomas are explored because either great vessels, or pancreas/duodenum are likely to be injured.

Expanding haematomas
Expanding haematomas must always be explored, but this can be daunting, even if the patient is 'stable'. Experienced help should be summoned.
- Control inflow by compression or cross-clamping of the aorta at the hiatus.
- Combine with local digital control until the injury is more clearly defined.
- Mobilize viscera by medial rotation from the left if the supracolic compartment is involved.

- Then more adjacent proximal and distal control is secured and repair accomplished in a bloodless field.

Non-expansile flank haematomas

Non-expansile haematomas around the kidneys are best left unexplored as it may lead to the unnecessary loss of a kidney.

Splenic preservation

To preserve the spleen completely, its whole surface must be accessible and intact capsule must be present.

- The splenic artery should be isolated above the pancreas.
- Small tears which result in a raw bleeding surface can be controlled by local tamponade using an absorbable thrombogenic matrix, e.g. microfibrillar collagen.

Suture repair

Suture repair is applicable in about 15% of adult injuries.

- Localized cracks in the splenic pulp can often be closed by a series of 2/0 or 0 chromic catgut mattress sutures passed on curved atraumatic needles.
- Tying these sutures over Teflon buttresses, or over a roll of omentum, may diminish the tendency to cutting-out as the capsule, except in children, is not robust.
- Mesh splenorrhaphy has gained acceptance for burst injuries. It holds the segments of spleen together with a mesh of polyglycolic acid wrapped firmly round it.
- Haemostasis must be satisfactory at the end of the procedure.

Minor liver injuries

Between 60% and 75% of liver injuries are minor.

- Many have stopped bleeding when they are found, and should not be disturbed, as the clot may be dislodged and bleeding may recur.
- For active bleeding, an 0 or 1 chromic catgut suture can be passed beneath the fracture on a 50 mm or 75 mm curved atraumatic needle without leaving any dead space. If these sutures are gently tied, bleeding should be controlled.
- Access to some cracks and fissures on the posterior and superior aspects of the liver is restricted and if they are dry it is right simply to provide drainage to the area.

- Some argument continues over this, but provided a soft silicone tube drain is led into a sterile closed bag via a stab incision there is no evidence that this promotes sepsis, and it can be removed in 24–48 hours if no bile drains.

The extrahepatic biliary tree

Although rare, extrahepatic biliary tree injuries may be isolated or associated with injury to the vascular structures in the free edge of the hepaticoduodenal ligament.

- Control of brisk haemorrhage takes priority. The whole area may be contused and haemorrhagic, and the clue to the diagnosis is bile staining.
- If the injury is not clearly identifiable, it is safer to create a controlled fistula by intubating the biliary tract and placing a drain adjacent to the injury site and returning at a later stage for a definitive restoration of bilioenteric continuity.
- Tangential injury of less than one third of the circumference can be sutured over a T-tube inserted through an untraumatized part of the duct to both stent and decompress the repair.
- If there is a complete transection and the patient is stable, then duct jejunal anastomosis is the preferred reconstruction in experienced hands. The inexperienced should create a controlled biliary fistula.

Urological injuries

(See the section on urinary tract injuries)
All general/trauma surgeons should be able to repair the intraperitoneal bladder rupture and fashion a spatulated stented ureteric repair with 6/0 chromic catgut interrupted sutures. All repairs to the urogenital tract should be drained.

Abdominal closure

At the end of the operation the peritoneal cavity should be irrigated, with large quantities of warmed isotonic saline until all the lavagate is removed, clean, and free from particulate matter. Look everywhere again.

- Intraperitoneal drains are not used routinely.
- Complex pancreatico-duodenal and urinary tract injuries always require drainage.
- Entry and exit wounds into the peritoneal cavity should be closed from the inside with one polyglycolic acid suture incorporating at least tranversus abdominus.

- Mass closure of the abdominal wall is performed with a continuous 0 loop nylon, polypropylene, or polydiaxanone suture.
- Closure of the skin and subcutaneous tissues should not be performed if gross contamination of the wound has occurred during laparotomy.
- The external traumatic wounds should be debrided and left open.
- Injuries from high-velocity missiles should be debrided of all doubtfully viable muscle and the skin laid open or incised to allow free drainage.

Pitfalls

- Not using packs until the source of bleeding has been found.
- Inadvertent damage to the capsule of the spleen.
- Inadvertent damage to the tail of the pancreas.
- Not securing ligatures on short gastric vessels and the main splenic pedicle, as they are at risk of slipping off.
- Omitting to recognize that serosal haematomas should be deroofed and underlying injury appropriately repaired.
- Not searching for entrance and exit wounds of every injured structure.
- Not including all layers in the suture line, as haemostasis may not be secured, especially in the stomach.
- Not considering the mechanism and pattern of injury. This will indicate the injuries to be suspected and allow identification and repair of all injuries.
- Not recognizing that laparotomy may be necessary as an integral part of the resuscitation.
- Not recognizing that the operative solution for individual organ injuries requires a sound anatomical knowledge, surgical judgement, and standard technical expertise. This will lead to successful single-stage treatment for the majority of trauma victims requiring laparotomy.

Recommended reading

Baker, L. W. 1990. Trauma of the abdomen, blunt and penetrating. In C. J. Mieny and U. Mennen (eds.) *Principles of surgical patient care*, Vol 2. Pretoria: Academia.

Demetriades, D., Rabinowitz, B., Hatzitheofilou, C. 1988. Penetrating wounds of the abdomen, in K. L. Mattox, D. V. Feliciquo, E. E Moore (eds.) *Trauma surgery*. Fourth Edition. Chapters 23–35. New York: McGraw Hill.

Thomson, S. R., Baker, L. W. 1998. Abdominal injuries, Chapter 10, in P. F. Jones, Z. H., Krukowski, G. G. Youngson (eds.) *Emergency abdominal surgery*, Third Edition. London: Chapman and Hall Medical, pp 417–475.

23 Splenic injuries

Pradeep H Navsaria

The management of the injured spleen has been revolutionized by the recognition of the immunologic functions of the spleen in host defence, and the improvement and advancement of radiological modalities in visualizing the injured spleen, particularly CT scanning. Conservative, non-operative management with the view to splenic preservation is the current treatment of choice.

Mechanism of injury

The spleen is the organ most commonly injured in blunt trauma. The two other mechanisms of splenic injury are:

1   Penetrating – stab and gunshot wounds
2   Iatrogenic – traction during laparotomy, inadvertent placement of chest drains through diaphragm, percutaneous catheter drainage of intra-abdominal abscess.

Splenic function

The haemotologic funtions include:

- Removal of red cell inclusions
- Remodelling of red cell membranes
- Destruction of abnormal red cells
- Compensatory haemopoiesis
- Storage of platelets, iron, factor VIII

The immunologic functions include

- Production of opsonins: tuftsin and properdin, assist with phagocytosis and complement activation
- IgM antibody formation

Anatomy

- The spleen is the second biggest reticulo-endothelial organ.
- It receives 5% of the cardiac output.
- It lies in the left upper quadrant, posterior, behind ribs 9, 10, 11.
- There are suspensory ligaments to the diaphragm, left kidney, splenic flexure of colon, stomach, and pancreas.

Initial assessment and management

Airway

Breathing – left-sided fractured lower ribs and pleural effusion

Circulation – suspect with:

- Abdominal distension
- Transient or no response to fluid resuscitation
- Positive diagnostic peritoneal lavage
- Abdominal ultrasound showing free fluid with or without splenic injury
- Unexplained low Hb/drop in Hb

High index of suspicion

The following are indications of splenic injury:

- Shock, not responding to resuscitation
- Unexplained blood loss
- Low Hb / gradual drop in Hb
- Positive DPL
- Left lower fractured ribs
- Pelvic fractures, particularly with concomitant chest injuries
- Contusions, abrasions, penetrating injury to lower chest, upper abdomen, and flank

History

Determine the mechanism of injury – blunt or penetrating?

Examination

Examination includes the following:

- Physical examination – neither sensitive nor specific for splenic injury
- Shock (about 30% of patients) – with/without response to fluid resuscitation
- Stable with/without peritonism – localized to left upper quadrant or diffuse

Special investigations

Chest radiograph: non-specific

- Fractured left lower ribs
- Elevated left hemidiaphragm
- Left pleural effusion

Abdominal radiograph: non-specific
- Fractured lower ribs
- Loss of splenic shadow
- Medial displacement of gastric bubble
- Loss of psoas muscle shadow on the left
- Large soft tissue density mass in left upper quadrant

Diagnostic peritoneal lavage
- Extremely sensitive to the presence of haemoperitoneum, but non-specific.

Computerized tomography (CT)
- The accuracy of CT is over 95% for splenic injuries.
- It grades splenic injury, associated haemoperitoneum, and other abdominal abnormalities.
- CT grading cannot decide which patient can be treated conservatively and which patient requires surgery.
- Contrast blush on CT scanning suggests active bleeding, ideally one should proceed to angiography and embolization, though this is not often feasible.

Radio-isotope scintigraphy
- Technetium-99m sulphur colloid scans are 98% sensitive for acute injuries.
- It has been replaced by CT scanning.

Ultrasound
- The primary goal of ultrasound is the detection of intra-abdominal fluid.
- It can identify splenic injury.

Diagnostic laparoscopy
- Diagnostic laparoscopy has not gained acceptance for blunt trauma.

Non-operative splenic salvage

Inclusion criteria for non-operative management of splenic injuries

- It is appropriate *only* for haemodynamically stable patients.
- CT scan diagnosis – ultrasound is accepted in some centres.
- Absence of associated intraperitoneal/retroperitoneal injuries requiring intervention.
- Limited blood transfusion, i.e. less than 2 units of blood in 24 hours.

Management of patient undergoing non-operative treatment

- Admit to a high care or ICU for minimum of 72 hours.
- Prescribe bed rest for 2–3 days.
- Insert nasogastric tube.
- Perform six-hourly serial physical examination for first 24 hours.
- Do six-hourly Hb estimation for first 24 hours, thereafter 12 hourly.
- To remain in hospital at least one week.
- Restrict activity for six weeks.

Factors predictive of failure for non-operative management of splenic injuries

- Age older than 55
- Haemodynamic instability
- Pre-existing splenic disease
- Severe grade
- Size of haemoperitoneum
- Contrast blush on CT

Apart from haemodynamic instability and contrast blush on CT, the above factors fail to individually preclude non-operative treatment.

Complications of non-operative treatment

- Delayed haemorrhage
- Splenic artery pseudoaneurysm
- Splenic abscess
- Splenic pseudocyst

Risk of infection following operative treatment

Overwhelming post-splenectomy infection (OPSI)

- Incidence: children < 5 years 10%, adults < 1%
- Clinically present with fever, nausea, vomiting, headache, confusion, coma, and death within 24 hours
- Disseminated intravascular coagulopathy, acidosis, hypoglycaemia
- Blood cultures: 50% cryptic in origin, 50% pneumococcus, meningococcus, haemophilus, E. coli.

Vaccination against a variety of encapsulated organisms to prevent OPSI has become the standard of care. Vaccination regimes are variable but should include:

- Pneumococcal vaccination
- *H. influenza* Type B vaccination
- Meningococcal vaccination
- Antibiotic prophylaxis

Each unit should determine its own policy. At least all patients should receive pneumococcal vaccination.

Timing of pneumococcal vaccination is variable. Delayed vaccination (7–14 days) appears to have a better immune response.

Operative management

Splenectomy

Splenetomy is indicated in failure of non-operative management, development of peritonitis, haemodynamic instability, and evidence of infection related to splenic trauma.

- Midline incision as for all laparotomies.
- Slide right hand over the convex of the diaphragmatic surface of the spleen down to lienorenal ligament – gently excise any adhesions encountered.
- Substitute left hand for the right and gently pull spleen into abdominal incision.
- Excise lienorenal ligament: posterior surface of spleen and hilar contents should now be in the wound.
- Divide short gastric vessels in gastrosplenic ligament passing to upper pole of the spleen.
- Dissect tail of pancreas off hilum.
- Divide splenic artery and vein and ligate separately.
- Turn spleen over and excise remaining portions of gastrosplenic ligament and colosplenic ligament to lower pole.
- Ensure adequate haemostasis.
- Pressure suction drain to splenic bed.

Splenorrhaphy

Splenorrhaphy is indicated for superficial and deep lacerations.

- Mobilize spleen to midline as for splenectomy.
- Place abdominal packs in splenic bed.
- 'Snare' can be applied to splenic artery to minimize blood loss.
- Place interrupted atraumatic 3–0 Prolene® sutures to splenic tissue.
- Deep lacerations may need further division of injured part to facilitate individual ligation of bleeding vessels with ligaclips or figure of eight 5–0 Prolene®.

- Reapproximate laceration with Prolene®. Teflon pledgets or omentum can be used to support sutures.
- Mesh splenorrhaphy: large denuded areas can be salvaged by use of application of microfibrillar collagen on the raw splenic surfaces and the use of an absorbable mesh tightly wrapped around the spleen, thus creating a tamponade effect.

Partial splenectomy

A partial splenectomy is indicated when there are devitalized upper or lower segments.

- The segmental arterial supply of the organ permits ligation of the arterial supply to the involved segment.
- Injury to upper pole: ligate short gastric vessels, await demarcation.
- A fish-mouth incision is used to amputate the involved segment.
- Bleeding vessels from raw surface ligated with Prolene® or ligaclips.
- Repair edges with catgut or Prolene®.

Splenic artery ligation

Splenic artery ligation is indicated for failed splenorrhaphy or partial splenectomy, and splenic artery injury.

In 95% of cases, the collateral circulation prevents splenic necrosis. Ligation may be done at the hilum or through the lesser sac along the upper border of the pancreas.

Pitfalls

- Non-operative management of splenic injury may fail to diagnose and treat concomitant intra-abdominal injuries. Therefore, regular serial examination is required. Conservative management of a splenic injury requires that the patient be in a high-care unit or in the intensive care.

Recommended reading

Esposito, T. J., and Gamelli, R. L. 1999. Injury to the spleen. Chapter 31. In K. L. Mattox, D. V. Feliciano, E. E Moore (eds.) *Trauma*, New York: McGraw-Hill. 683–711.

Figure 23.1 Algorithm for management of splenic trauma

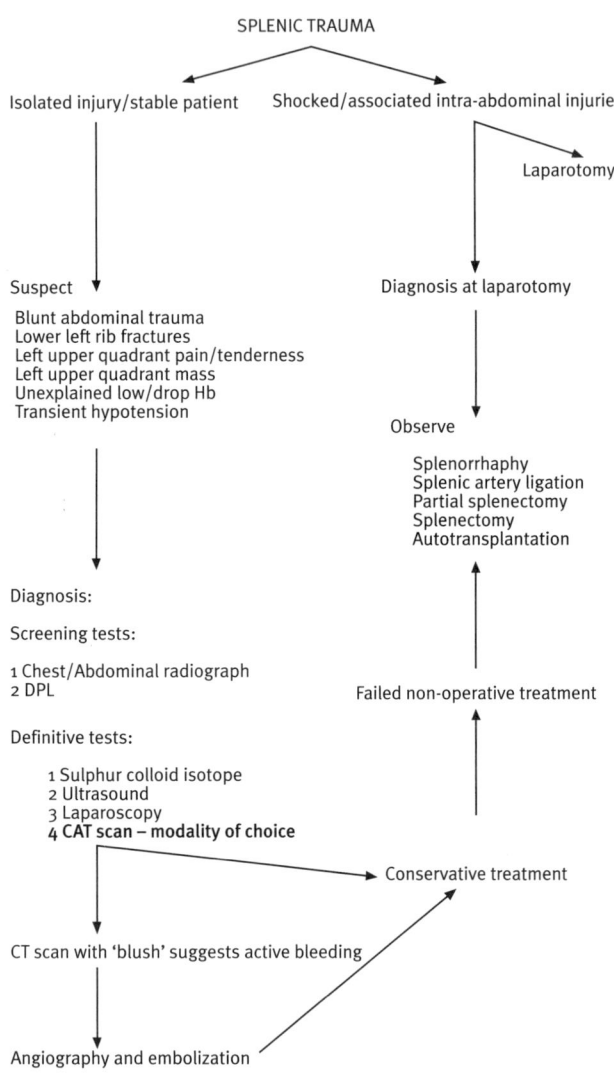

24

Liver trauma

Jake Krige

The liver is the most commonly injured intra-abdominal organ in adults. The magnitude of the injury, management requirements, and complexity of the operative procedure are determined by the cause, mechanism of injury, anatomic location, and extent of parenchymal and vascular damage. A broad spectrum of injuries are encountered, from minor lacerations with minimal bleeding that stop spontaneously and require no intervention, to major crush injuries and lacerations of the retrohepatic vena cava or hepatic veins that are often lethal. Failure to recognize or correctly manage serious abdominal injuries is an important cause of preventable death.

Mechanism of injury

Blunt liver trauma

Blunt liver trauma is a result of road traffic accidents, assaults, or falls from heights.

A stellate, bursting injury may occur in high-speed car accidents. This tends to affect the posterior superior segment of the right lobe because of its relatively fixed position. It results in deceleration injuries with shearing stresses, which may tear the hepatic veins where they enter the liver substance, producing a major retrohepatic injury in an area difficult to expose and repair surgically.

Penetrating liver injuries

High-velocity projectiles and close-range shotgun injuries cause marked fragmentation of the hepatic parenchyma with laceration of vessels and major intraperitoneal bleeding.

Penetrating injuries due to civilian violence, such as stab or gunshot injuries, cause bleeding, usually without much devitalization of liver parenchyma.

The management of liver trauma

Management is divided into four sequential phases:
1   Immediate resuscitation
2   Evaluation

3   Initial management
4   Definitive treatment

Immediate resuscitation

The resuscitation follows standard ATLS® principles.

- Immediate attention should be given to conditions that cause death within minutes (primary survey A, B, C, D, E), hypoxia, hypovolaemia, etc.
- Effective venous access should be obtained and volume replacement started immediately.
- Nasogastric tube and urinary catheter must be inserted.
- The patient's blood must be grouped and cross-matched, and blood samples sent for urgent analysis of haemoglobin concentration, white cell count, urea, creatinine, electrolyte concentrations, and blood gas levels.

Evaluation

The clinical evaluation of the patient with multiple trauma and major abdominal and suspected liver injury must be thorough and organized.

- A liver injury should be suspected in patients with evidence of blunt trauma, knife, or gunshot wounds in the right upper quadrant or epigastrium.
- Initial physical signs may be minimal.
- Gunshot entry and exit wounds can be deceptively distant from the liver.
- The clinical features of a major liver injury are hypovolaemic shock and abdominal distension.
- Diagnostic difficulties may occur in obtunded patients with an altered sensorium, or head or spinal cord injuries.

Initial management

The most important decision after initial resuscitation is whether urgent surgery is needed. Patients who respond to fluid resuscitation and remain stable can be observed closely, investigated, and re-evaluated (see Figure 24.1).

- Awake patients with increasing abdominal distension and tenderness, who remain shocked after 3 litres of intravenous fluid, usually have continued bleeding and need an urgent laparotomy.
- Patients with a head injury (where evaluation of the abdomen is difficult), and increasing abdominal distension with evidence of blood loss,

Figure 24.1 Management algorithm of major abdominal trauma

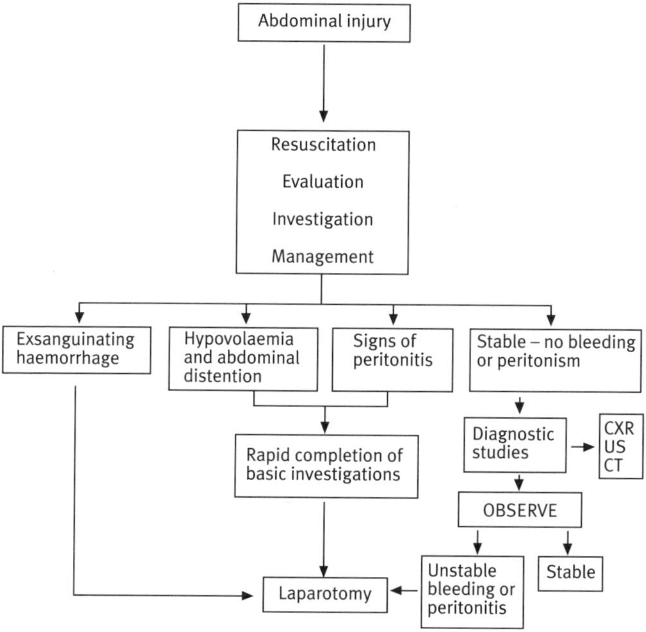

require either a diagnostic peritoneal lavage or an emergency room ultrasound of the abdomen to detect if the abdominal cavity is the source of the occult blood loss.

Definitive treatment

Non-operative management
- A liver injury with a large intrahepatic haematoma and an intact capsule can in a stable patient often successfully be treated non-operatively, with surgery reserved for complications.
- Liver injuries with limited capsular tears, and small volumes of blood in the peritoneal cavity can also be treated non-operatively. Larger capsular tears with continued intraperitoneal bleeding require surgery.
- CT scan of the abdomen is useful in haemodynamically stable patients

suspected of having a major liver injury. This shows the extent of injury, parenchymal lacerations, subcapsular, and intrahepatic haematomas, and the amount of intraperitoneal blood loss. These findings are useful for triage as minor injuries seldom require operation, whereas patients who are haemodynamically unstable with major injuries often do. An ultrasound is a valuable alternative.

- Patients who are initially managed conservatively require careful observation in a high-care environment and repeated physical examination.

The criteria for non-operative management of liver injuries are:

1 No persistent or increasing abdominal pain or tenderness
2 No other intra-abdominal injuries that require laparotomy
3 Less than 4 unit blood transfusion required
4 Haemoperitoneum < 500 ml on CT scan
5 Simple hepatic parenchymal laceration or intrahepatic haematoma on CT scan
6 Haemodynamically stable after resuscitation

Operative management

The indications for laparotomy are:

- Stab or gunshot wounds that have penetrated the abdomen with signs of peritonitis and those patients with unexplained shock, uncontrolled haemorrhage, or clinical deterioration during observation.

Principles of surgical management

The priorities in surgical management are to stop the bleeding, remove devitalized liver tissue, and to oversew or repair damaged blood vessels and bile ducts. Most liver injuries are simple and can be treated without difficulty. The few complex lesions need to be diagnosed early and may require major surgery by experienced hepatic surgeons. Apart from death due to associated injuries, bleeding is the major cause of death in patients with liver injuries.

Operative approach

- Prepare the patient and drape from the xiphoid to the pubic symphysis.
- Use a midline abdominal incision.
- If the liver is actively bleeding, the first step is to control the bleeding by manual compression using packs. Pack pressure on the liver is maintained until the anaesthetist has fully restored intravascular volume. Effective intra-operative resuscitation is crucial.
- Premature attempts to evaluate the extent of the injury and mobilize

the liver before adequate resuscitation may lead to catastrophic blood loss and unnecessary death.

- Suture any bowel perforations rapidly to minimize contamination. Once other intra-abdominal injuries have been repaired, a thorough exploratory laparotomy is performed.
- Most liver injuries have stopped bleeding spontaneously by the time the operation is performed. These wounds do not require suturing but a drain should be placed to prevent bile collections.
- If the liver is bleeding this can usually be stopped by compressing the liver wound with abdominal packs (see Figure 24.2). If bleeding continues after release of pressure, identifiable vessels in the laceration are carefully looked for and sutured.
- If visibility is obscured by continued bleeding, the hepatic artery and portal vein should be temporarily clamped with a vascular clamp

Figure 24.2 Manual compression of a liver injury using packs to control the bleeding

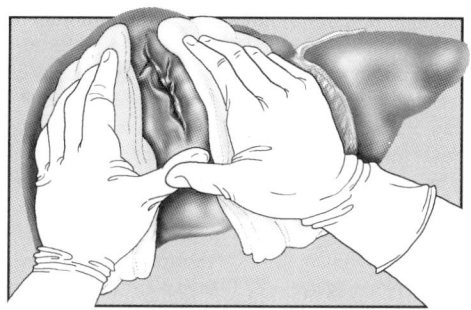

Figure 24.3 Vascular inflow occlusion of the portal triad (Pringle manoeuvre)

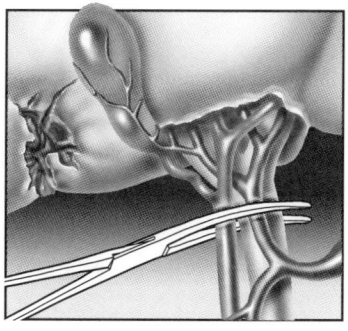

(Pringle manoeuvre) to allow accurate identification of the bleeding site (see Figure 24.3). Intermittent inflow release and effective suction allow identification of deeper bleeding sites, which are controlled by either direct suture, ligation, parenchymal suture, or a mattress liver suture.

- If bleeding cannot be stopped the liver injury should be packed, the abdomen closed, and definitive treatment deferred until a surgeon who can perform the required surgery is available or the patient can be transferred to a major trauma or hepatobiliary centre.
- Even for the experienced surgeon, if bleeding is controlled, discretion and packing may be the better part of valour. Other factors also influence the decision to pack. If the patient is acidotic (pH < 7.2), hypothermic (body temperature < 32 °C), coagulopathic, or has had a massive transfusion (> 10 units of blood), the liver should be packed, the abdomen closed, and the patient returned to the intensive care unit.

Perihepatic packing

The technique of perihepatic packing is important. Sufficient packs should be used to provide effective uniform pressure. A 'six pack' technique is generally used. An attempt should be made to restore the liver contour to normality by closing the defect and providing tamponade by external pressure with packs above and below the liver (see Figure 24.4). Too many packs may cause increased intra-abdominal pressure, caval compression, and acute renal failure. An important practical point is to avoid intrahepatic packing because packs forced into a liver fracture may aggravate the

Figure 24.4 Placement of gauze packs around the liver to compress and tamponade a bleeding liver injury

Figure 24.5 Total hepatic vascular control with vascular clamps across the vena cava above and below the liver and portal inflow occlusion of the portal triad

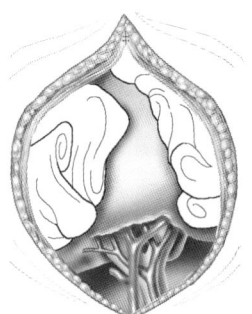

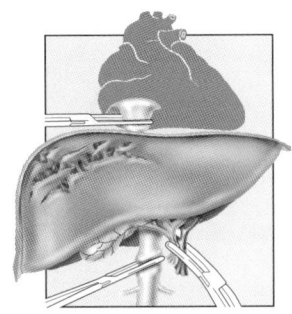

injury by increasing the size of the rent as well as tearing small hepatic veins. The abdomen is then closed without drainage and the packs removed under general anaesthesia in the operating theatre two days later. Packing is also used if a coagulopathy develops or to allow the patient to be transferred from a peripheral hospital with limited facilities to a referral unit for definitive management.

'The ten commandments' of the liver packing technique:

1 Use dry gauze packs.
2 Pack above and below the liver.
3 Avoid packing into the fracture.
4 Use sufficient packs ('6 pack' – six abdominal swabs).
5 Restore liver contour to normal by re-approximating the edges of defect.
6 Avoid excessive packs, which may cause abdominal compartment syndrome.
7 Ventilate the patient until the packs are removed.
8 Anticipate sepsis especially if there is: bile leak/bowel contamination.
9 Give intravenous antibiotics while packs are in place.
10 Remove packs in the operating theatre within 48 hours once coagulation abnormalities have been corrected.

Blunt trauma

Patients with blunt liver injuries and substantial parenchymal ischaemia may require resectional debridement. Rarely, a severe crushing injury necessitates a hepatic lobectomy.

The most difficult problems are lacerations of the vena cava and major hepatic veins behind the liver. If packing does not control bleeding, advanced operative techniques, including total hepatic vascular isolation and clamping of the portal vein, vena cava above and below the liver, may be required (see Figure 24.5).

Advanced operative techniques

Advanced techniques for control of bleeding from the liver include:

1 Hepatorrhaphy with absorbable sutures for compression
2 Hepatotomy with selective vascular suture
3 Resectional debridement
4 Segmentectomy
5 Lobectomy
6 Perihepatic packing
7 Absorbable mesh wrap
8 Total hepatic isolation

Post-operative complications

The following post-operative complications should be kept in mind:

- Rebleeding from the injury site, bile leaks, ischaemic segments of liver, and infected fluid collections are the main post-operative complications associated with liver trauma.
- If major venous bleeding continues, coagulation abnormalities should be corrected and the abdomen re-explored and visible vessels sutured.
- Angiography (with selective embolization) is useful if recurrent arterial bleeding or haemobilia occur.
- CT is used to identify intra-abdominal fluid collections, which are best drained by ultrasound guided needle aspiration or a percutaneous catheter.
- Sepsis develops in about a fifth of cases, usually related to bile leaks, ischaemic tissue, undrained collections, or undetected bowel injury.
- The sites of bile leaks are best identified by ERCP and treated by endoscopic sphincterotomy or stenting, or both.

Prognosis

The overall mortality after liver injury ranges from 10–15% and depends largely on the type of injury and the extent of associated injury to other organs.

- Only 1% of penetrating civilian wounds are lethal, whereas the mortality after blunt trauma exceeds 20%.
- The mortality in blunt hepatic injury is 10% when only the liver is injured.
- If three major organs are injured, mortality approaches 70%. Bleeding causes more than half of the deaths.

Figure 24.6 CT scan showing a gunshot injury to the right lobe of the liver

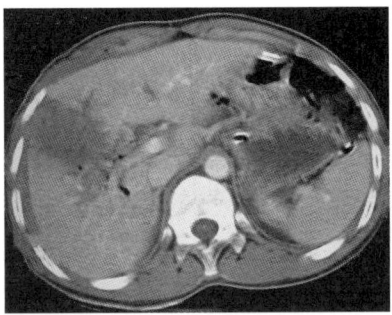

Conclusion

Liver trauma constitutes a broad spectrum of injuries from simple lacerations to avulsion of the liver. Modern management of severe liver injuries has evolved to provide a multidisciplinary approach with increasing reliance on ultrasonographic, angiographic, and interventional endoscopic techniques to drain septic collections, embolize intrahepatic bleeding, and stent bile leaks.

- The resuscitation of the patient follows standard advanced trauma life-support principles.
- Stable patients can be observed closely.
- Shocked patients require laparotomy.
- Most liver injuries are simple and can be treated with standard surgical procedures.
- Complex injuries are uncommon and may require advanced operative techniques.
- Post-operative complications are frequent.

Pitfalls

- Conservative management of a liver injury in the ward instead of a high-care unit, where any ongoing bleeding or rebleeding will be missed.
- Not suspecting a liver injury in penetrating right-sided thoracic trauma.
- A gastro-intestinal bleed after liver trauma is usually a result of haemobilia and requires an angiogram and embolization.

Recommended reading

Krige, J. E. J., Bornman, P. C., Terblanche, J. 1992. Therapeutic perihepatic packing in complex liver trauma. *Br J Surg*, 79:43–46.

Krige, J. E. J., Bornman, P. C., Terblanche, J. 1997. Liver trauma in 446 patients. *S Afr J Surg*, 35:10–15.

Marr, J. D. F., Krige, J. E. J., Terblanche, J. 2000. Analysis of 153 gun shot wounds of the liver. *Br J Surg*, 87:1030–1034.

Terblanche, J., Krige, J. E. J. Hepatobiliary trauma. In J. Bireger, J. P. Benhamon, N. McIntyre, M. Rizzetto, J. Rodes (eds.) *Oxford textbook of clinical hepatology.* 1998. Oxford Medical Publications, 2029–2038.

25

Pancreatic trauma

Jake Krige

Injuries to the pancreas are uncommon and account for 1–4% of severe abdominal injuries.

Mechanism of injury

Penetrating trauma

Simple lacerations are usually the result of stab wounds, which also often injure surrounding vessels or the bowel. High-velocity missiles produce devastating and often lethal injuries.

Blunt trauma

Blunt trauma is the result of a direct blow to the upper abdomen caused by assault, pedestrian road traffic accidents, or torso deceleration in unrestrained drivers or passengers without seat belts. In children, blunt trauma due to bicycle handlebars, falls, and car accidents are most commonly encountered.

Classification of injuries

The Lucas classification system is the most widely used (see Table 25.1).

Management

The initial management of the patient with pancreatic trauma is similar to that of any patient with severe abdominal injury. The priorities of primary management include maintaining a clear airway, urgent resuscitation, and ventilatory and circulatory support.

Indications for emergency laparotomy

Urgent laparotomy is required in all patients with evidence of major intraperitoneal bleeding and clinical findings suggesting peritonitis.

In patients who are stable without obvious clinical signs of intraperitoneal injury, careful observation and repeated clinical abdominal examination can be performed, with selective exploration if signs deteriorate.

Table 25.1 The Lucas classification system

Class 1	Contusion or peripheral laceration with minimal parenchymal damage. Main pancreatic duct intact
Class 2	Major laceration, perforation, or transection of body or tail with or without duct injury
Class 3	Severe crush, perforation, or transection of the pancreatic head with or without duct injury
Class 4	Combined pancreatico-duodenal injury:
a	Minor pancreatic injury
b	Severe pancreatic injury with duct disruption

Diagnosis of pancreatic injury

The diagnosis is often delayed because clinical signs may be subtle and late in onset due to the retroperitoneal location of the pancreas.

- An *abdominal X-ray* may show retroperitoneal air present in duodenal rupture.
- *Serum amylase levels* are unreliable and correlate poorly with the presence or absence of pancreatic trauma.
- *Contrast-enhanced CT scanning* is the investigation of choice. Features of pancreatic injury include pancreatic oedema or swelling, free intraperitoneal, retroperitoneal, or lesser sac fluid collections.
- *Endoscopic retrograde cholangiopancreatography (ERCP)* is used in stable patients to assess major duct integrity.

Intra-operative evaluation

Failure to recognize a major pancreatic duct injury is the principal cause of pancreatic injury-related post-operative morbidity. Clues suggesting a pancreatic injury are:

- Retroperitoneal bile staining
- Haematoma at the base of the transverse mesocolon or in the gastro-hepatic ligament
- Metastatic fat necrosis

Surgical exposure of the pancreas

- The lesser sac is entered through the gastrocolic omentum outside the gastroepiploic arcade. Retract transverse colon downward and stomach upward.
- Expose the anterior surface, and the superior and inferior borders of the body and tail of the pancreas. If the posterior surface of the pancreas requires exposure, the pancreas is mobilized upwards by dividing the inferior avascular peritoneal attachments.
- Spleen, tail, and body of the pancreas are reflected forwards and medially by developing a plane between the kidney and the pancreas. This manoeuvre allows full exposure and bimanual palpation of the tail and body of the pancreas.
- For full inspection of the pancreatic head and uncinate process, the Kocher manoeuvre is necessary to mobilize the second part of the duodenum medially toward the superior mesenteric vessels.
- The dissection and downward reflection of the hepatic flexure of the colon and the mesocolon further improve exposure of the second portion of the duodenum and uncinate process.
- All penetrating wounds should be traced through their entire intra-abdominal course to exclude pancreatic or other visceral injury.

Operative cholangio-pancreatography

Several radiological methods of intra-operative pancreatography to delineate the pancreatic duct have been recommended. The easiest and simplest method is to inject contrast medium into the gallbladder to obtain a cholecystocholangiogram. An alternative method is to perform a cholangiogram by direct puncture of the common bile duct with a 23-gauge needle. Small incremental volumes of contrast are injected to obtain a cholangiogram. The objective is to define the distal and intrapancreatic bile duct, as well as the integrity of the ampulla.

Treatment

Class 1: Contusions and lacerations without duct injury

- Seventy per cent of pancreatic injuries are minor without any underlying major ductal injury.
- Control of bleeding and simple external drainage without repair of capsular lacerations are sufficient treatment. Either a Penrose drain or a soft closed suction or sump drain is used. Drains should be removed only when drainage ceases or when a well-established tract has formed. If the drainage volume is large and the amylase concentration elevated,

the drain should be left in place until the nature, location, and extent of the pancreatic fistula are defined.

- Sinography is the simplest radiological investigation and may demonstrate a communication with the main pancreatic duct.
- An ERCP is indicated when there is a persistent leak for more than 10 days.

Class 2: Distal injury with duct disruption

Injury to the neck, body, or tail of the pancreas with major lacerations or transection and associated duct disruption is best treated by distal pancreatectomy. A splenectomy is usually necessary.

Class 3: Proximal injury with probable duct disruption

- Injuries to the head of the pancreas that do not involve the main pancreatic duct are best managed by simple external drainage.
- Even if there is a suspected isolated duct injury (as with a localized sharp penetrating injury) and a distal resection is not justified, external drainage of the injured area is often the safest option. A controlled fistula thus created either settles spontaneously or may later require elective internal drainage after definition of the exact site of duct leakage.

Class 4: Combined major pancreatico-duodenal injuries

These injuries usually result from gunshot wounds or blunt trauma with other associated intra-abdominal injuries.

- It is crucial to define the integrity of the common bile duct, pancreatic duct, and ampulla, and the viability of the duodenum.
- A cholangiogram performed through the gallbladder or bile duct may provide the information. If the common bile duct and ampulla are shown to be intact, the duodenal laceration is repaired and the pancreatic injury treated according to the site of the injury.
- The presence of bile staining in the retroperitoneum or around the lower bile duct in the hepatoduodenal ligament is confirmation of bile duct injury or ampullary avulsion.
- Penetrating injury in the pancreatic head without devitalization is best treated by careful drainage of the area.
- Where there is loss of tissue of the duodenum, a controlled fistula via a lateral or side-duodenostomy using a T-tube or a small Foley catheter with an inflated bulb has been recommended to reduce tension at the suture line.

Several complex and innovative techniques have been described to deal with *severe* injury to the duodenum in association with a lesser pancreatic head injury. Diversion can be accomplished by a duodenal 'diverticulization' procedure, which employs primary closure of the duodenal wound, a vagotomy, an antrectomy with an end-to-side gastrojejunostomy, a T-tube common bile duct drainage, and a tube duodenostomy. The aim is to convert a potentially uncontrolled lateral duodenal fistula into a controlled end-fistula by diversion of gastric and biliary contents away from the duodenal injury, while making provision for early enteral nutrition via a gastrojejunostomy.

An alternative option avoiding a vagotomy and antrectomy is the 'pyloric exclusion' procedure. The pylorus is closed with an absorbable suture performed through a gastrotomy, and a side-to-side gastrojejunostomy provides temporary diversion of gastric flow away from the duodenum while the duodenal and pancreatic injuries heal. The pylorus opens when the sutures dissolve three or four weeks later, or the sutures can be removed endoscopically after an intact duodenum has been confirmed. In selected patients, pyloric exclusion has proved useful in managing severe duodenal injuries combined with pancreatic head injuries in which a Whipple procedure is not justified.

The same objectives can be achieved by less complex procedures using primary duodenal closure, external catheter drainage near the site of the repair, a diverting gastrojejunostomy without closure of the pylorus, and a fine-bore silastic nasojejunal feeding tube.

Whipple's procedure

Reconstruction may not be possible in combined injuries of the proximal duodenum and head of the pancreas with devitalization, complete disruption of the ampulla involving the proximal pancreatic duct, and distal common bile duct or avulsion of the duodenum from the pancreas. In this situation, the only rational option is resection.

- The need for resection is usually obvious when there is massive destruction with gross devitalization, or pancreatobiliary, duodenal and ampullary disruption requiring debridement that results in a near complete pancreatico-duodenectomy.
- Technical problems arise in the reconstruction of pancreatic and biliary anastomoses due to the small size of the ducts. For the pancreatic anastomosis, invagination of the end of the pancreas into a Roux-en-Y jejunal loop is the most widely used technique.
- Biliary-enteric continuity is usually restored by a side-to-side choledochojejunostomy or hepaticojejunostomy using a high bile duct reconstruction technique with preplaced sutures.

- In unstable patients with serious associated injuries, simple controlled drainage and delayed reconstruction may be the most judicious and appropriate procedure (damage control procedure).

Post-operative care

A prolonged ileus and pancreatic complications may preclude normal oral intake in severely injured patients.

- The standard composition of regular tube feeds increases pancreatic secretion. The low-fat and higher pH (4.5) formulation of an elemental diet is less stimulating to the pancreas, and should be tried before instituting parenteral nutrition.
- A catheter jejunostomy using a submucosal needle technique or a fine bore silastic nasogastric tube with a weighted tip placed at the initial operation in all complex pancreatic injuries allows the option of early post-operative enteral feeding rather than total parenteral nutrition. The enteral route is more efficient for nitrogen utilization and may be more effective in restoring immune competence. The morbidity and cost of enteral nutrition are considerably less than for parenteral nutrition.

Complications

Fistula

Between 10 and 20% of major injuries to the pancreas result in a pancreatic fistula. Most fistulas are minor and resolve spontaneously within one or two weeks of injury, provided that adequate external drainage has been established.

Figure 25.1 ERCP after blunt abdominal trauma revealing a leak from the pancreatic duct in the region of the tail

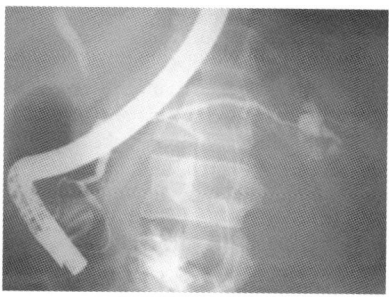

- High-output fistulas (> 700 ml/day) usually indicate major pancreatic duct disruption and are less likely to close spontaneously.
- An ERCP is indicated to establish the cause and site of the fistula, as well as to plan further therapy if a high-output fistula fails to progressively decrease in volume or persists more than 10 days.
- Persistent fistulas without evidence of obvious downstream duct narrowing may require internal drainage into a Roux-en-Y jejunal loop, or resection, if near the tail.

Pseudocysts

Pseudocysts may be a late presentation of isolated pancreatic trauma in up to 10% of patients and should be suspected when a palpable mass is noted in the epigastrium or left upper quadrant or where persistent elevation of the serum amylase level occurs.

- Non-operative treatment options include percutaneous ultrasound-guided aspiration or catheter drainage and endoscopic drainage.
- ERCP is useful in planning management strategy and identifying the site and extent of ductal disruption.
- Post-traumatic pancreatic pseudocysts can be treated by percutaneous aspiration or catheter drainage provided there is no major duct injury, stricture, or demonstrable communication with the main pancreatic duct present on ERCP.

Abscesses

Peripancreatic, subhepatic, and subphrenic fluid collections are commonly seen on U/S or CT after pancreatic trauma. Clinical evidence of intra-abdominal sepsis mandates guided aspiration to obtain fluid for bacteriology and amylase content. In contrast, pancreatic abscesses are uncommon and usually result from inadequate debridement of devitalized pancreatic tissue or ineffective drainage of the lesser sac and pancreatic bed in the presence of ongoing duct leakage.

- An abscess should be suspected in any patient who develops an elevated temperature, raised white cell count, prolonged ileus, or unexplained upper abdominal tenderness in the post-operative period.
- US or CT scan are necessary to confirm the diagnosis.
- Pancreatic abscesses require prompt drainage.
- Empiric broad-spectrum parenteral antibiotic therapy should be instituted to cover the full bacterial spectrum until definitive culture results become available.

- Percutaneous aspiration or catheter drainage is usually effective in patients with accessible unilocular collections and no evidence of pancreatic necrosis. The presence of necrotic pancreatic tissue generally mandates surgery with debridement of non-viable tissue and generous external catheter drainage.

Pitfalls

- Early diagnosis of isolated blunt pancreatic injury is hampered by the retroperitoneal location, which may conceal the clinical features.
- Surrounding haematoma and oedema may mask an injury and unless carefully evaluated at operation, a serious pancreatic injury may be overlooked.
- Pancreatico-duodenectomy (Whipple's) is reserved for maximal injuries to the head of pancreas and duodenum in which salvage is not feasible.
- With careful assessment of the injury by inspection, and judicious use of pancreatography, pancreatic complications can be reduced without the need for complex resections, enteric diversions, and pancreatico-enteric anastomoses.

Recommended reading

Jurkovich, G. J., Carrico, L. J. 1990. Pancreatic trauma. *Surgical clinics of North America*, , 70:575–593.

Krige, J. E. J., Bornman, P. C., Beningfield, S. J., Funnell, I. 1994. Pancreatic trauma. In: H. Pitt, D. L. Carr-Locke, R. Ferrucci (eds.) *Hepatobiliary and pancreatic disease*. Boston: Little, Brown and Company.

Lewis, G., Krige, J. E. J., Bornman, P. C., Terblanche, J. 1991. Traumatic pancreatic pseudolysis. *Br J Surg*, 78:1196–1202.

26 Vascular trauma

Frank Plani

Vascular trauma is often considered the most surgically challenging and least forgiving of all injuries. There are many reasons for this:

- Associated injuries may complicate surgery, cause contamination, or increase risks.
- Spinal injuries may prevent ideal positioning of the patient.
- Active bleeding from uncontrolled vessels may reduce visualization.
- Unfavourable time of the day: most penetrating injuries present after hours.
- The environment is high risk despite universal precautions such as double gloves and visors.
- The surgeon and theatre staff may be unfamiliar with vascular surgery.

The following management modalities need consideration:

- Damage control principles and techniques
- Temporary shunts as used in damage control and complex extremity injuries
- Conservative treatment
- Endovascular modalities used either as an adjunct to surgery, such as in providing proximal control, or to avoid open surgery, by the use of stent-grafts
- Delayed surgery may be an option when prioritizing the management of polytrauma patients
- Unsalvageable situations, where the decision to save life over limb has to be taken rapidly and often without consultation with the patient or other specialists

Once surgery is undertaken, it has to be technically perfect anywhere on the vascular tree, almost always followed by post-repair angiograms and frequently accompanied or preceded by generous fasciotomies.

This chapter aims to give a practical overview of the principles of the management of vascular trauma, and to describe the vascular surgery of the neck, thorax, abdomen, pelvis, and extremities.

Mechanism of injury to blood vessels

Blunt trauma

- Direct blow caused by a blunt object, strangulation, dog bites (beyond the area of penetrating injury), impact against vehicular parts or the ground, seat belts, direct injury from displaced bone, or compression against bony structures, etc.
- Indirect injury such as acceleration-deceleration forces, causing rupture of the descending aorta, avulsion of mesenteric vessels and portal vein, seat-belt aorta (intimal tear and thrombosis at aorto-iliac bifurcation), and dissection of carotid arteries (mainly internal carotid artery, about 2 cm above its origin). Traction injury occurs at points of bony instability, such as posterior knee dislocation, supracondylar humeral fractures, hip dislocations, etc.

Penetrating trauma

- Stabs, low-energy transfer gunshot wounds (velocity less than 600 m/s) passing through soft tissues.
- High-energy transfer gunshot wounds, such as high velocity, hollow point rounds that dissipate their energy in the body, and any projectile that hits bone.
- Shotgun injuries are associated with high-energy transfer, extensive cavitation, and multiple vessel perforations.

Blast injuries

- Primary blast effect leads to direct tissue damage and cavitation from shrapnel.
- Secondary effects include acceleration-deceleration injuries to vessels as body is hurled against solid surfaces.
- Tertiary effects are due to moving objects causing direct penetration or blunt damage to vessels.

Iatrogenic and self-inflicted injuries

- Inadvertent puncture of posterior wall or large anterior wall puncture laceration caused by arterial cannulation
- Thrombosis and distal embolization from indwelling balloon pumps and sheaths
- Intra-arterial injection of contrast agents and medications
- Intra-arterial injection of recreational drugs

Types of vascular injuries

- Lateral wall defect or laceration due to penetrating injury
- Complete transaction of vessel
- Defect with loss of tissue due to high- and low-energy transfer gunshot wounds, especially if associated with fractures
- Arterio-venous fistula after penetrating injuries
- Intimal tear or flap, due to proximity of gunshot wound, joint dislocation, acceleration-deceleration, or Fogarty catheter over-distension
- Pseudo-aneurysm occurring at the site of a vessel wall defect or intimal tear in a large artery
- Arterial spasm may compound already compromised distal perfusion
- Delayed thrombosis may occur at the site of arterial repair, or due to a neglected intimal tear

Assessment and investigations

Although all modalities are not always available in developing world health facilities, assessment for vascular injury can be approached in various ways.

Suspect certain injuries based on particular mechanisms of injury

- Restrained individuals may be susceptible to carotid and abdominal aortic injuries.
- Injuries found in the proximity of gunshot wounds include delayed thrombosis, venous lacerations, or thrombosis and intimal tears.
- Dislocations (knee, elbow) have a high risk of associated vascular injury.
- Blunt effects on vessels may occur beyond the obvious extent of large animal bites.
- Trans-mediastinal gunshots cause multi-vessel injuries.
- Shotgun wounds cause injuries at various levels.
- Blunt injuries to carotid arteries may be caused by contact or stick sports.

Repeated physical examination

- Not only should all pulses be assessed routinely in a trauma victim, but frequent reassessment is mandatory.
- Certain vascular injuries may be present despite palpable distal pulses

(subclavian, brachial artery injuries, intimal injuries, partial wall injuries).

- Search for early signs of raised compartmental pressures.

Doppler or digital pressures with contra-lateral comparison

Quite commonly, Doppler's are not available in emergency rooms; comparison of blood pressure can then be done digitally, with a baumanometer.

Ankle-brachial index for suspected thoracic aortic injury

A significant difference in blood pressure between upper and lower limbs is indicative of advanced thoracic aortic injury, with near-complete obstruction, and will often prevent a transfemoral angiogram, but mandates fine cuts (2–3 mm) dynamic contrast CT instead.

Duplex Doppler

When available, duplex Doppler provides excellent information, especially where closed or intimal injuries are suspected, for example, carotid or renal artery injuries.

Contrasted spiral CT-scan

For rapid evaluation of large vessel injury in polytrauma patients, the contrasted spiral CT scan may be useful if the patient needs to be taken to the operating theatre urgently, and needs assessment of possible intra-abdominal injuries.

Angiography

- Angiograms are frequently overutilized where hard signs of vascular trauma exist, while subtle and potential injuries still go undiagnosed.
- Emergency room angiograms are best carried out using the Seldinger technique with arterial line catheters or CVP (central venous pressure) lines, in view of the easy displacement of peripheral venous catheters from forceful contrast injections. They can demonstrate proximal lesions as well (subclavian, iliac injuries) if a blood pressure cuff is inflated immediately distally.
- Formal angiography may cause delays, but when indicated, yields detailed information.
- On-table angiograms are for rapid assessment of specific areas.
- Completion (post repair, on-table) angiograms are indicated in almost all cases.

Magnetic resonance (MR) scanning

MR (magnetic resonance) scanning is rarely indicated for vascular injury alone.

Indications for surgery

Reliable follow-up is often difficult to obtain in South Africa and many parts of the developing world. Therefore, treating minimal vascular injury conservatively, with serial follow-up angiography or duplex Doppler investigations, is not always feasible. Similarly, because of the widespread shortage of intensive care beds, minimally invasive procedures, such as percutaneous stent grafting, should be applied whenever indicated and available. Extensive crush injuries, with fixed staining and muscle rigidity, may require early amputation, in many instances.

In practice, we recommend operating on almost all vascular injuries, using endovascular methods if possible, and taking early decisive action regarding amputations.

Principles of management

Haemorrhage control

Inadequate haemorrhage control in the pre-hospital and emergency room setting continues to cost lives.

- Direct pressure, maintained digitally, or by applying tight dressings capable of exercising preferential pressure on the bleeding area rather than circumferentially, should be effected from the time the patient is first seen, up to surgical repair.
- The concept of direct pressure can be stretched to axillary, subclavian, and to a lesser extent, iliac vessels.
- Foley and Fogarty catheters for proximal control, aortic cross-clamping in the chest or abdomen, and pulmonary pedicle clamping all help to minimize bleeding prior to surgical correction.

Immediate surgery

Unless direct pressure has completely arrested the bleeding, the patient needs to be taken to the operating room immediately. This also applies to most other patients without active bleeding, unless:

- The nature of the injury, such as suspected mediastinal or multiple arterial or arterio-venous injuries, mandates an angiogram.
- Angiographic interventions may make further surgery less traumatic (Fogarty occlusion of major proximal vessels prior to exploration).

- Angiographic embolization can avoid vascular surgery altogether (facial, vertebral, profunda femoris, gluteal, splenic arteries, etc.).
- Angiographic stent grafting is felt to be safe and appropriate (thoracic and abdominal aorta, subclavian, carotid, etc.).
- Conservative treatment is contemplated (distal common carotid, thoracic aorta in some cases, certain venous injuries, etc.).

Access, incisions, and exposure

There is no place for keyhole surgery in vascular trauma, unless secure angiographic intraluminal occlusion guarantees proximal control. Some areas of major difficulty are described below.

Superior mediastinum and base of the neck

- Perform full median sternotomy, with extra-pericardial control of the arch of the aorta (intra-pericardial control only in very proximal lesions), slinging of innominate vein, and of each root, starting away from the injury.
- Follow this with distal control, the intermediate steps being dictated by the site of injury (resection of medial clavicle/standard neck exposure/supra-infra-clavicular incision, etc.).

Upper abdominal aorta and celiac plexus

Despite an extended Mattox manoeuvre (left rotation of all viscera from the diaphragm to the pelvis) the very high abdominal aorta may be difficult to control, in which case it should be cross-clamped in the lower left chest after opening the hiatus or left diaphragm.

Distal internal carotid artery

- The standard neck incision should be extended upwards and posteriorly behind the mastoid, denuding the styloid process, and shaving the origin of the sternocleidomastoid muscle from the mastoid process, which may be removed if necessary.
- A very distal anastomosis can be carried out by sliding the vein graft over a size 2 Fogarty, occluding the distal internal carotid intraluminally, and effecting the distal anastomosis over the Fogarty.

Infra-genicular popliteal artery and trifurcation

Whether this vessel needs to be exposed for a distal anastomosis, or for exposure and control of the bifurcation, a fasciotomy will have probably been done already as a first step, and the trifurcation can be exposed by dividing a constant branch of the popliteal vein overlying it.

Distal iliac vessels and pre-sacral venous plexuses

- The distal aorta is cross-clamped just above the bifurcation, the distal IVC is controlled in a similar position, with direct pressure on the femoral vessels at the groin and progressive control closer to the areas of injury, sometimes dividing the inguinal ligament for distal control.
- Suturing, ligating, stapling, packing, etc. may control venous bleeding, but deep sacral bleeding carries a high mortality, irrespective of methods used.

Retro-hepatic inferior vena cava

- Injuries to the retro-hepatic IVC may vary from minor posterior tears, controllable by pressure, packing, and natural haemostatic mechanisms, to exsanguinating hepatic vein avulsion injuries.
- Where packing alone or simple suturing does not work, the use of intra-caval shunts has proven useful in the hands of experts.
- A standard Pringle manoeuvre with aortic cross-clamping is done, followed by a median sternotomy to open the pericardium. A large Wishard catheter is prepared with an extra side opening, positioned to lie just inside the atrium, while the distal opening lies in the infra-hepatic IVC. The auricle of the right atrium is entered through a purse string suture, with slings tightened around the infra-hepatic IVC, and the proximal end of the catheter is either clamped, or used as vascular access for rapid fluid administration. The retro-hepatic IVC can then be repaired.
- The operative mortality is prohibitive, but there are no alternatives at present.

Vascular repairs

A substantial proportion of vascular injuries seen in the South African context present late, with multiple injuries and often in shock, following major energy transfers (from rifles or handguns with hollow-point bullets and accompanied by fractures), in well-muscled young individuals, who are often going to be lost to follow-up, and may be in advanced stages of Aids. This is compounded in the Highveld by high altitudes, and subsequent decreased oxygen tensions. For these and other reasons, complications are to be expected and avoided by aggressive surgery.

- *Lateral suture* – only for very large vessels, to avoid narrowing.
- *Vein or Gore-Tex patching* – for all other vessels, especially where intimal tearing has only affected one side of the vessel, and resection and anastomosis or grafting is difficult.
- *End-to-end anastomosis* – possible for most stabs and some gunshots and bony damage: mainly using interrupted sutures (at least one half), sometimes with a partial posterior intraluminal suture.

- *Ligation* – used for branches of the external carotid, profunda femoris, internal iliac (preferably unilateral), inferior mesenteric artery, etc. This can be necessary in any vessels in the context of damage control, or in the presence of such massive contamination as to render extra-anatomical bypass necessary.

Fasciotomies

Fasciotomies are to be carried out whenever a delay of more than six hours from injury to flow restoration (or four hours in Johannesburg and the Highveld) is expected.

Fasciotomies have to be re-assessed in the operating room, under GA, every 48 hours, until closed or skin-grafted, to exclude deep-sited sepsis and ischaemia.

In cases of delays requiring fasciotomies, we recommend exposing the bifurcations of the brachial and popliteal arteries, for embolectomy and flushing of each end vessel.

Temporary shunts

Temporary shunts are encouraged in complex injury, requiring orthopaedic interventions or damage control, for arterial and venous injuries. Surgery will often start with fasciotomies, followed by complete vessel explorations, clearing of the distal tree, exposure of injured vessels, temporary shunting, and orthopaedic surgery, followed by definitive bypass grafting in most cases.

Bypass grafting

Most gunshot injuries and many stab/blunt injuries from bony fragments will require short bypass grafting, preferentially using contra-lateral saphenous vein, other than for very proximal vessels such as aorta, common iliacs, and subclavians.

In inexperienced hands, and for vessels equal or smaller than popliteal or brachial arteries, interrupted sutures are preferable.

Venous injuries

Most venous injuries should be repaired, to avoid the serious morbidity of life-long venous hypertension. Direct suture, often with a transverse suture line, vein patch repairs, or venous grafting are the methods to utilize.

This holds particularly true for veins below the groin, the azygos vein, and forearm veins.

Suprarenal IVC ligation will lead to renal failure, and must be avoided, as are the ligation of the portal and superior mesenteric veins.

A combined arterial and venous injury mandates a fasciotomy of the affected limb, even with a satisfactory arterial and venous repair.

Vein ligation is justified mainly in the context of exsanguinating haemorrhage and damage control.

The clinical picture will dictate whether patients so managed should have venous reconstruction once stabilized.

Arteriovenous fistulae

These occur in an acute or delayed fashion, require angiographic identification, and lend themselves to open surgery, embolization (proximal and distal), or endoluminal stent grafting. Spontaneous venous thrombosis will follow arterial stenting.

General patient management

- Delayed revascularization predisposes to renal failure. Once the bleeding is controlled, aggressive fluid resuscitation and forced diuresis are mandatory in all late presentations.
- Standard low molecular weight heparin is sufficient after most successful arterial injuries, but early deep venous thrombosis (DVT) and pulmonary embolism (PE) prophylaxis may be necessary after complex venous repairs.
- Careful haemodynamic monitoring, with a normal blood pressure and a haemoglobin concentration of between 8 and 10 g%, is ideal after vascular surgery.

Vascular injuries in specific areas

Neck and superior mediastinum

There are no 'minimal' arterial injuries in this region, and most venous injuries must be repaired as well.

- Median sternotomy is the preferred incision, even for access to the origin of the left subclavian artery.
- Intraluminal shunts during internal carotid repair are rarely indicated in young patients with good collateral circulation.
- Intimal injuries of the internal carotid are easily missed, and the liberal use of carotid angiograms (or duplex Doppler's in good hands) is mandatory.
- Proximal vertebral artery injuries are treacherous, and often require

sternotomy for control, while distal injuries require imaginative surgery, ranging from plugs of muscle or sterile matches into the canal, to nibbling away at transverse processes in order to clamp once the artery becomes visible.

- In the superior mediastinum, when faced with a large haematoma immediately after dividing the sternum, it may be safer to control vessels from within the pericardium, while digital pressure for distal control is applied to the neck and upper limb root.

Upper and lower limbs

- The main problems here are missed injury, exsanguinating haemorrhage from a seemingly noncompressible portion of the limb, lack of run-off after technically perfect repairs, and decision-making regarding repairs of crushed limbs vs primary amputation.
- Missed injuries can be avoided by remembering the dangers of posterior dislocations of the knee and the elbow, the risk of intimal tears from clavicular and 1st rib fractures, and retaining a high index of suspicion in all penetrating injuries.
- The use of tourniquets, while dangerous, can be life saving. Adequate direct pressure against the clavicle and the 1st rib, the groin, and the pelvis can often allow control of seemingly uncontrollable haemorrhages.
- Fasciotomies, shunts, and meticulous flushing of all distal vessels minimizes the occurrence of poor run-off. Intra-arterial thrombolytic agents, judiciously used by experts, may improve run-off in isolated limb trauma without excessive bleeding.
- Crushed limb scoring systems may be useful, but the presence of fixed staining in more than one compartment should encourage primary amputation.
- Embolization, angiographic proximal control, and endoluminal stenting have been the main advances in limb vascular trauma in the past few years.

Intrathoracic great vessels

The management of blunt injuries of the thoracic aorta has probably undergone the greatest changes of all, going from mandatory surgery to selective non-operative management to endoluminal stent grafting. Likewise, many penetrating injuries, all requiring operative intervention previously, can now benefit from endovascular procedures, although at present no data on the long-term outcomes is available.

Blunt aortic injury

The main management dilemmas and pitfalls in blunt aortic injury, which is often associated with other major injuries, are:

- Effects of controlled hypotension for non-operative treatment on severe head injury
- Effects of cross-clamping and subsequent possible drop in blood pressure on severe head injuries
- Clearing the entire spine prior to a postero-lateral thoracotomy
- The use of contrast CT scan as definitive anatomical diagnosis or just an adjunct to angiography
- The need to re-evaluate the abdomen thoroughly after re-vascularization of the distal thoracic aorta
- The use of intraluminal stents

Penetrating aortic injury

- Contrast CT and MRI (magnetic resonance imaging) scans have proven particularly useful in the evaluation of projectile trajectories, often avoiding any further investigations of transmediastinal gunshot wounds once the tract could be reconstructed radiologically.
- Where surgery is required for penetrating thoracic trauma, we advocate the use of the median sternotomy for all injuries above the nipple line, medial to the anterior axillary lines, bilateral chest injuries, or combined thoraco-abdominal injuries where the use of extra-corporeal bypass or intra-caval shunts are contemplated.
- Posterior injuries should be treated with an antero-lateral thoracotomy, extended contra-laterally to a clamshell incision if necessary.
- We advocate aortic cross-clamping in the chest in all cases of emergency thoracotomy, even with injuries above, in order to perfuse the brain and the heart while the injury is sought and repaired.
- Massive bleeding from the lungs should be addressed by immediate cross-clamping of the pulmonary hilum within the pericardium upon entering the chest.
- Cell saving should be used in all cases of chest trauma requiring blood transfusion.

Abdominal and pelvic vascular trauma

- Abdominal vascular injury must be suspected in all penetrating trauma between the nipples and the knees.
- Auto-transfusion must be considered for all patients who are unstable, irrespective of the possibility of enteric contamination.
- In blunt abdominal trauma, compression of the aorta, renal vessels, and superior mesenteric artery (SMA) is more likely to cause injury than acceleration-deceleration, as is the case in blunt thoracic aortic injury.

- Where the patient does not need immediate surgery, dynamic CT scans may identify vascular injuries amenable to angiography, embolization, or stenting.
- In cases of major enteric contamination together with a retroperitoneal haematoma, one should control the contamination, wash out, and then explore the retroperitoneal structures if indicated.
- If massive bleeding and contamination are present, obtain temporary control of bleeding, with shunting if necessary, control contamination, followed by vessel repair or damage control.
- All central haematomas are explored, lateral haematomas are mostly watched in blunt trauma, explored in penetrating trauma, and pelvic haematomas are explored if bleeding already, otherwise packed, and investigated thoroughly prior to the next operation.
- Aortic grafts are placed with proximal end-to-end and distal end-to-side anastomoses.
- Only the infra-renal IVC can be ligated, but at the risk of major morbidity.
- Portal vein should be repaired, but hepatic artery can be ligated.
- In pelvic injuries with suspected vascular injuries, the sequence of events we recommend is: sheet around the pelvis, sometimes MAST suit (military antishock trousers), followed by theatre, packing and repair, angiography and embolization after theatre, only then external fixation.
- If there is no contamination, and bleeding can be repaired and controlled: internal fixation is preferred for better function and patient comfort.

Pitfalls

- Neglecting to assess all the pulses repeatedly in a polytrauma patient.
- Not doing fasciotomies early when indicated.
- Omitting post-operative on-table angiography.
- Insufficient haemorrhage control in the emergency room.
- Over-resuscitation of the actively bleeding patient.
- Missed vascular injuries associated with joint dislocations.
- Venous damage during arterial repair.
- Inappropriate ligation of vein and arteries.
- Occlusion from graft thrombosis.
- Graft infection from abdominal sepsis (rare).
- Aorto enteric fistulae (rare).
- Artero-venous fistulae after conservative management, ligations, or suture lines.
- Missile embolism (acute or delayed).
- Iatrogenic vascular trauma.

Recommended reading

Clarke, D. L., Madiba, T. E., Muckart, D. J. 1999. Inferior vea caval injury in the firearm era. *South African Journal of Surgery,* Nov, 37(4):107–9.

Greenhalgh, R. et al. 2001. *Vascular and endovascular surgical techniques.* Fourth edition. Philadelphia: WB Saunders.

Mattox, K. 1997. Red River anthology. *Journal of Trauma,* March, 42(3).

Moore, E. E., Mattox, K. L., Feliciano, D. V. 1991. *Trauma.* Third edition. Connecticut: Appleton & Lange.

Nair, R., Robbs, J. V., Muckart, D. J. 2000. Management of penetrating cervicomediastinal venous trauma. *European Journal of Vascular and Endovascular Surgery,* Jan, 19(1):65–9.

Ouriel, K. & Rutherford, K. 1998. *Atlas of vascular surgery: Operative procedures.* Philadelphia: WB Saunders.

Rich, N., Mattox, K., & Hirshberg, A. 2004. *Vascular trauma.* Second edition. Philadelphia: WB Saunders.

Rob & Smith's operative surgery, Trauma surgery. 1989. Part 2, Fourth edition. London: Arnold.

Rutherford, R.B. (ed.) 1999. Vascular surgery. Fifth edition. Philadelphia: WB Saunders.

27 Injuries to the urinary tract

Chris Heyns

Renal trauma

Renal injuries can vary from minor contusions with subtle signs to major life-threatening injuries requiring emergency surgery. Due to the anatomical location, the kidneys and ureters are rarely injured in isolation. Conservative management, where possible, has become the trend.

Causes

Blunt trauma: the kidney may be crushed against the ribs or vertebral column.

Penetrating trauma: gunshot or stab wounds may involve the kidney and surrounding structures.

Deceleration injury: (e.g. fall from a height) may cause avulsion of the renal vessels due to the mobility of the kidney within the perinephric fat.

Figure 27.1 Classification of renal injuries

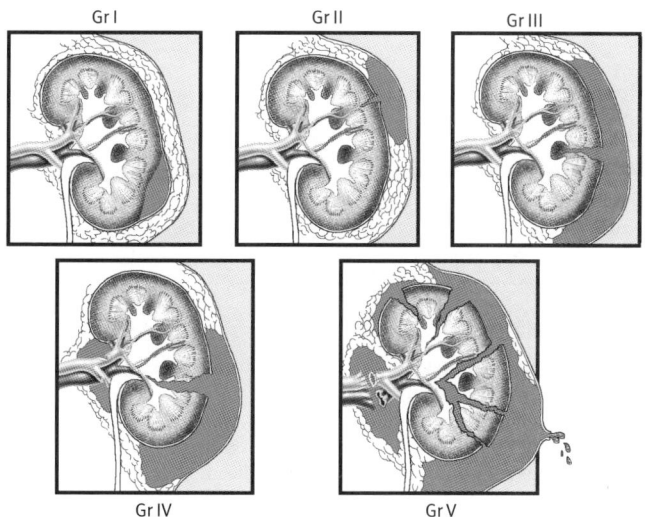

Gr I   Gr II   Gr III

Gr IV   Gr V

Classification

See box below.

Classification of renal injuries

Grade I
Contusion of the renal parenchyma, often with significant haematuria and a subcapsular haematoma, but no laceration of the renal cortex or capsule.

Grade II
Superficial laceration (less than 1 cm) of the renal capsule and cortex, causing a perinephric haematoma as well as haematuria, but the collecting system remains intact.

Grade III
Laceration more than 1 cm, but without involving the collecting system.

Grade IV
Deep laceration involving the larger intrarenal vessels and/or the collecting system, leading to a perinephric haematoma as well as urinoma, due to extravasation of urine (avulsion of the upper or lower pole can occur, due to a deep laceration transecting the kidney).

Grade V
Rupture (fragmentation or 'shattered kidney') consists of multiple deep lacerations, and/or pedicle injuries, such as avulsion of the renal artery and/or vein with severe blood loss, a large perinephric haematoma and devascularization of the kidney, or an intimal injury, where only the inelastic intima of the renal artery is torn, leading to thrombosis of the artery and infarction of the kidney, but without any perinephric haematoma.

Pathophysiology

- An abnormally large kidney (e.g. with hydronephrosis or a tumour) is more easily injured than a normal kidney.
- A child's kidney is more vulnerable, as the adult kidney is well protected by rigid ribs and stronger posterior abdominal wall muscles.
- Renal injuries are often associated with head, chest, and abdominal trauma, as well as major limb fractures.

- Mortality is often due to associated injuries and not to the renal trauma, thus it is important to diagnose and treat such injuries promptly.

Clinical presentation

- Pain presents in the flank, back, or abdomen.
- Abrasion or bruising of the skin occurs in the flank area.
- Any skin laceration in the vicinity of the kidneys must raise the suspicion of renal injury.
- There may be signs of haemorrhagic shock.
- On abdominal examination there may be:
  - distension (ileus due to perinephric haematoma or urinoma)
  - tenderness in the flank
  - muscle rigidity
  - a palpable mass or dullness to percussion in the flank (perinephric haematoma)
  - shifting dullness (free blood in the abdomen)
  - a rebound sign and absent bowel sounds (intraperitoneal leakage of bowel content, urine, or bile).
- Urine should always be examined with dipsticks and microscopy, because myoglobinuria may give a false-positive test for blood.
- Haematuria in a trauma patient indicates urinary tract injury.
- However, there is a poor correlation between the degree of haematuria and the severity of urinary tract injury:
  - patients with microscopic haematuria may have a major renal injury
  - those with macroscopic haematuria may have a minor renal injury.
- The haematuria may be due to a cause other than trauma.
- Severe renal trauma may occur without detectable haematuria.

Imaging

Chest X-ray (CXR)

CXR is essential in all patients with suspected renal trauma. It may show rib fractures, haemo- or pneumothorax.

Abdominal X-ray (AXR)

AXR may show fractures of the ribs or vertebral transverse processes, indicating significant trauma which may also have injured the kidney. Scoliosis concave towards the injured kidney is usually due to pain. The psoas line may be obliterated by a perinephric haematoma or urinoma, which may cause a visible soft tissue mass (opaque area) displacing the bowel from the renal area.

Intravenous pyelogram (IVP) (excretory urogram, EUG)

This is still the most readily available screening study for suspected renal trauma. Although not very accurate in showing the precise extent of renal injury, it will exclude severe trauma, and demonstrate the presence of a normal contralateral kidney. A high dose of contrast medium should be used. Nephrotomograms are extremely valuable to delineate the kidney in the nephrogram phase and to confirm the absence of devascularized areas (grade IV–V injuries).

The following abnormalities may be seen on the IVP in renal trauma:

Contusion – slightly delayed nephro- or pyelogram, filling defects (blood clots) in the collecting system, otherwise normal kidney

Superficial laceration – signs of a perinephric haematoma including an obliterated psoas line, bowel displaced from the renal area, ureter stretched and displaced medially, kidney displaced anteriorly (on nephrotomogram one kidney remains 'out of focus')

Deep laceration – part of the kidney not visible in the nephrogram phase of the IVP and/or there is extravasation of contrast (i.e. leakage of urine)

Figure 27.2 Intravenous pyelogram (IVP) showing extravasation from left renal pelvis due to penetrating injury (stab wound)

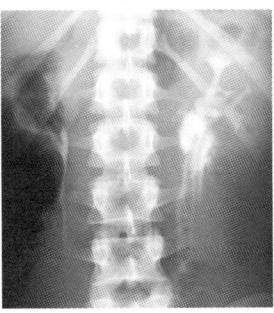

Figure 27.3 IVP showing a non-functioning left kidney in patient with blunt trauma

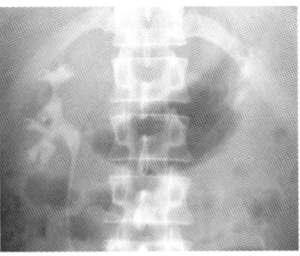

Rupture of the kidney or avulsion of the renal vessels – non-functioning kidney (absent nephrogram, no contrast excretion in the pyelogram phase) with signs of a large perinephric haematoma.

Intimal injury – non-functioning kidney, no perinephric haematoma.

Contraindications to IVP are:

- Haemorrhagic shock (patient cannot be resuscitated)
- Iodine allergy
- Renal failure (elevated serum creatinine)
- Pregnancy

Computerized tomography (CT)

This is unquestionably the imaging study of choice in abdominal trauma, but it is costly and not always readily available. It provides excellent imaging of the kidneys, liver, spleen, and other abdominal structures. However, spiral CTs are completed so rapidly that there may not be sufficient time for the collecting system to fill with contrast, thus extravasation may be missed. Ideally, the spiral CT should be done immediately after IV contrast injection to demonstrate the vascular and cortical structures, and then repeated after 20–30 minutes to look for contrast extravasation from the collecting system. If the IVP is abnormal but does not adequately demonstrate the extent of the renal injury, CT is indicated.

Ultrasound

This may demonstrate a cortical laceration, perinephric haematoma or urinoma, but it provides no indication of renal function. Ultrasound is a

Figures 27.4 and 27.5 Computerized tomography (CT) scan showing (A) rupture of spleen and (B) non-functioning left kidney due to renal artery thrombosis (intimal injury)

A

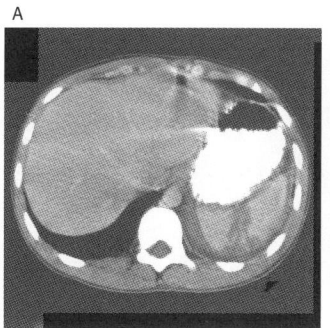

B

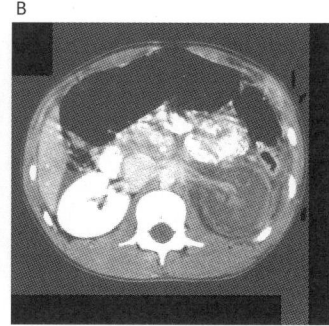

useful screening study in children with abdominal trauma, but its reliability is highly dependent on the quality of the equipment and experience of the operator.

Renal arteriography
When IVP demonstrates no function in the region of an ultrasonically present kidney, arteriography may confirm occlusion of the renal artery (intimal injury). In patients with secondary haemorrhage after renal trauma, arteriography is the study of choice, as the most common cause of secondary haemorrhage is arterio-venous fistula (AVF) or traumatic aneurysm.

Radio-isotope renography
This involves less radiation than an IVP, and is of value in children.

Management

Most renal injuries are relatively minor (grades I–III) and can be managed non-operatively, since the kidney has a remarkable ability to heal spontaneously. Major renal injuries, although rare, may be life-threatening and require immediate surgery.

- If the patient with suspected renal trauma is haemodynamically unstable and cannot be resuscitated, immediate laparotomy is indicated.

Figures 27.6 and 27.7 CT showing (A) subcutaneous air (surgical emphysema) due to rib fracture and pneumothorax, with a large left perinephric haematoma (note anterior displacement of the left kidney by the haematoma), and (B) shattered left kidney with contrast extravasation (grade IV injury)

A

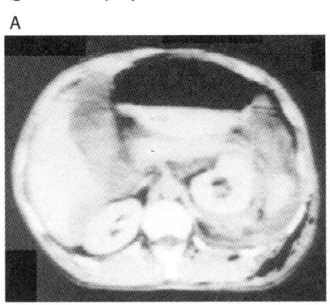

B

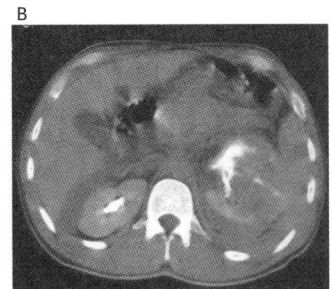

- A 'single shot' IVP on the operating table (10–20 minutes after contrast injection) is not very accurate in defining the nature or extent of the renal injury, but may be valuable in demonstrating a normal contralateral kidney.
- If the patient is haemodynamically stable, imaging (CXR and IVP or CT) is obtained immediately.
- In all cases of penetrating trauma with haematuria (even if only microscopic) an IVP or CT is essential.
- Immediate imaging is not necessary in the following situation: blunt trauma, with microscopic haematuria, no haemodynamic instability, and no abdominal signs on examination, provided the patient returns 2–3 weeks later for imaging studies if there is persistent microscopic haematuria.

Non-operative (conservative) management

The following renal injuries can be managed non-operatively:
- Contusion and superficial laceration (grades I–III)
- Deep laceration with slight extravasation (most grade IV injuries)
- Stab wounds posterior to the anterior axillary line, provided there is no evidence of severe blood loss, no acute abdomen, and no significant abnormality on IVP (adequate imaging is essential).

Non-operative management consists of:
- Monitoring vital signs
- Giving intravenous fluids and blood as required
- Regular re-evaluation of abdominal signs
- Serial monitoring of the amount of haematuria
- Bed rest for 2–3 weeks after macroscopic haematuria has cleared up

In the haemodynamically stable patient, a transurethral catheter is only indicated if there is clot retention for which bladder washout is required. Antibiotics are indicated in penetrating, but not in blunt renal trauma.

Follow-up at six weeks is essential, and should include blood pressure measurement, abdominal examination, auscultation for bruits over the renal areas, urine dipstick testing, and a repeat IVP (unless the initial study was completely normal).

Operative (surgical) management

Surgery is indicated in:
- Deep lacerations with significant extravasation
- Non-functioning of half or more of the kidney (severe grade IV injuries)
- Pedicle injuries (avulsion of the renal vessels/grade V)

- Associated intra-abdominal injuries (liver, spleen, bowel, etc.)
- Penetrating injuries with signs of severe blood loss, acute abdomen, or significant abnormality on the IVP

If pre-operative IVP or CT shows a normal contralateral kidney, and there is no reason to suspect other intra-abdominal injuries, an extraperitoneal flank approach to the injured kidney may be used, as it has a lower morbidity than laparotomy.

If there has been no imaging, or if there are signs of other abdominal injuries, laparotomy is required, in order to explore both kidneys and abdomen.

Exploring a retroperitoneal haematoma involves the risk of releasing the tamponade effect provided by the perinephric (Gerota's) fascia, with the risk of severe haemorrhage and unnecessary nephrectomy.

Figure 27.8 Renal angiogram showing a false aneurysm due to laceration of a large renal artery branch

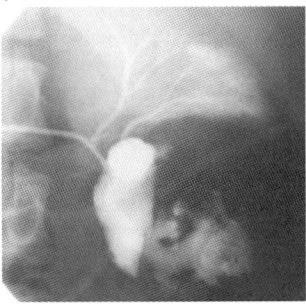

Figure 27.9 Renal angiogram showing an arterio-venous fistula (AVF) due to a stab wound – note catheter in renal artery, with rapid filling of renal vein immediately after contrast injection

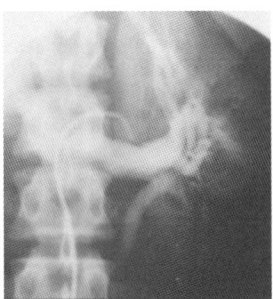

If there has been no pre-operative imaging, and a retroperitoneal haematoma is found at laparotomy, the following guidelines apply:

- For penetrating trauma, explore the haematoma for large vessel injuries.
- For blunt trauma, explore a lateral haematoma only if it is pulsating or rapidly enlarging.
- Central haematomas due to blunt trauma should be explored to exclude large vessel or duodenal injury.
- Surgery requires early vascular control of the renal vessels, debridement of devascularized tissue, suturing of the parenchyma and/or collecting system, adequate haemostasis, and placement of a large-bore drain.
- Suturing of the collecting system and small bleeders in the parenchyma can be performed with absorbable sutures (e.g. chromic or polyglactin 4/0 or 3/0).
- Suturing of the renal parenchyma may be difficult, as the sutures tear out if tied too tightly. Interrupted chromic 2/0 or 0 sutures on a large tapered (non-cutting) needle may be buttressed by placing perinephric fat or omentum into the parenchymal defect before tying the sutures.
- Heminephrectomy or nephrectomy is indicated to remove devascularized tissue.

Complications

- Primary haemorrhage can lead to haemorrhagic shock and death.
- Ileus may result from a large retroperitoneal haematoma.
- Secondary haemorrhage (macroscopic haematuria recurring 2–3 weeks after the injury) is the most common late complication of renal trauma:
  - the cause is usually an arterio-venous fistula (AVF) or traumatic aneurysm
  - the management is resuscitation and, if more than 3–4 units of blood are required to restore the haemoglobin, renal arteriography should be performed
  - if an AVF or bleeding from a large vessel is demonstrated, selective embolization of the involved segmental artery is performed, using a coil or other thrombogenic material.
- Perinephric urinoma with infection and abscess formation may occur. This can often be treated with percutaneous catheter drainage alone.
- Hypertension may be due to renin hypersecretion by a segment of hypo-perfused kidney, or due to compression of the kidney by a perinephric haematoma (Page kidney).
- Stone formation as a result of renal injury is rare.

Ureteric trauma

Ureteric injuries are relatively rare as the ureters are fairly well protected in their retroperitoneal location. When present, however, they may be difficult to diagnose.

Causes

- The most common cause of ureteric trauma is inadvertent iatrogenic injury.
- Most ureteric injuries are caused by urologists during ureteric stone removal, but these injuries are usually recognized immediately and treated appropriately.
- Unrecognized ureteric injury can occur during procedures such as hysterectomy, caesarean section, colo-rectal resection, and aorto-iliac bypass grafting.
- Such injuries can lead to serious complications, as well as litigation, especially if the diagnosis is delayed.
- Penetrating trauma (especially gunshot wounds) may involve the ureter.

Figures 27.10 and 27.11 Intravenous pyelogram showing (A) left hydro-ureteronephrosis due to iatrogenic injury of the distal ureter during hysterectomy and (B) contrast leakage from the dilated distal ureter (the patient presented with incontinence due to a uretero-vaginal fistula)

A

B

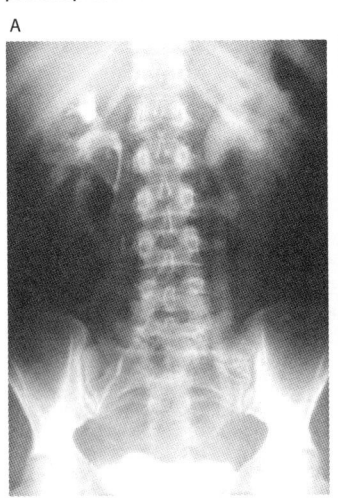
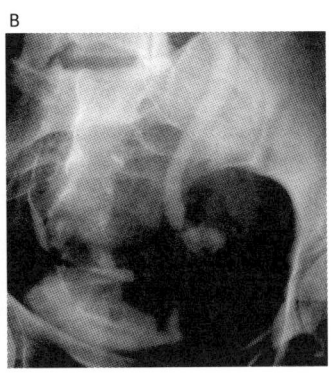

Mechanism

- Iatrogenic injury to the ureter usually comprises an accidental cut or laceration, leading to urine leakage, or the ureter may be inadvertently caught up in a ligature, leading to hydro-ureteronephrosis.
- Quite often necrosis occurs at the point where the ureter was tied off, leading to hydronephrosis as well as urine leakage, e.g. uretero-vaginal fistula with ipsilateral hydro-ureteronephrosis after hysterectomy.
- Ureteric injury due to gunshot or stab wounds can be easily missed at laparotomy if pre-operative imaging of the urinary tract with an intravenous pyelogram (IVP) was not performed.

Clinical presentation

- The only sign may be haematuria, usually microscopic, but this may be absent if the ureter is completely severed.
- An IVP or CT usually shows leakage (extravasation) of contrast from the ureter.
- If imaging has not been obtained, and ureteric injury is suspected at laparotomy, methylene blue or indigo carmine can be given intravenously, which colours the urine blue and may demonstrate the point of leakage.
- Late (post-operative) signs of ureteric injury include abdominal or flank pain, tenderness in the lumbar area, fever, symptoms of urinary tract infection, and blood, pus cells or organisms on urinalysis.
- Symptoms may be vague and obscured by post-operative pain and unless the surgeon maintains a high index of suspicion, may lead to delayed diagnosis.
- Anuria will be present only if both ureters have been tied off, or if there is only one functioning kidney.
- Urine leakage may occur via a drain or surgical incision, or through the vagina (the typical picture is a woman who becomes 'incontinent' after hysterectomy, due to a uretero-vaginal fistula).
- Fluid from the vagina, drain, or surgical incision may be sent for urea and creatinine assay to determine if it is urine or serum.
- Abdominal distension may occur due to urinary ascites or because of a retroperitoneal urinoma causing ileus.
- Delayed diagnosis may lead to severe hydro-ureteronephrosis and eventual loss of kidney function.

Imaging

Intravenous pyelogram (IVP)

IVP will usually show leakage of contrast from the ureter injured by penetrating trauma. In the post-operative patient with suspected ureteric injury, an IVP is the best imaging study to demonstrate hydronephrosis, as well as contrast extravasation.

Ultrasound
This is a convenient modality for demonstrating hydronephrosis or a urinoma in the post-operative patient, but it cannot accurately localize the point of ureteric injury.

Computerized tomography (CT)
CT with intravenous contrast may show extravasation from the ureter, but it is important that delayed films be obtained, since spiral CT scans may be completed so rapidly that contrast extravasation may be missed.

Retrograde uretero-pyelography
This is very useful in the post-operative patient for showing the precise level at which the ureter was cut or tied off.

Prograde pyelography via percutaneous nephrostomy
This is useful if there is hydronephrosis, as it will relieve pain and prevent pyonephrosis and deterioration of kidney function.

Figure 27.12 End-to-end anastomosis of spatulated ureter with absorbable 4/0 sutures over an F5 double-J ureteric stent

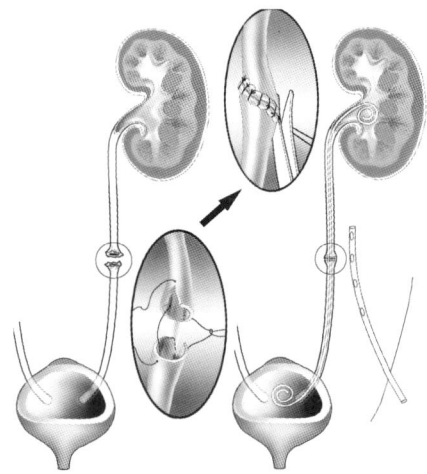

Management: Pre- or intra-operative diagnosis

- If the ureteric injury is recognized pre-operatively or during laparotomy, primary repair is the best option.
- The ends of the severed ureter are debrided, if necessary, and spatulated (cut open with 5 mm long V-shaped incisions on opposite sides of the two ends) so that a wide lumen end-to-end anastomosis can be performed.
- Absorbable suture material should be used to prevent stone formation (chromic or polyglycolic acid 4/0).
- It is important to insert a ureteric stent (JJ or double pigtail ureteric catheter).
- A wide-bore tube drain and/or nephrostomy tube should be placed to divert urine from the anastomotic site.
- Interrupted rather than running sutures are preferable, since it is more important to retain blood supply to the ureteric tips than to produce a water-tight anastomosis.
- In an unstable patient or where primary repair is not technically feasible, an F5 or F8 nasogastric tube or JJ ureteric stent can be inserted into the proximal ureter, fixed with a suture around the ureter, and brought out through a separate skin incision (ureterostomy-in-situ). This allows free drainage of the kidney so that delayed repair can be performed when the patient's condition allows.

Delayed (post-operative) diagnosis

- If ureteric injury is diagnosed post-operatively, cystoscopy and retrograde pyelography is required, and an attempt should be made to pass a double-J ureteric stent.
- If a stent can be passed, this is left in situ for six weeks, after which it is removed and an IVP or ultrasound obtained 1–2 weeks later to see if the ureter has healed without stricture.
- If double-J stenting is not possible, a percutaneous nephrostomy may be placed to relieve pain and preserve kidney function prior to definitive surgery.
- If inadvertent iatrogenic ligation of the ureter is diagnosed early, re-laparotomy and deligation with ureteric stenting can be performed.
- If the distal ureter has been injured, re-implantation can be done, either directly into the bladder, or with the aid of a psoas hitch or bladder flap (Boari flap).
- Trans-uretero-ureterostomy (where the injured ureter is brought across to the opposite side and anastomozed end-to-side to the non-injured ureter) is an option if re-implantation into the bladder is not possible.

- Post-traumatic stricture of the ureter can be treated with:
  - balloon dilatation
  - open surgical ureterotomy, with insertion of a double-J-stent and omental wrapping
  - ureteroplasty using a free patch graft of buccal mucosa wrapped with omentum
  - endoscopic ureterotomy, e.g. using a holmium laser.
- Ileal interposition may be used to replace the whole ureter if a very long segment has been injured.
- Auto-transplantation of the kidney into the iliac fossa can be performed if the ureter is irreparably damaged.
- Nephrectomy is indicated if the kidney is non-functioning or has less than 10–20% of the differential renal function as shown on isotope renography.

Complications

- A common complication of ureteric injury during hysterectomy is a uretero-vaginal fistula.
- Urinoma, urinary ascites, peritonitis, intra-abdominal abscess, and septicaemia may occur.
- Ureteric stricture leading to hydronephrosis, pyonephrosis, and loss of function of the involved kidney may occur.
- Penetrating injury of the ureter associated with bowel and large blood vessel injuries may result in dehiscence of bowel and vascular anastomoses, therefore it is very important to adequately divert and drain the urine after ureteric repair.

Bladder trauma

Causes

- Blunt injury to a full bladder usually causes intraperitoneal rupture at the fundus, the weakest part of the detrusor, which is not supported by the pelvic side walls.
- Pelvic fracture often causes extraperitoneal bladder rupture. This is probably due to a bursting mechanism caused by severe compressive force on an empty bladder, rather than to shearing forces or direct laceration of the bladder by pelvic bone spiculae.
- Penetrating trauma (gunshot or stab wounds) and iatrogenic trauma (e.g. during hysterectomy, caesarean section, bladder biopsy, or transurethral resection of bladder tumours) are causes of intra- or extraperitoneal bladder rupture.

Figure 27.13 Pelvic fracture; note displacement of pubic rami and symphysis, with soft tissue swelling of penis and scrotum due to perineal haematoma

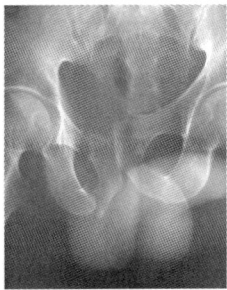

Figure 27.14 High-pressure cystogram showing intraperitoneal bladder rupture (note Foley catheter in bladder)

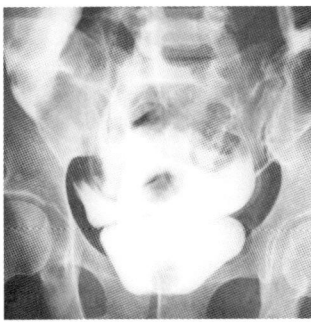

Classification

Contusion of the bladder – there is haematuria, but no extravasation of urine.

Intraperitoneal rupture – blunt trauma on a full bladder usually causes rupture of the bladder fundus, with extravasation of urine into the peritoneal cavity.

Extraperitoneal rupture – pelvic fracture or penetrating trauma may lacerate the extraperitoneal part of the bladder, usually the lateral walls near the bladder neck and trigone, causing leakage of urine into the perivesical fat and fascia.

'Spontaneous' bladder rupture – occurs without a history of trauma, and is usually due to underlying pathology (urethral stricture with chronic retention, tuberculosis or carcinoma of the bladder), or the patient was intoxicated or unconscious at the time of sustaining bladder trauma.

Clinical presentation

- The patient may present with suprapubic pain, tenderness, and inability to urinate, because the bladder cannot fill.
- If the patient is able to urinate, there may be dysuria and gross haematuria.
- Clinically significant bladder injury always causes macroscopic (and not just microscopic) haematuria.
- Urine in the peritoneal cavity causes abdominal distension, ileus (tympanic abdomen on percussion), and shifting dullness ('ascites').
- Intraperitoneal rupture causes the abdominal cavity to fill up with urine, and a transurethral catheter may pass through the ruptured fundus into the peritoneal cavity, thus rapidly draining a very large volume of urine (more than 2 litres). This should raise suspicion of bladder rupture.
- Within 12–24 hours after intraperitoneal rupture, the serum urea and creatinine may be elevated ('renal failure') due to absorption of urine from the peritoneal cavity.
- With iatrogenic laceration of the bladder during hysterectomy there may be incontinence due to a vesico-vaginal fistula.

Imaging

Abdominal X-ray (AXR)

AXR may show a pelvic fracture, dilated bowel loops (ileus), or an opaque, 'ground glass' appearance due to urine in the abdomen.

Figures 27.15 and 27.16 Cystograms showing (A) a pelvic haematoma displacing the bladder superiorly, with extraperitoneal extravasation on the left, and (B) a large extraperitoneal bladder rupture (note diastasis of pubic symphysis)

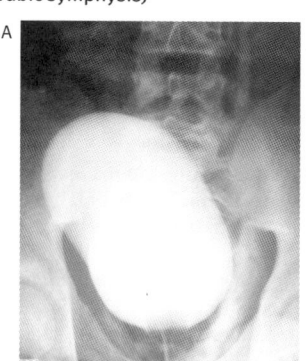 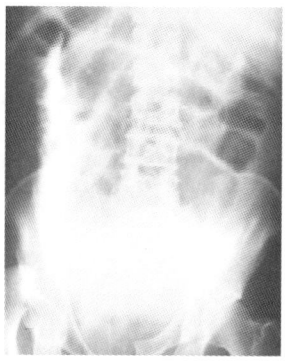

Cystography

This is the best imaging study to demonstrate bladder rupture. Water-soluble contrast medium is instilled through a transurethral catheter. It is important to use an adequate volume (300–400 ml) at sufficient pressure (50–100 cm water). This is done by using a bladder (Toomey) syringe, or by connecting the catheter to a bottle of contrast medium hanging 50–100 cm above the level of the bed. Oblique views are useful, but often impossible due to pain in patients with a pelvic fracture. Post-voiding views are important in order not to miss a small leakage in the pouch of Douglas. An inverted 'tear-drop' appearance of the bladder is seen in pelvic fractures where the haematoma due to bleeding from torn vessels compresses the bladder from both sides. Extraperitoneal rupture is demonstrated by a flame-like, wispy, or 'sunburst' pattern of contrast leakage in the fat and fascia layers around the bladder.

Intraperitoneal rupture leads to contrast leakage into the abdominal cavity, showing up the smooth outlines of bowel loops.

The cystogram phase of the IVP

This may show a bladder rupture, but it is often false negative if the bladder is not adequately filled. In the trauma patient with gross haematuria, who may have both renal and bladder injuries, it is reasonable to perform an IVP first and if this demonstrates bladder rupture, a cystogram is obviated. However, if the bladder appears normal on the IVP, a cystogram is still required to rule out bladder rupture.

Computerized tomography (CT)

CT is often false negative for bladder rupture; unless the bladder is filled as for a high-pressure cystogram before the CT scanning is commenced.

Cystoscopy

This is rarely necessary to confirm bladder rupture, but may be required if the cystogram is not diagnostic.

Indications for surgical management

- All cases of intraperitoneal bladder rupture
- All penetrating bladder injuries (to exclude bowel injuries, and to prevent infection and fistulae)
- Extraperitoneal rupture with:
  - severe bleeding (which may block the catheter and thus prevent spontaneous healing of the ruptured bladder)
  - a large amount of contrast leakage
  - a bone fragment protruding into the lacerated bladder.

- Concomitant laceration of the vagina or rectum (primary repair is required to prevent fistula formation).

Management of intraperitoneal bladder rupture

- Laparotomy, suturing of the bladder (using an absorbable suture, e.g. 3/0 polyglycolic acid or 2/0 chromic)
- Suprapubic and/or transurethral catheters (if there is gross haematuria, two catheters provide better drainage and quicker healing of the bladder)
- Drain in the pouch of Douglas
- Some authors advocate two or even three layers of suturing, but a single layer is just as effective.

Management of extraperitoneal bladder rupture

- Extraperitoneal bladder rupture with minor contrast extravasation can be managed non-operatively with the placement of a transurethral catheter only, but it is important to ensure that the catheter does not become blocked with blood clots, because leakage of urine can lead to complications.
- If laparotomy is required for another reason, extraperitoneal bladder rupture should be repaired at the same time.
- Surgical repair of extraperitoneal bladder rupture is best performed by laparotomy, opening the bladder in the midline between stay sutures, passing F5/F8 infant feeding tubes or ureteric catheters to identify and protect the ureters, and suturing of the laceration(s) from the inside of the bladder, using absorbable sutures.
- Attempts to suture the lacerations from outside the bladder increases blood loss by disrupting tamponade of the pelvic haematoma, and increases the risk of ureteric injury.
- In penetrating trauma involving the bladder or urethra as well as the rectum, it is important to perform primary repair of the lacerations with omental interposition, diverting colostomy, distal rectal washout, and presacral drainage.

Complications

- Peritonitis, pelvic, and intraperitoneal abscesses may result from intraperitoneal leakage of infected urine, and may lead to mortality.
- Perivesical urinoma, osteomyelitis (due to contamination of a pelvic fracture with infected urine), and abscess formation may result from extraperitoneal bladder rupture.
- Urinary fistulae to the vagina, abdominal wall, or bowel may occur in penetrating trauma.

- Ureteric injury may occur during operative suturing of extraperitoneal bladder rupture.

Urethral trauma

Causes

- Iatrogenic trauma (catheter, dilator, cystoscope) is the most common cause, and usually leads to injury of the narrowest parts (penile urethra and external meatus).
- Pelvic fracture causing displacement of the pubic rami leads to distraction and laceration or complete avulsion of the bulbomembranous junction, which is attached to the inferior pubic rami via the urogenital diaphragm.
- Straddle injury (falling on the perineum with legs apart) causes trauma of the bulbar urethra, which is crushed against the pubic symphysis.
- Penetrating trauma (gunshot or stab wounds) may cause direct injury to any part of the urethra.
- Urethral injury may be associated with bladder rupture in 35–40% of patients with pelvic fracture.
- Pelvic fracture is often associated with other severe and life-threatening injuries, which take precedence over repair of the urethral injury.

Figures 27.17 and 27.18 Retrograde urethrogram showing (A) slight extravasation from an incomplete rupture of the bulbar urethra and (B) complete rupture of the bulbomembranous urethra with extravasation of contrast above and below the urogenital diaphragm

A

B

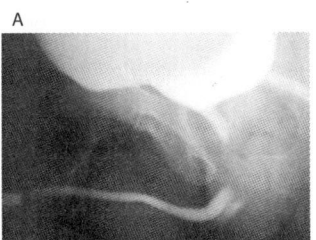
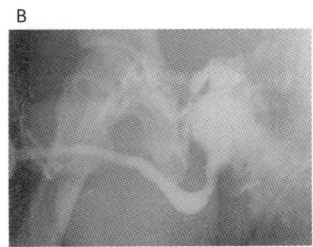

Figures 27.19 and 27.20 Prograde urethrogram showing (A) bulbar urethral rupture due to straddle injury and (B) complete rupture of the bulbomembranous urethra due to pelvic fracture

A

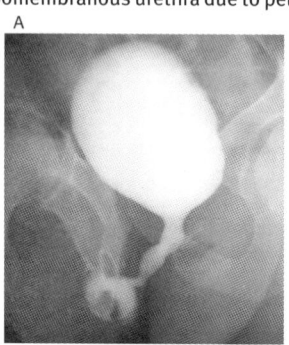

B

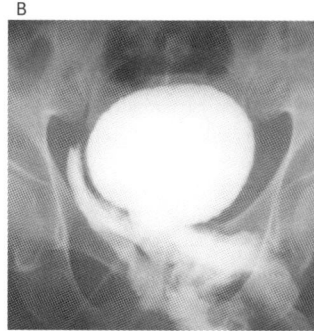

Classification

Urethral rupture may be incomplete (partial) or complete.

Class I: Posterior urethra stretched but intact
Class II: Prostatomembranous urethra torn above the urogenital
          diaphragm
Class III: Tear of both anterior and posterior urethra, with disruption of
          the urogenital diaphragm
Class IV: Injury of the posterior urethra as well as the bladder neck or
          base
Class V: Anterior urethral injury.

Clinical picture

- Bleeding from the external meatus is virtually diagnostic of urethral
  injury.
- If the patient is able to pass urine, there will be pain and haematuria
  (note that this is not the same as free bleeding from the meatus).
- There may be urinary retention (usually in patients with a complete
  membranous urethral rupture).
- There may be swelling or discoloration (haematoma) of the perineum
  and lower abdomen (the 'butterfly' pattern of discoloration is due to the
  attachment of Colles' fascia in the perineum).
- On rectal examination there may be upward displacement of the
  prostate, or it may be impalpable due to a large pelvic haematoma.

- Rectal examination is extremely important in patients with pelvic fracture and those with penetrating trauma – blood on the glove indicates a rectal or colonic laceration.
- Although urethral injury in the female is rare, vaginal examination should always be performed in women with pelvic fracture to exclude urethral laceration.

Special investigations

- An abdominal and pelvic X-ray may show a pelvic fracture.
- Retrograde urethrography is performed by inserting the tip of a bladder (Toomey) syringe or Foley catheter into the external meatus, inflating the balloon with 2–3 ml water to hold the catheter in place, and injecting 10–30 ml of water-soluble contrast medium under radiological screening to delineate the urethra and demonstrate extravasation. Ideally, oblique views of the urethra should be obtained by tilting the patient's pelvis 45 degrees to the horizontal, but this may be impossible due to pain in patients with pelvic fracture. With incomplete urethral rupture there will be extravasation, but contrast will also pass into the bladder.

Prograde urethrography. If a suprapubic catheter has been inserted, prograde urethrography can be performed by filling the bladder with contrast and asking the patient to void under X-ray screening.

Figure 27.21 Re-alignment of the ruptured posterior urethra by using a suprapubic catheter passed through the bladder neck to pull a transurethral catheter into the bladder

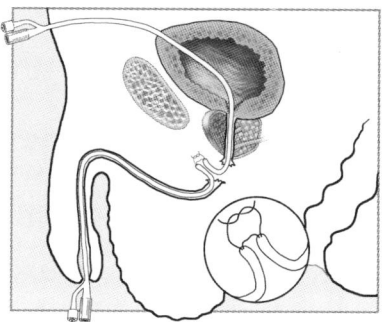

Management

- If urethrography shows a urethral rupture, the best option is to place a suprapubic catheter to divert urine away from the area of injury. If the bladder is full and clearly palpable, a suprapubic stab catheter can be placed under local anaesthesia. If the bladder is not clearly palpable or percussable (e.g. due to haematoma associated with pelvic fracture) a syringe with a long, thin needle may be used to aspirate urine before the suprapubic stab catheter is inserted.
- If the patient has to undergo laparotomy for some other reason (e.g. liver or spleen injury) an open (formal) suprapubic cystostomy is done.
- Careful insertion of a transurethral catheter may be successful, but an unsuccessful attempt may convert an incomplete to a complete urethral rupture, and it may lead to infection and osteitis.
- If a transurethral catheter has been placed, it is important to inject contrast first and obtain X-ray confirmation that the catheter tip is in the bladder, before the balloon is inflated. The fact that bloody urine is passed through the catheter does not mean that the catheter tip is in the bladder, since it may be lying in the urinoma/haematoma outside the bladder.
- Primary re-alignment of the urethra: At laparotomy the bladder is opened through a median incision and F16 or F18 catheters placed pro- and retrograde through the bladder neck and urethra, respectively. With minimal dissection in the retro-pubic space of Retzius, the tips of these catheters are then pulled out through the urethral defect. The tips of the catheters are sutured together so that the transurethral catheter can be pulled into the bladder (so-called railroading). Metal sounds should not be used for this, since there is a risk of causing a false passage into the bladder.
- Delayed re-alignment: In the unstable patient, the above procedure can be performed 5–10 days later, when active bleeding from the pelvic haematoma is much less likely. The advantage of transurethral catheterization is that the torn edges of the urethra are aligned and approximated so that the subsequent stricture is shorter and easier to treat. Traction on the transurethral catheter in an attempt to improve approximation is probably best avoided.
- Primary suturing of a urethral rupture in the acute stage is very difficult, due to active bleeding from the torn pelvic vessels, and is not recommended. It may also increase the risk of subsequent incontinence and erectile dysfunction, due to neurovascular damage during placement of the sutures.
- Orthopaedic reduction of unstable pelvic fractures with external or internal fixation is useful to limit blood loss and to facilitate later repair of the urethra. However, open reduction and internal fixation incurs a

high risk of infection if a suprapubic catheter is left indwelling, whereas the risk is significantly lower with a transurethral catheter. Therefore, primary re-alignment with railroading of a transurethral catheter is preferable when internal fixation of the pelvic fracture is performed.

Complications

- Urine leakage may lead to para-urethral infection and abscess formation or necrotizing fasciitis (Fournier's gangrene).
- Bladder infection or epididymo-orchitis may occur.
- Urethral stricture is very common, regardless of the primary management, although the stricture may be shorter if primary re-alignment was possible.
- Erectile dysfunction (impotence) is quite common in men with a pelvic fracture and membranous urethral injury, probably because of damage to the nerves and blood vessels supplying the corpora cavernosa, which are located close to the prostatic apex and membranous urethra.
- Management of the urethral stricture, which virtually always occurs, may consist of dilatation with filiform dilators, or optical (direct vision) internal urethrotomy (Sachse procedure), or urethroplasty. Dilatation or optical urethrotomy may be attempted at any time after development of the stricture, but urethroplasty is usually done after 3–6 months of suprapubic catheter drainage to give the peri-urethral inflammation and fibrosis time to settle down.

Penile trauma

Causes

- Circumcision (especially the ritual type) may lead to excessive skin loss, injury to the glans and urethral meatus, infection, or gangrene of the penile shaft due to constrictive bandages used for haemostasis.
- Fracture of the penis usually occurs during vigorous sexual activity, and consists of a tear in the tunica albuginea of the corpus cavernosum. This may be associated with a tear in the urethra.
- Penetrating trauma (gunshot or stab injury, animal bites) may cause penile injury.
- Avulsion of skin from the penile shaft usually occurs when the penis is caught in machinery.
- Strangulation is caused by a constricting band or ring placed around the base of the penile shaft, usually in an attempt to attain or prolong erection.
- Complete severance of the penis with a sharp instrument is usually an act of vengeance or mental derangement.

Clinical picture

- There is usually a history of trauma, with pain, swelling, tenderness, and discoloration due to haematoma formation.
- Penile fracture is characterized by sudden, severe pain, loss of erection, swelling, and discoloration of the skin over the area of the tear in the tunica albuginea.

Management

- Avulsion of the skin is treated with primary or secondary suturing.
- With extensive skin loss, scrotal skin, or a split thickness skin graft, can be used.
- If there is skin loss from the proximal shaft, with full-thickness skin remaining on the distal shaft, primary suturing may lead to lymph-oedema of the distal skin. Thus, it is better to remove the distal skin and cover the defect with a split-thickness skin graft.
- Penile fracture is treated by suturing of the laceration in the tunica albuginea to prevent the complication of erectile dysfunction. If there is an associated urethral tear, this should be sutured over an F14/F16 transurethral catheter.
- Strangulation is a dire emergency treated by removal of the constricting object.
- Gangrene of the penis requires debridement of devitalized tissues to prevent severe infection and possible mortality due to septicaemia.
- Complete severance of the penis necessitates micro-surgical re-anastomosis.

Scrotal and testicular trauma

Causes

- Blunt trauma may cause a subcutaneous scrotal haematoma, avulsion of the scrotal skin, rupture of the testis, or a haematocele (blood inside the tunica vaginalis).
- Penetrating trauma can cause lacerations of the scrotal skin or testes.

Clinical picture

- With a clear history of scrotal trauma, the diagnosis is usually obvious, although it may be impossible to distinguish clinically between a scrotal haematoma and testicular rupture with haematocele.
- Patients with torsion of the testis, epididymo-orchitis, or a testis tumour sometimes give a misleading history of trauma (usually minor), which may be coincidental, or may direct the patient's atten-

tion to a pre-existing scrotal swelling. Thus, a history of relatively slight trauma followed by severe pain or a large scrotal swelling should be regarded with a high index of suspicion.

- Ultrasound imaging of the scrotum is useful, but if the diagnosis is uncertain, surgical exploration is necessary.
- If there is suspicion of a testis tumour, exploration through an inguinal approach is indicated.

Management

- Slight injuries can be managed with bed rest, scrotal elevation and support, analgesics or non-steroidal anti-inflammatory drugs.
- Rupture of the testis is best managed with surgical exploration, debridement, suturing of the tunica albuginea of the testis, and drainage of the scrotum.
- If a testis tumour is suspected, an inguinal incision is preferable to a trans-scrotal approach (due to the risk of tumour recurrence in the scrotal wall, which can lead to lymph node metastases in the inguinal as well as the para-aortic areas).
- With complete avulsion of the scrotum, the testes can be buried subcutaneously in the inguinal areas, and reconstruction of the scrotum with a split thickness skin graft or full-thickness flap can be done later.

Pitfalls

- In patients with renal trauma, mortality is most often due to associated injuries; if present, these should be managed urgently and appropriately.
- If the urine is not examined, urinary tract injury will remain unrecognized.
- Failure to obtain pre-operative renal imaging may lead to incorrect management of an intra-operatively discovered injury.
- Unnecessary nephrectomy may result if superfluous exploration of an injured kidney is performed.
- Although ureteric injury is rare in patients with penetrating abdominal trauma, a high index of suspicion is required in order not to miss the diagnosis.
- Missed ureteric injury and delayed diagnosis may lead to serious complications.
- Iatrogenic injury of the ureter may occur during pelvic procedures, is easily missed, and may lead to costly litigation.
- An IVP or CT alone is not reliable in demonstrating bladder rupture – this requires a correctly performed high-pressure cystogram.
- Undiagnosed bladder rupture, especially in the presence of pelvic fracture, may lead to serious complications and even mortality.

- In patients with pelvic fracture, passing a transurethral catheter which drains bloody urine does not guarantee that the catheter tip is inside the bladder – it may just be draining the extravesical urinoma/haematoma. The position of the catheter has to be confirmed by contrast injection before its balloon is inflated.
- Urethral injury may be associated with bladder rupture (especially in patients with pelvic fracture). A suprapubic stab catheter should only be inserted after confirmation (by needle aspiration or ultrasound) that the bladder is full.
- Re-alignment of a ruptured posterior urethra using metal sounds may result in a false passage being made into the bladder.
- Not examining genitalia in pelvic injuries.
- Not distinguishing between trauma and pre-existing scrotal swelling or a torsion of the testis.

Recommended reading

Carlin, B. I., Resnick, M. I. 1995. Indications and techniques for urologic evaluation of the trauma patient with suspected urologic injury. *Seminars in Urology*, 13(1):9–24.

Chapple, C. R. 2000. Urethral injury. *British Journal of Urology International*, 86:318–326.

Koraitim, M. M.1999. Pelvic fracture urethral injuries: The unresolved controversy. *Journal of Urology*, 161:1433–1441.

Santucci, R. A., McAninch, J. W. 2000. Diagnosis and management of renal trauma: Past, present, and future. *Journal of the American College of Surgeons*, 191(4):443–451.

Watnik, N. F., Coburn, M., Goldberger, M. 1996. Urologic injuries in pelvic ring disruptions. *Clinical Orthopaedics Rel Res*, 329:37–45.

Pelvic fracture resuscitative management

Gordon Siboto

The type of injuries incurred dictates the specific management of pelvic fractures. Life-threatening pelvic fractures are commonly associated with serious injuries in other systems.

Primary management

Primary management is according to ATLS® protocols and is directed at:
- Maintaining airway with C-spine control
- Maintaining breathing
- Stopping bleeding, which may come from more than one source
- Preventing secondary damage to the central nervous system and other systems

Pelvic management

Pelvic management is directed at:
- Determining the site of the blood loss
- Stabilization of the pelvic skeleton

Site of bleeding in a patient with a pelvic fracture

The majority of patients with pelvic fractures are haemodynamically stable. Those who are haemodynamically unstable are often associated with other serious injuries. The site of bleeding may be extra-pelvic or intra-pelvic.

Extra-pelvic:
Chest	haemothorax
	ruptured thoracic aorta
	blunt cardiac tamponade
Abdomen	intraperitoneal (spleen, liver, mesentery)
	retroperitoneal (aorta, pancreas, kidney)
Limbs	femur fracture

Intra-pelvic: Severe bleeding occurs in a small number of patients. There are many sources of bleeding within the pelvis, which may bleed alone or in combination. The treatment must be directed to the source. An external fixator cannot treat all.

Large named vessels (Iliac or femoral arteries and veins)

The patients often die at the scene or soon after arrival in hospital. They need massive blood transfusion (more than ten units).

Treatment

Proceed as follows:

- Check femoral pulses early as part of general assessment. Sometimes angiography and/or venography have to be done to make a diagnosis.
- Direct surgical control and repair of the vessels where possible is the only hope to save a few of these patients.
- Hemi-pelvectomy may be required.

Small named vessels

One of the internal iliac artery branches (inferior gluteal, pudendal, obturator, vesical arteries but commonly involved is the superior gluteal artery). Many of these vessels are closely applied to the pelvic bones. Fracture of the bone or dislocation of the sacro-iliac joint may cause damage to one of them. If this is the only source of bleeding, blood transfusion usually restores the blood pressure to normal for a while only to drop again. It ends up with massive blood transfusions.

Treatment

If all other causes are excluded, angiography must be done in order to embolize the damaged vessel.

Small unnamed vessels

These are injured with disruption of the pelvic floor muscles and venous plexus. The severity of bleeding relates to the extent of soft tissue disruption, which in turn corresponds to the extent of pelvic ring disruption (typically open-book type fracture) (see Figure 28.3), and gross disruption anywhere in the posterior sacro-iliac segment (ilium posterior to the acetabulum, sacro-iliac joint, and sacrum) (see Figure 28.1).

Treatment

External fixator helps by:

- Increasing the interstitial pressure, thus stopping the bleeding
- Stopping excessive soft tissue movement, thus preventing blood clots dislodging
- Stabilizing the pelvis for nursing care though the reduction may not be adequate

Figure 28.1 Shaded area represents the posterior sacro-iliac segment

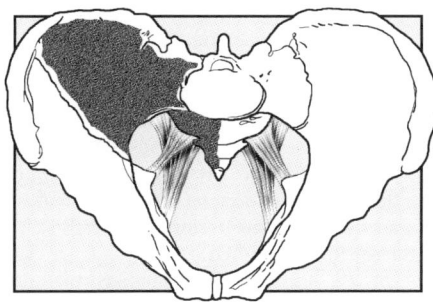

Cancellous bone fracture
Alone this source is unlikely to cause massive blood loss.

Pelvic fracture classification

For diagnostic and resuscitative purposes, the fracture can be classified as follows:
- Open or closed
- Mechanically stable or unstable

Closed. Closed pelvic fractures are in the majority with 10.5% mortality.

Open. The fracture directly communicates with the skin laceration, perineum, and vaginal or rectal tears. These are in the minority, yet the mortality is 50% due to:
- Increased blood loss (the most common cause of early death)
- Sepsis from the injured soft tissues
- Multiple organ failure

Treatment of open fractures
 Proceed as follows:
- Control bleeding from the source.
- Administer tetanus toxoid.
- Give prophylactic antibiotics (penicillin, gentamycin, and metronidazole).
- Divert faeces when there is a perineal, vaginal, or/and rectal wound by doing a sigmoid colostomy. Vaginal wound must be cleaned and referred to a gynaecologist.

Mechanical instability

Clinical assessment

By gently but firmly pushing in and out at the iliac crest, a diagnosis of a stable or grossly unstable pelvic fracture can be made.

Radiological assessment

For making a diagnosis for resuscitative purposes an antero-posterior (AP) X-ray is adequate. Inlet and outlet views (Pennel views) which give further information on the direction and extent of displacement, should be done only when the patient has become haemodynamically stable. An AP view will show that the pelvic ring is either:

- Intact (in which case serious bleeding is unlikely to be from the pelvis)
- Disrupted
  Where? (anterior, posterior, or both segments)
  How much? (this may be misleading, because the X-ray may look normal due to soft tissue recoil)

Figure 28.2 Application of the Pelvigrip® to the pelvis

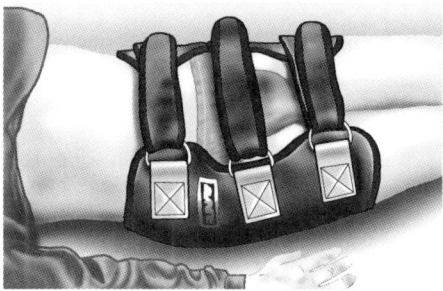

Figure 28.3 Open-book pelvic fracture

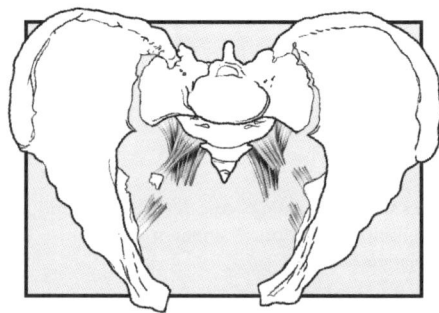

The direction of deformity implies the direction of force applied (lateral or antero-posterior compression, or a combination). This classification helps in alerting the attending doctor to look out for the associated injuries commonly seen with each type of pelvic fracture. Any fracture type can bleed excessively depending on the extent of the pelvic soft tissue damage and the caliber of vessels involved.

Treatment of instability
If the pelvis is mechanically as well as haemodynamically unstable, stabilize it by using:

- Sheet wrapped around the pelvis, a Pelvigrip®, MAST suit, or similar garment as a temporary measure
- External fixator. It must be positioned such that a laparotomy may still be performed.

Figure 28.4 Lateral compression fracture

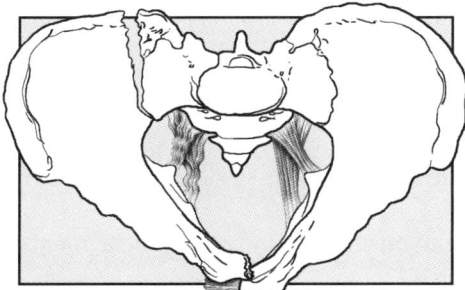

Figure 28.5 Vertical shear fracture

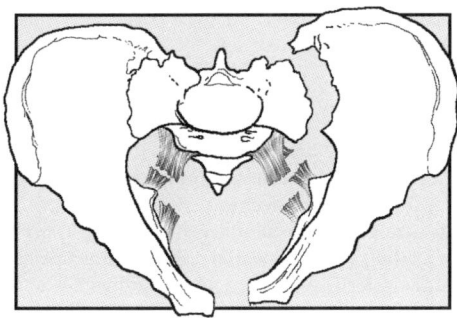

Management according to mechanical stability fracture pattern

Open-book pelvic fracture

The open book involves the anterior part of the ring opening out, whilst the posterior segment remains relatively intact. This implies that the perineal skin, pelvic floor muscles, and vessels may be torn depending on the amount of force applied.

Treatment – if haemodynamically unstable
- Check femoral pulses
- Close the pelvis (sheet, Pelvigrip®, external fixator, etc.)
- If the patient remains unstable and extra-pelvic bleeding is excluded, do angiogram and embolize if indicated.

Lateral compression

The pelvic bone is displaced medially. The pelvic floor muscles, organs, and vessels are compressed during the impact, consequently the source of bleeding is most likely to be extra-pelvic. A bone spike may cause damage to the bladder and/or vagina.

Treatment
The external fixator may be useful for nursing care and pain relief.

Gross disruption anterior and posterior segments of pelvis (vertical shear)

This implies severe pelvic soft tissue disruption. The extent of damage depends on the amount of energy dissipated. Bleeding can be from:
- Soft tissue
- Small named vessels, e.g. superior gluteal artery
- Large named vessels, e.g. iliac vessels
- A combination.

Treatment
Treatment depends on whether the fracture is closed or open:
- Stabilize the pelvis in order to increase interstitial pressure that will help stop the bleeding by external fixation.
- Perform an angiogram once all other sources have been excluded and embolize if it is the small calibre artery, and surgical repair for large vessels like the iliac artery.

Summary of pelvic fracture management

Fracture management is summarized in the diagram below.

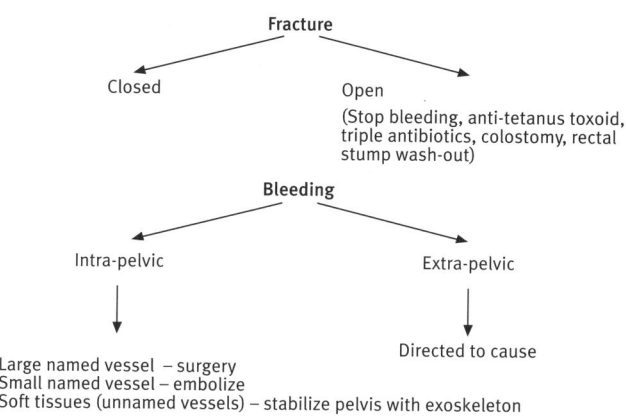

Summary of pelvic fracture management

Fracture

Closed

Open
(Stop bleeding, anti-tetanus toxoid, triple antibiotics, colostomy, rectal stump wash-out)

Bleeding

Intra-pelvic

Extra-pelvic

Directed to cause

Large named vessel – surgery
Small named vessel – embolize
Soft tissues (unnamed vessels) – stabilize pelvis with exoskeleton

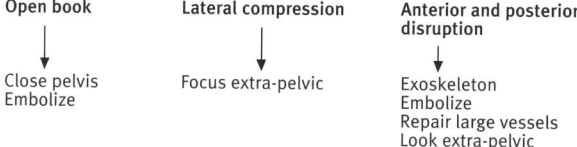

Fracture pattern/stability

Open book

Close pelvis
Embolize

Lateral compression

Focus extra-pelvic

Anterior and posterior gross disruption

Exoskeleton
Embolize
Repair large vessels
Look extra-pelvic

Pitfalls

- A diagnosis of the source of bleeding must be made, then treated accordingly.
- Haemodynamically unstable patients with pelvic fracture commonly have other associated injuries that also bleed.
- There are few patients with pelvic fracture that bleed from the pelvis alone.
- Intra-pelvic bleeding may come from more than one source.
- External fixator controls bleeding coming from the pelvic floor tissues by increasing the interstitial pressure and by limiting tissue movement that may dislodge already formed clots.
- Antero-posterior X-ray is adequate for making a diagnosis of pelvic fracture for resuscitation purposes.

Recommended reading

Cryer, H. M., Miller, F. B., Rouben, L. R., Seligon, D. L. 1988. Pelvic fracture classification: Correlation with haemorrhage. *J Trauma*, 28:973–980.

McMurtry, R., Walton, D., Dickson, D., Kellem, J., Tile, M. 1980. Pelvic disruption in the polytraumatized patient: A management protocol. *CORR*, September, 22–30.

Pelvic ring injuries: Part I. *Injury*, 1996, 27, Suppl.1.

Rothenberger, D., Velasco, R., Strate, R., Fischer, R. P., Perry, J. F. 1978. Open pelvic fracture: A lethal injury. *J Trauma*, 18:184–187.

29 Extensive soft tissue and crush injuries

Jan Pretorius

Extensive soft tissue injury is associated with various local and/or systemic clinical problems. Local complications of significant soft tissue injury, such as crushing injury, sjambok injury (extensive lashing or caning), or limb ischaemia, include compartment syndrome, muscle ischaemia-reperfusion injury, and rhabdomyolysis. The common denominator is myonecrosis, which, if present in large areas, may lead to myoglobinuria, myoglobinaemia, hyperkalaemia, hyperphosphataemia, hypocalcaemia, cardiovascular instability, and acidosis. Sequelae of the release of these potentially toxic substances into the circulation include acute renal failure and disseminated intravascular coagulation. These systemic manifestations of a local muscle injury are known as crush syndrome.

Skeletal muscle

- Skeletal muscle accounts for 40–50% of total body weight, which makes it the largest organ of the body.
- Muscle represents the single largest pool of body water.
- Muscle contains about 70% of body potassium and the largest concentration of Na/K-ATP-ase pumps.
- Skeletal muscle is highly susceptible to mechanical trauma and rhabdomyolysis.
- Muscle injury may unleash extreme disturbances in body fluids, acid-base balance, and electrolytes, leading to hypovolaemic shock and circulatory collapse.
- Extensive muscle injury is associated with pigment nephropathy, leading to acute renal failure.

Causes of skeletal muscle injury

Mechanical or biological injuries

Various mechanisms of injury may affect soft tissue, notably also prolonged pressure, compression, and immobilization.

- Multiple trauma
- Crush injury

- Vascular or orthopaedic surgery (ischaemia-reperfusion injury)
- Coma
- Immobilization
- Electric shock
- Thermal injuries: burns
- Hypothermia

Exertional trauma

Exertional trauma may affect normal muscle in certain circumstances. These are:
- Extreme exertion (march myoglobinuria)
- Environmental heat illness
- Sickle cell trait
- Seizures, tetanus, status asthmaticus
- Hyperkinetic states

Exertional trauma of abnormal muscle may occur in the presence of:
- Metabolic myopathies
- Mitochondrial myopathies
- Malignant hyperthermia
- Neuroleptic malignant syndrome

Non-exertional trauma

Non-exertional muscle trauma could result from:
- Alcoholism
- Drugs and toxins
- Infections (including HIV)
- Electrolyte abnormalities
- Endocrinopathies, e.g. thyrotoxicosis
- Inflammatory myopathies
- Miscellaneous: toxins, CO, snake and other venom

Clinical syndromes associated with muscle injury

Compartment syndrome

Definition
Compartment syndrome consists of the local manifestations of nerve and muscle ischemia due to increased pressure within osteo-fascial compartments.

Cause

- Local soft tissue ischaemia-reperfusion injury
- Local extensive soft tissue trauma
- Crush injury, fracture, electric burn
- Intracompartmental haematoma

Clinical findings

- Tense, swollen compartment
- Increased pressure in the compartment
- Pain on passive stretching
- Paraesthesia
- Anaesthesia
- Paralysis/weakness
- Pallor
- Pulses may be present or absent
- Late – Volkman's contracture

Crush syndrome

Definition

Crush syndrome consists of the systemic manifestations of muscle injury after direct trauma or ischaemic reperfusion.

Cause

The causes of crush syndrome are extensive soft tissue trauma, compartment syndrome, snake bite, etc.

Clinical findings

- Tense, oedematous, painful limb
- Dark, tea-coloured urine; impending acute renal failure
- Circulatory shock and metabolic acidosis
- Raised serum lactate levels

Pathophysiology of muscle injury

Reperfusion injury

When ischaemic muscle is reperfused, a distinct pattern of histologic change is noted, with areas of normal muscle adjacent to areas of injury. This uneven distribution of injury may be related to heterogeneous derangements in the blood supply to the ischaemic muscle on reperfusion, with scattered areas of microcirculatory occlusion (focal endothelial injury and plugging of the microcirculation with polymorphonuclear leukocytes).

- Reperfusion may be more detrimental than the ischaemia.
- Calcium is a principal mediator of cellular injury.
- Reintroduction of oxygenated blood to ischaemic tissue paradoxically increases the severity of cellular damage.
- Excess free radicals are produced via xanthine oxidase. The free radicals cause local damage by initiating a cascade of cytokines and recruiting and activating neutrophils. This leads to increased capillary permeability, local inflammation and eventually to distant damage of lungs, gut and kidneys. (See Figure 29.1 and Table 29.1.)
- Focal injury to myocytes with the release of myoglobin and potassium, which leads to distant organ injury.

Clinical findings
- Local pain, oedema, function loss
- Hypovolaemic shock, acidosis, electrolyte disturbances
- Large volumes of fluid lost into muscle cells deplete the intravascular compartment

Rhabdomyolysis

Definition
This is a syndrome characterized by skeletal muscle necrosis and the release of intra-cellular constituents into the systemic circulation. Two distinct problems are identified: local muscle, vessel, and nerve injury, and systemic depletion of intravascular volume, electrolyte imbalances, and renal injury from myoglobins.

Clinical findings
- Rhabdomyolysis is a consequence of muscle injury associated with compartment syndrome, crush injury, and reperfusion injury. Myoglobinaemia and myoglobinuria are consequences of rhabdmyolysis.
- Findings are quantified by measuring plasma creatine kinase (CK) levels. The threshold for significant rhabdomyolysis has not been defined.
- Clinical consequences include a spectrum of problems, ranging from asymptomatic increase of muscle enzyme levels to life-threatening extreme enzyme increases, with electrolyte imbalance and shock.
- It is responsible for a significant percentage of all cases of acute renal failure in SA.

Myoglobinaemia

Free myoglobin present in the blood is due to saturation of the binding capacity of haptoglobin for myoglobin. It can be measured in the serum.

Figure 29.1 Mechanical and toxic effects of myoglobin on the kidney

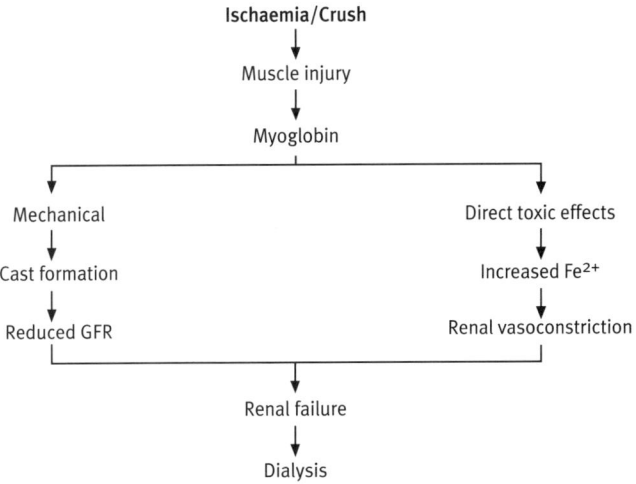

Myoglobinuria

- Myoglobinuria is the presence of myoglobin in the urine. The excretion rate depends on glomerular filtration rate, urine flow rate, and percentage of free myoglobin in plasma.
- Urine dipstick testing will be positive for blood despite absence of red cells on microscopy.
- It can be measured in the urine.

Diagnostic approach

Suspect rhabdomyolysis

- Consider the presenting disease or pathology as a cause for rhabdomyolysis.
- Notice red to brown urine.
- Centrifuge urine: examine sediment, supernatant – test for haeme.
- Look for source of rhabdomyolysis.
- Determine plasma creatine phosphokinase levels.
- Determine serum and urine myoglobin.
- Determine serum Na^+, K^+, and Ca^{++}.
- Determine serum lactate and acid-base status.
- Monitor high-risk limbs frequently.

Table 29.1 Flow of solutes and water across skeletal muscle cell membrane in rhabdomyolysis

Influx from extracellular compartment into muscle cells	Consequences
Water, sodium chloride, and calcium	Hypovolaemia and haemodynamic shock, prerenal and later acute renal failure, hypocalcaemia, aggravated hyperkalaemic cardiotoxicity, increased cytosolic calcium, activation of cytotoxic proteases.

Efflux from damaged muscle cells	Consequences
Potassium	Hyperkalaemia and cardiotoxicity aggravated by hypocalcaemia and hypotension
Purines from disintegrating cell nuclei	Hyperuricaemia, nephrotoxicity
Phosphate	Hyperphosphataemia, aggravation of hypocalcaemia, and metastatic calcification, including the kidney
Lactic and other organic acids	Metabolic acidosis and acidurea
Myoglobin	Nephrotoxicity, particularly with coexisting oliguria, aciduria, and uricosuria
Thromboplastin	Disseminated intravascular coagulation
Creatine kinase	Extreme elavation of serum creatine kinase
Creatinine	Increased serum creatinine: urea ratio

Source: From Better and Stein, *The New England Journal of Medicine*, 1990, 322:825–829.

Factors predisposing to compartment syndrome

- Duration of ischaemia
- Systemic hypotension
- Massive swelling
- Crush injury
- High-velocity injury
- Combined arterial and venous injury

Diagnosis of compartment syndrome

- When really in doubt, measure compartment pressure directly. Use pressure transducers from arterial or venous catheter monitoring equipment or even an ordinary central venous pressure manometer. Capillary perfusion pressure is 25–30 mmHg.
- When compartment pressures exceed capillary perfusion pressure, decompression by fasciotomy may be indicated.
- Absolute numbers may be misleading. Exercise clinical judgement – especially in hypotensive patients in whom lower absolute compartment pressures may produce profound muscle ischaemia in poorly perfused areas.

Treatment

Local treatment

- Remember that prevention is better than cure.
- Restore blood flow promptly. Ischaemic times longer than six hours are likely to have unfavourable outcomes.
- Arterial repairs or grafting should be performed promptly, with careful thrombectomy and embolectomy. Ligation of large arteries should be used as a last resort because this commonly leads to amputation.
- Orthopaedic injuries associated with vascular trauma should be managed initially with the application of external splinting and traction. The vascular injury should be repaired first, then definitive orthopaedic reduction and fixation can be achieved. Open fractures need thorough irrigation, debridement, and antibiotics.
- Fasciotomy involves rapid surgical decompression of the investing fascia of all affected compartments.
- Amputation is indicated for massive myonecrosis when limb salvage is no longer possible. The limb now threatens the patient's overall health.
- Physiologic amputation is an alternative in patients who are too critically ill to undergo amputation. Isolate the limb with tourniquets and then freeze it with ice. Pain is thus relieved and spreading of harmful infection and biological material is stopped. Amputate when stable.

Systemic treatment

- Treat shock early and vigorously. Restore intravascular volume first.
- Then add inotropic or other pharmacologic manipulation if indicated.
- Correct the underlying cause of shock or limb ischaemia rapidly.

The risk of myoglobinuric renal failure depends on:
- Significant soft tissue injury
- Delay in diagnosis
- Delay in treatment
- Dehydration
- Pre-existing renal disease
- Advanced age

Determine CK and myoglobin levels serially. These may be useful as components of risk stratification, as well as assessment of a patient's response to therapy.

Large-volume infusion of crystalloid can be used successfully to dilute the myoglobin load delivered to the kidneys and to cause a diuresis. It also reduces cast formation and flushes myoglobin out of the renal tubules.

Controversy exists about the optimal fluid composition and rate of administration. Early, large-volume infusion should be the first step in treating these patients.

Mannitol may be added for the following effects:
- Osmotic diuresis
- Intravascular volume expansion
- Reduction of blood viscosity
- Renal vasodilatation
- Hydroxyl radical scavenging
- It does not acidify urine as do loop diuretics

Note that mannitol can produce a hyperosmolar state and electrolyte abnormalities if used in large volumes or for prolonged periods.

Alkalinization of the urine is advised to minimize renal damage during rhabdomyolysis. Acidic urine promotes tubular cast development and renal injury.

Fluid management

- Choose the volume to be infused: 4 or 6 or 8 litre saline (0.9% NaCl) per 24 hours (according to body mass and fluid requirements).
- An average of 200–300 mmol Na^+HCO_3 is given per 24 hours.
- Mannitol maximum dose 200 g per 24 hours.

Pitfalls

- Take care not to sacrifice the patient to save a limb.
- Maintain a high index of suspicion for muscle ischaemia or compartment syndrome.
- Absolute numbers for compartment pressures may be misleading – primarily use clinical judgement.
- Perform fasciotomies earlier rather than later.
- Never underestimate the risks of subclinical hypovolaemia in a trauma patient.

Table 29.2 Ratios and volumes of fluids required for the management of acute rhabdomyolysis. Depending on the volume chosen, mix in saline:

Volume per hour:	Add Na$^+$HCO$_3$	Add 20% mannitol
4 000 ml/24 hours	300 mmol/4l	200 g/4l
= 166 ml/hour	= 75 mmol/1 000 ml	50 g/1 000 ml
	= 75 ml 8.5% Na$^+$ HCO$_3$/l	= 250 ml 20% mannitol/l
6 000 ml/24 hours	300 mmol/6l	200 g/6l
= 250 ml/hour	= 50 mmol/1 000 ml	= 33 g/1 000 ml
	= 50 ml 8.5% Na$^+$ HCO$_3$/l	= 165 ml 20% mannitol/l
8 000 ml/24 hours	300 mmol/8l	200 g/8l
= 333 ml/hour	= 37.5 mmol/1 000 ml	25 g/1 000 ml
	= 37.5 ml 8.5% Na$^+$HCO$_3$/l	= 125 ml 20% mannitol/l

- When serum sodium is elevated, mix:
  1 000 ml 0.45% NaCl

  +

  70 mmol 8.5% NaHCO$_3$ (70 ml)

  +

  37.5g 20% mannitol (± 190 ml)
  (3 amps of 12.5 g)
- Administer at 100–120–200 ml/h
- Aim:
  ± 300 ml urine/h
  Urine pH > 6.5
  Arterial pH < 7.5
- Stop when s-myoglobin is less than 300

Recommended reading

Abassi, Z. A., Hoffman, A., Better, O. S. 1998. Acute renal failure complicating muscle crush injury. *Seminars in Nephrology,* 18:558–565.

Slater, M. S., Mullins, R. J. 1998. Rhabdomyolysis and myoglobinuric renal failure in trauma and surgical patients: A review. *Journal of the American College of Surgeons,* 186:693–716.

Zager, R. A. 1996. Editorial review. Rhabdomyolysis and myohemoglobinuric acute renal failure. *Kidney International,* 49:314–326.

30 Hand injuries

Michael Solomons

The hand is the most commonly injured part of the body because it is involved in activities of daily living, work, and play. The huge representation of the hand in the cortex attends to the fact that the hand is of vital importance in our daily lives. The initial examination and primary care of the injured hand is critical. Maximum functional recovery must be the goal.

Early mobilization of the hand and the 'safe position' for immobilization

The function of the hand revolves around mobility and sensibility. Trauma causes an inflammatory response with resultant oedema. Oedema settles in the peri-articular tissue and resolves by fibrosis, resulting in stiffness. A stiff hand is a useless hand. Avoid or limit stiffness where possible by:

- Elevation
- Early movement – one full flexion and extension of the fingers is equal to six hours of elevation in oedema control.

If oedema is unavoidable, then the hand must be placed in a position of safety. The safe position consists of the hand immobilized in the following manner:

- Wrist 30 degree dorsiflexed
- Metacarpo-phalangeal joint (MPJs) 90 degrees flexed
- Inter-phalangeal joints (IPJs) straight.

The safe position is the opposite of the hand's position of comfort. Local wrist blocks may be used to push the hand into the 'safe position'. Hold this position with a dorsal plaster slab until oedema resolves or movement can be started.

Assessment of the injured hand

History

Ascertain the patient's history:

- Mechanism of injury
- Time of injury

- Work
- Hobbies
- Hand dominance
- Co-morbidities

Examination

Nowhere else in the body are motion and function more closely related to anatomic structures than in the hand. Meticulous assessment of all-important structures is required:

- Three nerves and their branches (radial, ulnar, median, and ten digital nerves)
- Eleven flexor tendons
- Twelve extensor tendons
- Bones and joints
- Muscles

Radial nerve function

- Sensory – dorsum 1st web space
- Motor – wrist extension, metacarpo-phalangeal joint (MPJ) extension. The interphalangeal joints (IPJs) are extended by the intrinsic muscles under median and ulnar nerve control.

Median nerve function

- Sensory – thumb and index finger tips
- Motor – Flexor pollicis longus (FPL) and Flexor digitorum profundus (FDP) to index (O sign), opposition

Figure 30.1 How to test for flexor digitorum superficialis (FDS) function

Figure 30.2 How to test for flexor digitorum profundus (FDP) function

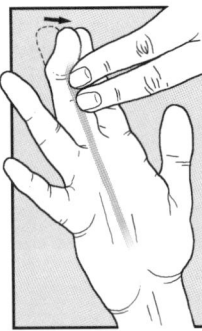

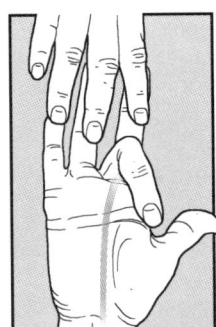

Figure 30.3 How to test for extensor digitorum function

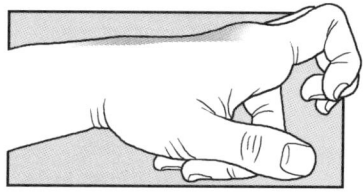

Ulnar nerve
- Sensory – tip of little finger
- Motor – 1st dorsal interosseous and abductor digiti minimi; test ability to cross fingers

Radiographic examination

Radiographic examination is essential in almost all hand injuries. Always perform a PA and lateral X-ray. An oblique X-ray is also often required.

Closed injuries

Nail-bed injuries

Nail-bed injuries are common and due to a crushing force.
- Subungual haematomas are very painful, and need to be drained. Use a heated paperclip.
- Nail avulsed or partially avulsed – *best to pull nail back* – to protect nail bed.
- Suture nail bed with 6/0 Vicryl (absorbable).
- Nail bed may be trapped in fracture site or in growth plate in children, and must be removed and sutured.

Mallet finger

- A mallet finger occurs when the extensor tendon to the terminal phalanx is disrupted. This results from forced flexion against resisted extension.
- It is common in sports, work, and domestic injuries.
- It causes an inability to extend the distal interphalangeal (DIP) joint.
- X-ray is necessary to exclude an avulsion fracture.
- Treatment is non-operative with a Mallet splint.

FDP avulsion – rugby jersey injury

FDP avulsion is uncommon and easily missed.
- Diagnosis – look for inability to flex the DIP joint.
- Delayed referral results in an untreatable situation.
- It requires operative re-insertion of the detached tendon by a hand surgeon.

Proximal interphalangeal joint (PIPJ) injuries

Collateral ligament injuries

These injuries are extremely common and most are not reported. They are characterized by a partial tear of collateral ligament – sprain. The PIPJ is stiff and swollen. The treatment is to buddy strap the finger to the adjacent finger for three weeks continuously and three weeks further when at risk. The patient must be warned that it could be painful for many months and swelling could persist for years.

PIPJ dislocation

These are usually dorsal dislocations and dislocation implies rupture of the volar plate.
Treatment:
- *Do not immobilize.*
- Buddy strap for three to six weeks.
- All should be X-rayed to exclude more serious fracture dislocation.

Boutonniere injury

A Boutonniere injury is a jamming injury of finger. The PIPJ is forced into flexion while actively extending, which avulses or tears the central slip of the extensor tendon. This is characterized by:
- An inability to actively extend the PIPJ.
- The deformity is exacerbated by lateral bands subluxing volarly and becoming 'flexor'.
- Rupture of the central slip is differentiated from the more common injury to the collateral ligament by location of maximal tenderness – dorsum for Boutonniere, medial or lateral for collateral, and inability to extend PIPJ. If the patient is unable to extend due to pain, then a digital block must be performed to confirm the ability to extend.
- Treatment is to splint *only* PIPJ in extension. Leave DIPJ free and actively mobilize.

Metacarpo-phalangeal joint (MPJ) dislocations

- The vast majority of these dislocations are dorsal.
- Simple dislocation: MPJ is hyperextended; articular surfaces are in partial contact – relatively easy to reduce. Reduction performed under wrist block. Hyperextend the MPJ, advance the proximal phalanx distally, and then into flexion.
- Complex dislocation: finger is parallel to palm; metacarpal head palpable in palm; wide gap on X-ray; sesamoid in joint pathognomonic. *Do not try closed reduction. Needs surgery.*

Fractures of metacarpals and phalanges

Try to differentiate between stable and unstable fractures:

Stable

Crack or minimally displaced fractures. Treatment is to buddy strap and move early.

Unstable

Comminuted or displaced fractures or a transverse fracture. This can usually be treated in dorsal plaster slab from forearm to finger tips in the *safe position*. It is important to check rotation by looking at fingernails in slight flexion. If still displaced it will need fixation.

Articular fractures

Undisplaced – early movement; displaced – open reduction and internal fixation (ORIF).

Thumb injuries

Bennett's fracture dislocation of the carpometacarpal (CMC) joint

- Small volar/ulnar fragment remains. Rest of thumb metacarpal and joint surface subluxes dorso-radially
- Undisplaced: thumb spica cast with thumb abducted
- Displaced: K-wire across joint

Ulna collateral ligament tear ('Skier's thumb')

- Tenderness and able to open the joint on the ulnar side
- Needs local anaesthetic to separate partial from complete tears
- Partial: plaster of Paris
- Complete: surgery

Figure 30.4 Bennett's fracture

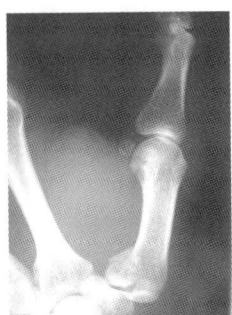

Figure 30.5 Ulnar collateral ligament tear

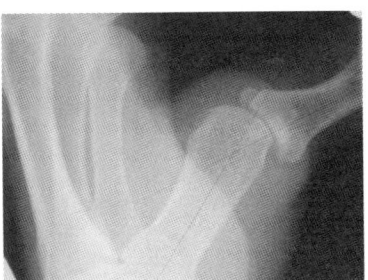

Scaphoid fractures

Forceful hyperextension occurs after a fall on the outstretched hand, and is characterized by tenderness in the anatomical snuff box and scaphoid tubercle at the base of the palm.

- Confirm with scaphoid series of X-rays.
- X-rays negative but scaphoid fracture suspected: scaphoid plaster for two weeks and then repeat X-rays out of plaster.
- Confirm scaphoid fracture – undisplaced or displaced.
  Undisplaced: Scaphoid plaster and refer
  Displaced: Will need ORIF.
- Scaphoid plaster: Below elbow, wrist extended 30 degrees, thumb abducted and included in plaster up to but not including IPJ (so-called holding a wine glass position).

Figure 30.6 Undisplaced scaphoid fracture

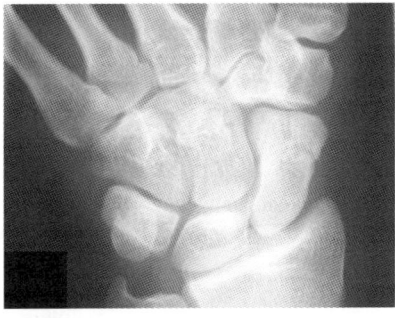

Open injuries

- Cutaneous barrier has been violated.
- Risk of infection.
- Clinical assessment followed by primary wound management is the key.

Assessment

- Deep laceration to dorsal aspect of hand or wrist invariably will damage extensor tendons.
- Do not be fooled by the ability to extend IP joints under intrinsic muscle control.
- Flexors: assess all nine long flexors to the digits.
- Nerves: test all nerves with pin prick and eyes closed (NB: Before injecting local anaesthetic).

- All open injuries should be X-rayed to exclude skeletal injury and/or foreign bodies.

Primary wound management

- Avoid the ubiquitous hand bath, which results in swollen hand with poor function.
- Remove all rings.
- Pour 2 litres of Ringer's lactate or at worst normal saline over and into wound.
- Cover with a sterile dressing.
- *Elevate* early – pillowslip hanging from a drip stand will suffice.
- Remember antibiotics and tetanus prophylaxis.

Management of the amputated part

- Wrap in a sterile gauze. Enclose and seal in sterile plastic bag.
- Place in container with water and *some* ice.
- Do not place human tissue in direct contact with ice – tissue destruction will occur and render part non-replantable.

Pitfalls

Avoid pitfalls by taking the following precautions:

- Refer all cut tendons and nerves.
- An open wound with an underlying fracture needs to be treated like any other compound fracture.
- If both digital nerves are cut on a digit, then suspect that both digital arteries have been transected – assess distal perfusion.
- *Never* blindly clamp a suspected arterial injury – nerves are always in close proximity.
- *Beware* the small laceration on the dorsum of the MPJs (knuckles) – suspect a human tooth laceration with penetration into the joint.

Recommended reading

Green, David P. (ed.) 1993. *Operative hand surgery.* Edinburgh: Churchill Livingstone.

31 Fractures and dislocations

Rory Harvey

A fracture can be defined as any breach of a bone's architecture.

Classification of fractures

Fractures can be classified in a number of ways, as described below.

Open or closed

'Open' refers to a fracture that communicates directly with the environment via a breach in the overlying skin and 'closed', which does not. This is of major importance in the assessment and treatment of fractures, as 'open' fractures are exposed to all the pathogens (e.g. bacteria) in the environment and are therefore at great risk of becoming infected.

The term 'compound' to denote an open fracture is ambiguous and therefore no longer used.

Extra-articular or intra-articular

The term 'intra-articular' means a fracture that involves a joint surface, and 'extra-articular' is used when a fracture does not involve a joint surface.

This is of clinical relevance, as fractures involving joint surfaces need to be perfectly reduced to allow smooth and even joint motion which in turn delays/prevents early onset (or secondary) osteoarthritis.

Anatomical location

Proximal, middle, or distal are used when referring to diaphyseal (shaft) fractures. Supracondylar (femur or humerus), subtrochanteric (hip), are used when referring to the fracture in relation to an anatomical landmark (e.g. lesser trochanter).

Fracture pattern

Fracture patterns are referred to as transverse, spiral, oblique, comminuted ('multifragmentary'), or compression (typically vertebrae).

Displaced or undisplaced

Undisplaced fractures tend to resemble the normal bony alignment and displaced fractures do not. In general, displaced fractures need to be manipulated into a better position and held in that position by means of either a plaster or a fixation device.

Stable or unstable

'Stable' refers to the ability of a fracture to maintain its position under a physiological (normal) load. This is clinically important in that no special method of immobilization is required. A good example of this is a wedge compression fracture of a single vertebra involving less than 25% of the vertebral height.

'Unstable' is quite simply the opposite and a good example of this would be a 'vertical shear' fracture of the pelvis.

Pathological fractures

Any of the above fracture types can occur in normal or abnormal (pathological) bone. The most common causes of abnormal bone are tumours (benign or malignant) and infection. Obviously much less force is required to fracture abnormal bone, compared with normal bone. Due to the poor bone quality, stable operative fixation is the gold standard.

Diagnosis

History

Try and determine the mechanism of injury. In motor vehicle accidents, try to get an idea of a) the speed of the car, b) whether the patient was in the front or back seat, and c) if a seatbelt was used. Ejection from the vehicle or death of another passenger in the same vehicle significantly increases the chances of serious injury. Always find out the time of the accident, as it is vital in the treatment of open fractures.

Examination

General examination

- A general examination is done according to ATLS® guidelines and will not be covered in this chapter. Suffice to say that the ABC of trauma needs to be assessed first, followed by regional orthopaedic management.

- The two potentially life-threatening orthopaedic injuries that need attention in the 'Primary Survey' are the cervical spine (C-spine) and pelvic fractures.

Local examination

- Obvious fractures do not need any specific diagnostic tests, but subtler fractures can be picked up by swelling, local tenderness, movement at the fracture site, and crepitus.
- All wounds near the suspected fracture site must be documented, especially where there is communication with the fracture itself (i.e. an open fracture).
- Two good tests for picking up difficult neck of femur fractures in the elderly/infirm are 'rolling' the patient's leg with the flat of the hand on the thigh and asking the patient to 'straight-leg raise'. Inability to do this should result in the patient being fully investigated to exclude a suspected fracture.

Distal examination

- This examination should entail a detailed neurovascular examination, to assess whether any nerves or vessels have been damaged near the fracture site. Disruption of the circulation to either the arm or leg constitutes an orthopaedic emergency and the patient must be taken to theatre urgently to restore blood flow.
- In all cases of suspected/documented fracture the limb must be assessed for the presence of compartment syndrome. This is especially common in the forearm and lower leg.

Special investigations

X-rays

- X-ray is the investigation of choice in trauma patients.
- The 'rule of two' provides an easy way of remembering what views need to be done and when.

Two views – AP and lateral in all cases

Two joints – visualization of the joints above and below the injury is mandatory

Two sides – especially important in the interpretation of children's fractures around the elbow, where ossification centres can confuse the inexperienced. X-ray the other 'normal' side for comparison if there is any doubt.

Two times – before and after treatment, e.g. plaster application or operative fixation.

Bone scan

Bone scan is important in cases where patients have given a history of trauma, are clinically suspected of having a fracture, and yet have a 'normal' X-ray. The best example of this would be a fall in a 70-year-old lady, followed by an inability to weight bear and straight leg raise on the affected leg.

CT/MRI

CT/MRI are more sophisticated investigations used either to screen for occult fractures or to provide additional information on the anatomy of complex fractures of the spine, pelvis, and joints.

Principles of fracture management

Rule number one is that the patient must first be treated as a whole, and this means prioritizing the order of treatment as given below.

Life threatening

Namely the ATLS® protocol of managing the 'ABCDE' of trauma.

Limb threatening

- Damage to the vascular supply of a limb, which can either be direct (e.g. severed artery), or indirect (compartment syndrome). Urgent repair (for the former) or decompression (the latter) must be done as soon as possible.
- Open fractures are also classified as limb threatening, in that they are prone to infection, which if left untreated will eventually lead to amputation. For this reason, debridement and lavage of the fracture site will need to be done as an emergency in theatre and under general anaesthetic.

The fracture itself

- The fracture must first be categorized into fractures that are in an acceptable (stable and undisplaced/minimally displaced) position and those that are not (i.e. fractures that are shortened, shifted, rotated, or twisted).
- The exact point at which a fracture position goes from acceptable to unacceptable varies according to the anatomical location and an experienced orthopaedic opinion must be obtained.

Acceptable – these are best treated by simple immobilization, e.g. below elbow plaster for an undisplaced, distal ulna fracture and buddy-strapping for minimally displaced metacarpal fractures.

Unacceptable – these will need to be reduced and held in that position until bony union. Reduction can either be closed or open method. By far the more preferable is closed reduction, as open reduction exposes the fracture to environmental organisms and hence infection.

Methods of management

Closed reduction and application of plaster. This remains the treatment of choice for the most common fracture worldwide, i.e. the Colles' fracture. Most displaced forearm and tibial fractures in children are managed in this way.

Closed reduction and percutaneous pin fixation. This method is used when plaster alone is not sufficient to hold a fracture reduced until bony union. A good example of this would be an unstable Colles' fracture, but is probably more commonly used in displaced supracondylar (of the elbow) fractures in children.

Closed reduction and intramedullary nail fixation. This remains the gold standard for femoral shaft fractures and is also widely used in tibial fractures. Under X-ray guidance the nail is passed from the piriform fossa, past the fracture site, to a point 3 cm above the knee joint. The nail is then secured to the bone (to prevent rotation) by means of two 'locking bolts' above and below the fracture site. Flexible nails are also very effective in treating unstable midshaft fractures in children.

Open reduction and pin/nail fixation. These are done in (b) and (c) where closed reduction is not possible, e.g. old fracture with shortening or where soft tissue interposition precludes closed reduction.

Open reduction and internal fixation (ORIF). This constitutes the most invasive means of fracture stabilization, as it exposes the fracture to both the environment and to foreign material. Despite this, it remains the treatment of choice for almost all displaced intra-articular fractures, and midshaft radius and ulna fractures in adults. Prophylactic intravenous antibiotics must be given for 24 hours in all such cases.

Methods of reduction

Direct reduction

With direct reduction, fracture is manipulated into position under direct vision, using bone-reducing instruments, e.g. bone lever/holder.

Indirect reduction

Indirect reduction involves traction, which can be skin (neck of femur fractures in the elderly) or skeletal (Cone's calipers for C-spine injuries, Denham pin through proximal tibia for femur shaft/acetabular fractures). Both the above can be static (pulley plus weight over end of bed) or dynamic (Thomas splint with balanced traction).

Treatment of common fractures

Upper limb

Colles' fracture
- This is an extra-articular fracture of the distal radius (within 2.5 cm of the wrist joint) and is the most common fracture junior doctors will have to treat.
- The typical Colles' fracture occurs most commonly in osteoporotic ladies over the age of 50, and is almost always due to a fall on the outstretched arm.
- Clinically the injured wrist is swollen, painful, and has a 'dinner-fork deformity'. Neurovascular damage needs to be excluded in all cases, especially signs of acute carpal tunnel syndrome (median nerve entrapment). Symptoms include numbness/pins and needles in the radial three and a half fingers and signs are decreased sensation in these fingers, with or without weakness of opponens pollicis.
- AP and lateral X-rays of the wrist show the following deformities:
  a Dorsal angulation (tilt) and translation (shift). Seen on lateral X-ray.

Figure 31.1 Colles' fracture on AP X-ray

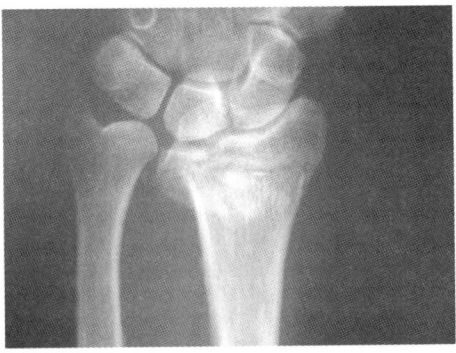

b Radial angulation and translation. Seen on AP X-ray.

c Impaction (shortening).

d Ulnar styloid fractures and disruption of the distal radio-ulnar joint (DRUJ) can occur.

- Treatment of displaced Colles' fractures is closed reduction and application of a below-elbow, moulded plaster. This is most commonly done under regional anaesthesia (Bier's block), but it can be done under general anaesthesia. Reduction involves the following steps:

  1 Sustain traction for 3–5 minutes.

  2 Increase the deformity to disimpact the fragments.

  3 Correct the deformities listed above by manipulating the distal fragment into slight flexion, ulnar deviation, and pronation.

- Failure to mould the plaster correctly after reduction will almost certainly lead to loss of reduction within one week. A post-reduction X-ray must be done in all cases to check the fracture position. It is even more important to check the neurovascular status of the hand within 12 hours, as the plaster does not allow for post-reduction swelling and compartment syndrome can lead to permanent neurovascular damage if left untreated. 'Splitting' the plaster while it is still wet is a very useful idea to avoid this complication.

- All patients will need to be X-rayed again at one week, as it is at this time that the swelling subsides and the fracture position is lost. Fracture union usually takes six weeks, but clinical signs of union (with the plaster off!) must be present before discharging the patient. Lastly, the patient should be referred to physiotherapy for gentle wrist mobilization.

Scaphoid fractures

- These fractures are common and a failure to recognize/treat them properly can lead to problems of delayed/non-union. Sixty-five per cent occur at the waist, 15% at the proximal pole, 10% distal pole, 2% distal articular surface, and 8% at the tuberosity.

- They typically occur in young adults after falling on the outstretched hand. The pathognomonic clinical sign is tenderness in the anatomical 'snuffbox' (at the base of the thumb, between the tendons of EPL on the ulna side and APB/EPB on the radial side).

- Standard X-rays of the wrist (AP and lateral) are not sufficient to view the scaphoid adequately. Special 'scaphoid views' must be requested.

- Treatment usually consists of eight weeks in a 'scaphoid plaster'. This comprises a below-elbow plaster with a thumb extension up to, but not including the interphalangeal joint (IPJ) of the thumb. To preserve the web-space between thumb and index finger, the plaster is applied with the hand in the 'glass-holding' position.

- A high index of suspicion is essential for diagnosing and treating this difficult fracture. In other words, any patient with wrist pain after a fall must be treated as a scaphoid fracture until proven otherwise.
- Never make the diagnosis of 'wrist sprain' in patients with snuffbox tenderness and a 'normal' X-ray. The gold standard of treating such patients would be to apply a scaphoid plaster and to repeat the X-ray in 10–14 days (with the plaster off!).
- At the same time the patient's wrist can be re-evaluated for snuffbox tenderness. If the X-ray is normal and the wrist is non-tender, no further treatment is required. However, if the X-ray is normal and the patient is still tender, further investigation is required (i.e. bone-scan, CT, or MRI).
- Due to the complexities of its blood supply, fractures of the scaphoid have a notorious reputation for delayed/non-union. These are either stable or unstable and are best treated by bone graft ± internal fixation.

Forearm fractures

Much like the pelvis, the radius and ulna (with the elbow joint above and wrist below) should be thought of as a 'closed loop'. Apart from a 'defence' fracture of the ulna, the loop is usually disrupted in two places (both bones or one bone and one joint).

1 Both radius and ulna

Midshaft fractures are generally displaced in the adult and are best treated by ORIF. In children, undisplaced fractures can be treated in an above-elbow plaster. Displaced fractures can still be reduced quite successfully under general anaesthetic. If the position can be maintained in plaster until bony union (three weeks), that is all that is necessary. If not, one further manipulation under anaesthesia can be tried, although insertion of flexible intramedullary nails may be a better option in cases where doubt over stability exists.

2 Ulna only

This fracture is also called a 'defence fracture' as it is usually caused by a direct blow to the raised forearm. Clinically it is very important to exclude an open fracture and to assess ulna nerve function. X-rays must include the joint above and below the injury, to exclude dislocations/damage to either the elbow or wrist. These fractures are normally stable and minimally displaced.

Distal third fractures (most common) can be treated with a below-elbow plaster, and fractures more proximally with an above-elbow plaster.

3 Ulna fracture and radial head dislocation (Monteggia)

Most cases involve a fracture of the proximal third of the ulna and anterior dislocation of the radial head (90%), but posterior dislocation (10%) also occurs. Clinically, injuries to associated nerves (radial and posterior interosseous) must be excluded, as they are damaged in up to 17% of cases. Closed reduction can be attempted in children, but ORIF is usually the treatment of choice in adults.

4 Radius fracture and DRUJ disruption (Galleazzi)

Here, the distal third of the radius is fractured and the distal radio-ulnar joint (DRUJ) is disrupted/dislocated. Clinically, neurovascular damage is rare, but one must look for signs of DRUJ disruption (prominent ulna head dorsally).

Closed reduction of this injury is very unsatisfactory and the treatment of choice is ORIF.

Figure 31.2 Monteggia fracture AP and lateral X-rays; note the ulna fracture (white arrow) and dislocation of the radial head (black arrow)

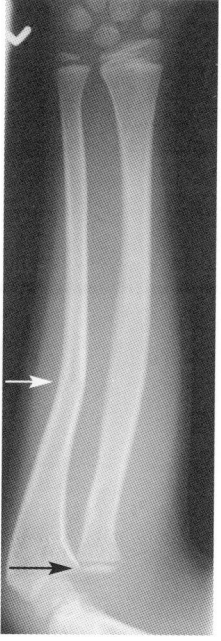 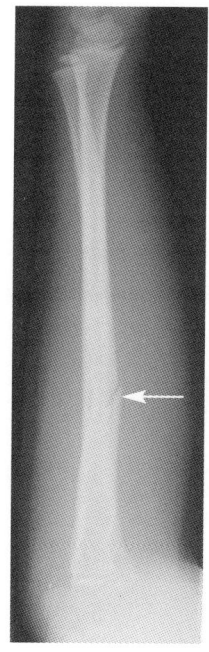

Elbow fractures

1 Radial head

This fracture usually causes far more pain around the elbow than one would expect for the size of the fracture. The most important signs clinically are tenderness directly over the radial head and pain when rotating the forearm.

The treatment for undisplaced/minimally displaced fractures is symptomatic only (analgesia and early mobilization). Cases that need operative intervention are best remembered by the 'rule of threes', i.e. 3 mm step in articular surface, > 30 degree tilt, and fracture involving more than 30% of the joint surface. Although modern fixation methods can be used in the simpler fractures, common sense must prevail in the complicated fractures and one should rather err on the side of replacing the radial head with a prosthesis.

2 Olecranon

Olecranon normally fractures transversely as a result of falling directly onto the elbow. Undisplaced fractures with an intact extensor mechanism can be managed conservatively. Displaced fractures with a disrupted extensor mechanism (patient is unable to extend elbow actively) are best treated operatively with tension band wiring.

3 Distal humerus

- Intra-articular fractures are usually seen in the over 50 age group and extra-articular fractures ('supracondylar') in children under the age of eight.

Figure 31.3 Galleazzi fracture AP and lateral X-ray; note fracture of the distal 1/3rd radius (white arrow) and dislocation of DRUJ

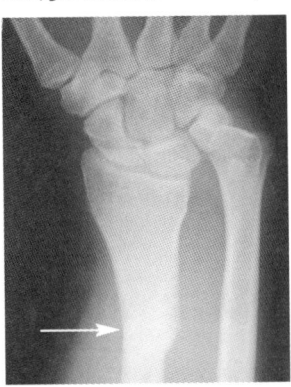
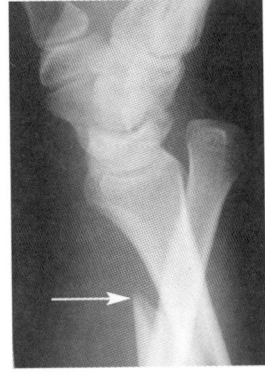

- Intra-articular fractures are best treated by ORIF, provided the bone is of sufficient quality for plate and screws.
- Extra-articular fractures in children are treated according to the grade of severity:

Grade one (minimally displaced) – i.e. posterior angulation of < 20 degrees. These can be managed conservatively in a collar and cuff.

Grade two (moderately displaced) – posterior angulation of > 20 degrees with discontinuity (separation) of the anterior cortex. These will need reduction under anaesthesia and if stable (and radial pulse present) after reduction, an above-elbow plaster can be applied with the forearm in full pronation. On the other hand, unstable fractures will need to be treated with 'cross K-wires'.

Grade three (severely displaced) – both cortices are not in continuity. The arm is usually very swollen. The median nerve and radial pulse need to be checked pre- and post-treatment. Treatment of choice here is closed reduction and cross K-wiring under general anaesthesia.

   Both grade two and three need to be treated *urgently* by an *experienced* orthopaedic surgeon.

Humeral shaft fractures
As an isolated injury, usually treated in a 'hanging cast' or 'U-slab'. If seen in a patient with other long-bone fractures, closed reduction and intramedullary nail fixation should be considered. Radial nerve function must be assessed (and documented!) before and after treatment.

Proximal humerus fractures
- Neer (1970) classified proximal humerus fractures into four 'parts':
   1   The humeral head
   2   The humeral shaft
   3   The greater tuberosity
   4   The lesser tuberosity.

In order for any of these to be considered 'a part', it must be more than 40 degrees rotated or more than 1 cm displaced. The axillary nerve must be evaluated in all cases.
- It is important to note that greater tuberosity fractures can be associated with anterior dislocations and lesser tuberosity fractures with posterior dislocations.
- In general, 85% of these fractures can be treated conservatively in a collar and cuff. The 2- and 3-part fractures need closed reduction and percutaneous K-wire (threaded) fixation. On the whole, 4-part fractures are best treated with a cemented hemi-prosthesis, where it is

absolutely essential to secure the fractured tuberosities onto the prosthesis, to preserve rotator cuff function.

Shoulder dislocations

- Shoulder dislocations are broadly categorized into anterior (90%) and posterior (10%). The lateral X-ray is of paramount importance in distinguishing which one of the two it is. Anterior dislocation can be caused by a direct blow to the humeral head, but is more commonly caused by forceful abduction and external rotation of the arm (seen in rugby tackles, kayaking, volleyball, etc).
- Diagnosis is made by the absence of the normal contour of the shoulder anteriorly and is confirmed on X-ray (AP, lateral, and axillary views).
- Treatment involves immediate reduction under sedation and a sling is used until pain free. Two common reduction methods are used:
  1 *Hippocratic method* – here the foot is placed in the patient's axilla and gradual longitudinal traction is applied to the arm (in full supination and 30 degrees abducted).

Figure 31.4 Anterior dislocation of the shoulder

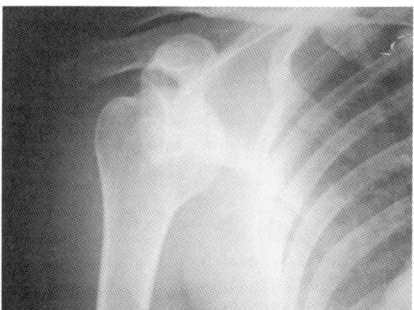

Figure 31.5 Basal fracture of the left femoral neck

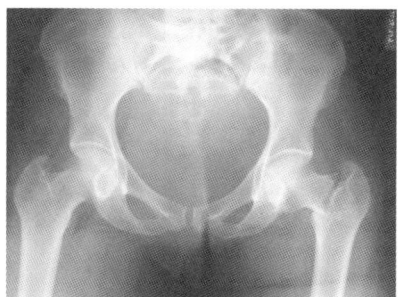

   2 *Kocher method* – traction is applied with the arm abducted and externally rotated. The arm is then adducted across the front of the body and internally rotated until a 'pop' is felt.

- Young patients who are actively involved in contact sport will often require operative stabilization at a later stage.
- Posterior dislocations are 1/10th as common and 10 times more difficult to diagnose. This is because the X-ray can look *normal* to the untrained eye. The give-away clinical sign is that the patient cannot externally rotate the arm past neutral. Two important X-ray signs are:
  1. The bulge of the greater tuberosity is lost and the humeral head looks like a 'light bulb'.
  2. Instead of the humeral head overlapping the glenoid on an AP X-ray, there is 'daylight' between the glenoid and the humeral head.

Lower limb

Femoral neck fractures

- These fractures are all intracapsular and are further sub-classified according to anatomical location:
  a   Subcapital
  b   Transcervical
  c   Basal.
- As most of these fractures occur in the elderly, the most important factor determining outcome is blood supply to the femoral head. In fractures where the blood supply is disrupted, avascular necrosis of the femoral head is much more likely to occur. The capsule of the hip joint attaches distal to the femoral neck and the main blood supply to the femoral head runs directly on the femoral neck. The direct correlation from this is that intracapsular fractures disrupt blood supply and extra-capsular fractures do not.
- As with all fractures, the patient must be assessed for other injuries and a proper neurovascular assessment of the affected limb must be done. As nearly 100% of these fractures are treated operatively, the patient's leg must be rested on a pillow and placed in non-adhesive skin traction, with a 5-pound weight over a pulley. This is purely for comfort and is not done to reduce the fracture. Non-adhesive material is used to prevent damage to the skin.
- All patients must be 'worked up' for a general anaesthetic, i.e. CXR, bloods for X-match, electrolytes, full blood count, and sometimes an arterial blood gas needs to be done.

A very brief outline of the orthopaedic management follows:

Subcapital – Undisplaced: Fixed with three partially threaded AO screws

Displaced: If patient is over 70 years and very frail, a Moore's hemiprosthesis is used. If between 50 and 70 years, a cemented 'bipolar' prosthesis is used. If under 50, an attempt is made to reduce the fracture (closed or open) and to stabilize with three screws.

Transcervical – Undisplaced: Dynamic Hip Screw ('DHS').

Displaced: Closed reduction and application of DHS. If closed reduction fails, treat as a 'displaced subcapital'.

Basal – Undisplaced: DHS

Displaced: Closed reduction and DHS.

Intertrochanteric fractures

- These are extracapsular fractures and therefore the femoral head is at very little risk of undergoing avascular necrosis. They occur in slightly younger patients compared with femoral neck fractures.
- They are subdivided into two main types:
  Stable – Two-part fracture with intact medial cortex. Ideally treated with a DHS.
  Unstable – Three- or four-part fracture with fragmentation of medial cortex. These are best treated with a DHS, DCS, or cephalomedullary nail.

Femoral shaft fractures

- These fractures mostly occur in young adults who have undergone major trauma. They are frequently associated with injuries elsewhere, e.g. knee ligaments and pelvis.
- At least 1–1.5 litres blood loss in isolated femoral shaft fracture, therefore haemorrhagic shock remains a very real risk. Intravenous access must be obtained and pulse and BP observations done regularly. An X-ray of the whole femur (including the hip and knee joint) must be done.
- If the patient is not going to theatre within the next 12 hours, skeletal traction must be applied. This is done by means of a Denham Pin placed through the proximal tibia. A Thomas splint is then applied and the limb placed into 'balanced traction'. This remains the method of choice for treating these fractures non-operatively, but this is rarely necessary with modern fixation techniques.
- Femoral shaft fractures are usually classified according to anatomical location:
  Proximal third – includes subtrochanteric fractures.

Middle third – includes midshaft fractures.

Distal third – includes supracondylar fractures.

- The 'Gold Standard' for treating both closed and open femoral shaft fractures is by means of an intramedullary nail (preferably with two locking bolts above and below the fracture to maintain length, alignment, and rotation). ORIF is used in the small percentage of fractures not amenable to an IM nail (a good example being a supracondylar fracture < 6 cm from the joint surface).

Intra-articular fractures distal femur

These fractures include condylar and intercondylar fractures. Both these require ORIF, as they involve the joint surface.

Patella fractures

- There are two mechanisms of injury:

  Direct trauma – mostly causes a multifragmentary/stellate fracture, where the patella is severely damaged, but the extensor mechanism can surprisingly be intact.

  Indirect trauma – resisted extension of partially flexed knee causes quadriceps muscle to transversely fracture the patella.

- By far the most important criterion governing the need for operative treatment is whether the extensor mechanism is intact or not (clinically tested by seeing whether the patient can hold his/her knee extended or not).

- A plaster cylinder is used in undisplaced fractures with an intact extensor mechanism. In displaced transverse fractures where the extensor mechanism is disrupted, operative stabilization is best done by means of tension band wiring. Displaced multifragmentary fractures with disruption of the extensor mechanism may be amenable to operative fixation, but if not, patellectomy remains a reasonable alternative (especially patients over 50).

Figure 31.6 Severe comminuted tibial plateau fracture

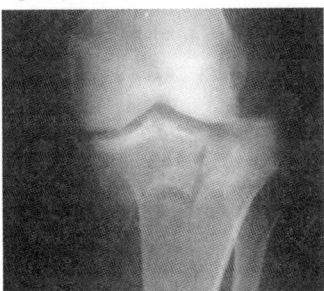

Tibial plateau fractures

- Usually caused by a direct valgus force to the knee, e.g. MVA or rugby/soccer tackle. For this reason, the lateral condyle is affected far more commonly than the medial. It is important to rule out damage to the lateral peroneal nerve and popliteal vessels, seen especially in medial condylar fractures Type (iv).
- Six types are described by Schatzker:
  1 *Vertical shear* – if displaced, best treated with two partially threaded cancellous screws. Undisplaced fractures treated with cast-brace.
  2 *Condylar depression* – more than 8 mm depression treated with bone graft, elevation, and fixation with buttress plate. Less than 8 mm requires cast brace.
  3 *Sheer and depression* – same as above.
  4 *Medial condyle* – if displaced, two partially threaded cancellous screws. Undisplaced fractures can be treated with a cast brace.
  5 *Bicondylar* – safest treatment is skeletal traction combined with early mobilization.
  6 Any of the above *plus* a fracture to the tibial shaft – important to fix the fracture fragments to the shaft with a plate and screws plus percutaneous screw fixation of the other condyle.

Tibial shaft fractures

- Almost the same management as femoral shaft fractures with the following important differences:
  a A significant percentage of closed tibial fractures can be managed successfully non-operatively (combination of plaster and cast brace).
  b Open tibial shaft fractures are better managed by means of an external fixator in inexperienced hands. IM nails can be used quite safely in open fractures, where there is no neurovascular damage (i.e. Gustilo grades 1, 2, and 3a).
  c Compartment syndrome is common in tibial fractures.
  d Vascularity and soft tissue cover is much less in the tibia, especially the distal 1/3. For this reason, morbidity (sepsis and non-union) is much higher in tibial fractures.
- In summary, closed tibial shaft fractures are best treated in plaster if an acceptable position can be maintained until bony union (at least 12 weeks). A good example would be a simple transverse midshaft fracture. A bad example would be a long oblique fracture which would ideally be treated with an IM nail.

- Open tibial fractures remain extremely common and are best treated by urgent wound debridement and stabilization of the fracture by either an external fixator or IM Nail, depending on the experience of the surgeon. Both these devices allow access to the soft tissues for dressings, skin grafting, and complex plastic reconstructive flaps.

Ankle fractures

- Probably the most common lower limb fracture. The stability of the ankle is determined by both bony and ligamentous structures. The distal tibia and fibula form an inverted 'U', into which the talus fits – allowing hinge movements in the AP plane. Ligamentous stability is provided medially by the deltoid ligament, laterally by the three bands of the lateral ligament, and between the tibia and fibula by the interosseous membrane and tibio-fibular syndesmosis.
- Ankle fractures and ligament injuries are ultimately caused by the talus and are most easily classified according to Weber. This is done very simply with the aid of an AP and lateral X-ray of the ankle and relies on the fact that a 'pull-off' injury causes a transverse fracture pattern, and a 'push-off' injury causes an oblique/spiral fracture pattern. Rupture of the syndesmosis is assumed when there is separation (diastasis) between the tibia and fibula.
- *Weber A* – The talus moves inwards as a result of an inversion/adduction injury. This causes a short oblique fracture of the medial malleolus and a tear of the lateral ligament. The syndesmosis remains intact.
- *Weber B* – The talus moves outwards as a result of an eversion/abduction injury. This is the most common type of ankle fracture and causes a transverse fracture of the medial malleolus and oblique fracture of the lateral malleolus. Part of the syndesmosis may be ruptured.
- *Weber C* – The talus moves out and around from an abduction and external rotation injury. The syndesmosis is always ruptured, and the fibula fracture is spiral and a few centimetres proximal to the ankle joint. The medial malleolus is fractured transversely at the level of the ankle joint.
- Tibial plafond fractures are caused by the talus moving upwards at a force, which is normally much greater than that seen in ankle fractures. Here, soft tissue swelling is often more dangerous than the fracture itself and is best dealt with by urgent orthopaedic referral.
- Non-operative treatment of ankle fractures involves:
  1 Reduction under sedation/general anaesthesia, and
  2 Maintenance of reduction by means of plaster until bony union (6–8 weeks). A below-knee plaster is used for Weber A and B fractures, and an above knee plaster is used for Weber C fractures. ORIF is necessary when an acceptable reduction cannot be maintained.

- An acceptable reduction of an ankle fracture involves the following:
  - Perfect tibio-talar congruity
  - Less than 3 mm fibular shortening
  - Less than 2 mm of diastasis
  - Posterior malleolar fractures of less than 20% can be ignored, even if displaced.

Management of open fractures

- By definition, open fractures communicate directly with the outside and therefore come into contact with all the bacteria etc. present in the environment. This subsequently places the fracture ends at significant risk of becoming infected. For this reason, all potentially 'open' fractures should be given antibiotics (for 24 hours) and tetanus toxoid, as well as have a betadine dressing placed on the wound before being taken to theatre.
- If open fractures are left untreated, they can lead to loss of limb/life. This, therefore, constitutes an orthopaedic emergency and the patient will need to be taken to theatre immediately for debridement (removing dead tissue from fracture site and irrigating with 6 litres saline) under general anaesthetic. This should preferably be accompanied by stabilization of the fracture, in order to place the fracture ends in the correct position whilst the soft tissues heal. The preferred methods of fracture stabilization in open fractures are IM (intramedullary) nails and external fixators. The use of a plate and screws should be avoided if possible as their placement often causes further devitalization of the fracture ends and they also act as foreign material at the fracture site. It is also very important not to try and close wounds that are > 2 cm at the first operation. This can lead to devitalization of the skin and/or sepsis.
- Plastic surgery (e.g. skin grafting and placement of flaps) is often essential in the treatment of open fractures as there is frequently insufficient skin to cover the fracture ends. These are usually done at the second operation, which is 48 hours after the first. Fracture stabilization is once again very important as it allows minimal movement at the fracture site and this in turn results in better healing and less infection.

Complications of fracture

Life threatening

Hypovolaemic shock
Bleeding can either be external, e.g. through a wound in an open fracture or internal, where the bleeding occurs into a body cavity (e.g. pelvis

fractures) or into a potential space, e.g. around the fracture in femoral fractures. Bleeding can be caused by the fracture ends itself or from an arterial/venous injury.

Damage to viscera
The bladder and bowel can easily be perforated by fracture fragments in pelvic fractures, and it is therefore important to look for haematuria and to do a rectal examination in all pelvic fractures.

Spinal cord damage
Spinal cord damage can cause death if there is an unstable high cervical fracture that is not identified.

Fat embolus syndrome (FES)
FES causes a TRIAD of: (1) hypoxia from ARDS, (2) confusion, and (3) petechiae 24–72 hours after a long-bone or pelvic fracture. The fat is thought to come from the fracture site and/or damaged adipose tissue. Any patient clinically suspected of having FES should have urgent blood gases and a CXR. If hypoxia is confirmed the patient should be transferred to an ICU for oxygenation and fluid resuscitation. Fracture stabilization is also vital in the treatment.

Limb threatening

Arterial injuries
- All fractures must be properly assessed for neurovascular damage before and after treatment. The absence of a pulse distally must be treated as an emergency. The first step in the management is to reduce the fracture and to reassess the distal perfusion. If this is still absent after 10–20 minutes, an urgent arteriogram (Doppler of no use!) must be requested and a vascular surgeon consulted.
- Fractures/dislocations at high risk of vascular injury:
  1. Knee dislocation
  2. Medial condyle tibial plateau fracture (Schatzker 4)
  3. Supracondylar humeral fracture.

Compartment syndrome
Compartment syndrome is defined as an increase in pressure within an osteo-fascial compartment to a level above that of the capillary perfusion pressure. If not relieved by fasciotomy, it will eventually result in necrosis of muscles and nerves within that compartment.

Outpatient plaster management and pitfalls

The Ten Commandments

1 Always use sufficient padding for the entire length of the plaster, with slightly more being necessary over bony prominences and potential pressure areas, e.g. the heel.

2 Day one after plaster application, check whether it is too tight. Swelling continues after plaster dries, leading to compartment syndrome.

3 In cases where the plaster is thought to be too tight, release the entire length of both the plaster *and* padding.

4 Week one after plaster application, check whether it is too loose! The swelling seen soon after a fracture tends to subside, leaving the plaster too big.

5 A plaster must *always* be changed if thought to be too loose.

6 X-rays must *always* be done after plaster application to check the position of the fracture.

7 *Never* ignore a patient who complains of pain underneath the plaster. There is *always* a legitimate cause for this.

8 Below-knee plaster is generally required for ankle fractures (Weber A and B) and fractures distal to the ankle. Weber C ankle fractures and fractures proximal to this require an above-knee plaster.

9 Likewise, a below-elbow plaster is necessary for wrist fractures, while fractures proximal to this require an above-elbow plaster.

10 *Never* apply a circumferential plaster to an elbow fracture. Swelling is particularly severe in fractures around the elbow, and the risk of compartment syndrome is too high to apply a plaster safely.

Reference

Neer, C. S. 1970. Displaced proximal humeral fractures. Classification and evaluation. *Journal of Bone and Joint Surgery*, 82:204–210.

Recommended reading

McRae, R., Kinninmonth, A. W. G. 1997. *Orthopaedics and trauma.* Edinburgh: Churchill Livingstone.

PART 3

Special patients and problems

32 Trauma in the elderly

Basil Bonner

Trauma in the elderly is a growing concern for a number of important reasons. In the USA, the elderly constitute 12% of the population, yet consume 33% of the health-care resources spent on the management of trauma and its consequences. Among South Africans over 65 years of age, trauma is the fifth leading cause of death and will become more prominent as the Aids epidemic takes its toll on the younger generation.

The elderly are, in general, less active, and are therefore less exposed to trauma. When injured, however, they suffer disproportionately worse complications, and are six times more likely to die from their injuries compared to younger patients with similar injuries. They therefore require a higher index of suspicion for injury, with more intense monitoring and resuscitation, in order to reduce morbidity and mortality. Their in-hospital mortality rate is 15–30% versus the 4–8 % for the younger population.

Factors that influence injury likelihood and outcome

Physical changes in the elderly

- Posture becomes stooped and the centre of balance is shifted.
- Balance is affected by different factors, which include peripheral proprioception, cerebellar function, and oculo-vestibular integrity.
- Motor strength diminishes with age, especially if exercise was insufficient in life.
- Coordination is primarily determined by the integrity of the cerebellar system and its connections.
- Deterioration of visual acuity due to degenerative changes of the lens, macula, and retina are often underrated, and may significantly affect the visual cueing that facilitates balance and coordination.

Commonly encountered co-morbidity in the elderly

Some diseases that may co-exist with the trauma are:

- Ischaemic heart disease
- Arrhythmias
- Metabolic conditions such as diabetes
- Conditions that result in impaired physiological compensatory mechanisms
- Postural hypotension

Pre-injury medications

Medications, especially those likely to aggravate the effects of hypovolaemia (beta blockers and anti-hypertensives), may interfere with physiological responses, or worsen the effects of trauma.

Reduced physiological reserves

Cardiac output in the old elderly (80+ years) is approximately 50% of that of a 20-year old, thus making compensation less effective, and the effects of blood loss more pronounced.

Causes of injury in the elderly

The types of injuries seen in the elderly are generally the same as those seen in younger patients, however, the causes and frequencies differ.

Motor vehicle accidents

The elderly are more likely to be involved in accidents closer to home, during the day, and during good weather. (They are also more likely to be at fault.) The over 75-year age group is second only to 16–25 year olds in the frequency of accidents (relative to the number of drivers).

They also show a much lower incidence of alcohol (6% vs 23%) usage than that found in younger drivers. Age-related physiological factors play a role instead.

Falls

Falls constitute the most common cause of injury in the over 75-year old age group. Twenty-five per cent of falls result in injury with resultant loss of function or loss of mobility. Approximately 50% of geriatric patients hospitalized for traumatic fractures die within one year.

Violence

Violence accounts for up to 14% of admissions in the elderly population of the USA, with a 4% elder abuse profile. In South Africa these figures are likely to be much higher, but accurate statistics are currently not available. One should maintain a high index of suspicion for elder abuse when assessing older patients presenting with trauma.

Recognizing elder abuse

The following factors may indicate abuse:
- A long delay between incident and presentation
- An inconsistent history of the events
- Caregiver dominance at the consultation
- Repeated admissions for similar incidents
- Cigarette burns
- Signs of restraint

Management

Factors that influence the management of trauma in the elderly

- Diminished cardiac reserve
- Decreased sensitivity to catecholamines, with reduced compensatory tachycardia
- Decreased pulmonary compliance with associated decreased mucociliary clearance
- 30–40% decrease in glomerular function by 65 years

Emergency Unit management

Follow ATLS® principles of resuscitation, bearing in mind the complicating factors given below.

Airway

Endotracheal intubation may be more difficult due to brittle or absent teeth, dentures, limited temperomandibular joint mobility and poor glottic visualization.

Breathing

- Smaller tidal volumes (6–8 ml/kg) are required, more frequent arterial blood gas and end-tidal CO_2 monitoring should be done.
- Chest injury is more devastating due to diminished TV, FEV_1, and decreased functional reserve.
- Osteoporosis and increased chest-wall rigidity implies an increased risk of rib and sternal fractures.
- Blunt chest trauma almost always requires admission, irrespective of how innocuous it seems at first.
- Atelectasis readily occurs from hypoventilation due to diaphragmatic splinting, resulting in the development of pneumonia.

- The side-effects of systemic analgesics may necessitate early thoracic epidural or paravertebral nerve block to ensure adequate pain control.
- Always consider early transfer to ICU, and have a low threshold for invasive monitoring.

Circulation
- Assessment of vital signs could be clouded by inappropriate physiological response to catecholamines.
- Systemic vascular resistance (SVR) may be increased even in the presence of hypotension.
- ECG must be done to differentiate between myocardial contusion and infarct.

Disability
- The elderly have a poorer outcome with head injury.
- Cortical atrophy implies greater likelihood of larger subdural haematoma and later presentation.
- Subdural haematoma in the elderly is three times more common than extradural haematoma.
- All anaesthetic induction agent doses need to be reduced by 20–40% (benzodiazepines, barbiturates, etomidate).

Outcome of blunt trauma

Mortality

In a sample of 100 geriatric trauma survivors, 65% were returned to good health, 50% went back to normal levels of activity, 50% returned to their own homes, 25% became permanently institutionalized, and 20% were financially ruined.

Factors that increase mortality

- Rising age (16% mortality in age 65–74, vs 21% if age > 74)
- Male gender
- Respiratory rate abnormal on presentation (< 10 or > 30)
- Hypotension on presentation is associated with 75% mortality
- Glasgow Coma Scale < 12 is associated with 50% mortality, while GCS < 6 has a mortality > 80%

Pitfalls

- Failure to prevent the complications of hospitalization (more common than in younger patients).

- Failure to prevent multi-organ dysfunction (MODS), which may lead to respiratory, renal, and cardiovascular failure.
- Failure to provide adequate pain control.
- Extubating too early.
- Delayed fracture fixation – fat embolism may be less common, but more devastating.
- Morbidity and mortality are higher in the elderly, and should be anticipated and prevented by having a high index of suspicion for injury.
- Each patient should be evaluated and managed aggressively, with the goal of early return to functional living.
- A low threshold is required for invasive monitoring and transfer to ICU.

References and recommended reading

Hazzard, W.R., Blass, J.P., Ettinger, W.H. Jr., Halter, J.B., (eds.) 1999. *Principles of Geriatric Medicine and Gerontology*. Fourth edition. New York: McGraw-Hill.

Linder, J., Fleming, A. 2001. Trauma in the elderly. *Clinical Geriatics*, 3.

Scalea, T., Kohl, L. 1991. Geriatric trauma, in D. Feliciano (ed.) *Trauma*. Third edition. Connecticut: Appleton & Lange.

Wright, A., Schurr, M. 1999. Geriatric trauma: Review and recommendations. *World Medical Journal*.

33 The injured child

A B (Sebastian) van As

The successful management of the injured child requires that there be an organized team approach with frequent review of the response to treatment, a designated team leader and adherence to advanced paediatric life-support principles (APLS®).

The injured child differs from an adult in three main respects:

1 Types and patterns of injury sustained
- Injuries are predominantly blunt trauma.
- Multiple and multi-system injury is common.
- Severe injuries are more often concealed than revealed.
- Be aware of non-accidental injury (medico-legal, social implications).

2 Anatomical features
The following features apply to children:
- Small size – requires appropriate resuscitation equipment and techniques (venous access).
- Fluid volumes and drug dosages – calculate according to weight.
- Relatively large head – frequently injured.
- Thin integument plus high surface:weight ratio – risk of rapid heat loss and increased oxygen demands.
- Immature upper respiratory tract – obligate nose-breathing under six months of age.
- Soft bones with poor protection of the viscera. Open epiphysis with a high incidence of growth-plate injuries until adolescence.

3 Physiological responses
- Ventilation – high oxygen consumption, low functional residual capacity (FRC), therefore increased right to left shunting.
- Circulation – increased physiological reserve, so vital signs (BP, pulse) are often normal despite significant fluid loss.
- Shock with lowering of the blood pressure is a pre-terminal event in children. Adequate perfusion is maintained for a long period. When the physiological condition has worsened to the extreme, collapse occurs and resuscitation is often futile.

- Post-paediatric trauma deaths are immediate. Survival in hospital depends on vigorous, adequate resuscitation, and diligent assessment of injuries performed simultaneously by the trauma team.

Initial assessment and resuscitation

Adapt the 'ABCD' approach to the specific needs of children.

Airway

Give supplemental oxygen early by nasal prongs (over six months of age) or mask (less than six months).

- With stridor or central cyanosis, check for inhaled foreign body – place head down, slap on back, perform the Heimlich manoeuvre in older children.
- Avoid over-extension of neck (kinking of trachea, possible cervical spine injury) and pressure on floor of mouth (tongue falls back).
- Insert an oral airway only if the gag reflex is absent.
- For endotracheal intubation, use a straight-blade laryngoscope for under one year; uncuffed endotracheal tube (ET) of size to allow small air leak.
- Use needle cricothyroidotomy (16-gauge cannula) if the upper airway is compromized (the airway is too small under 10 years to perform a surgical cricothyroidotomy).

Breathing

Assess the breathing clinically (respiratory rate, colour, auscultation), on blood gases and pulse-oximetry (oxygen saturation should be over 95%).

- When ventilation is inadequate, exclude aspiration (vomitus, foreign body), ET tube in oesophagus, tension pneumothorax (clinical diagnosis), flail segment, rupture of the diaphragm, or splinting of diaphragm from acute gastric dilatation.
- The most common cause of respiratory failure is a depressed level of consciousness from head injury.
- Place prophylactic intercostal chest drains on side of injury if the patient requires ventilation or general anaesthetic.

Circulation

Control any haemorrhage early where possible by splinting fractures and direct pressure over external bleeding.

- The normal systolic blood pressure (BP) = 80 mmHg + (2 × age in years).

- The pulse rate is often a better indicator than blood pressure.
- Note the trends in pulse rate and blood pressure rather than single values.
- Asystole – then external cardiac massage.
- Emergency room thoracotomy is not indicated in blunt trauma.
- Assess fluid loss according to peripheral colour, temperature, capillary refill, and sensorium.
- Blood pressure and haemoglobin are poor guides to degree of blood loss.
- Do not delay IV fluid replacement until vital signs deteriorate.
- IV access – peripheral cannula, femoral vein push-in, saphenous vein cut-down (ankle), intra-osseous (tibial) infusion.
- Avoid central venous catheterization – high morbidity unless CVP measurement required. (Internal jugular vein, never the subclavian vein.)
- Draw blood for X-match, full blood count, arterial blood gas and serum amylase if abdominal trauma suspected.
- Commence IV replacement with 20–40 ml/kg balanced salt solution – follow with packed RBC; immediate O-negative blood is seldom necessary.

Failure to respond to fluid resuscitation

- Consider pneumothorax, cardiac contusion, and exsanguinating intra-abdominal bleeding requiring urgent laparotomy.
- Monitor response to resuscitation – Hb, HR, BP, and urine output (+CVP if 40%+ blood loss). Place naso/oro-gastric tube, indwelling urinary catheter, and request X-rays of cervical spine, chest, and pelvis.

Disability

A closed head injury is common in children. Obtain an early baseline assessment of neurological status.

Is the patient Alert, responding to Vocal stimuli, only Painful stimuli, or Unresponsive? ('AVPU' scale).

Assess pupils for size, equality, and response to light in order to screen for focal injuries.

Normal paediatric values			
	Infants	Pre-school	Scholar
Heart rate/min	120–140	100–120	80–100
BP Systolic	70–90	80–90	90–110
Resp. rate/min	30–40	20–30	15–20
Blood Vol ml/kg	90	80	80

Secondary survey and management

General principles

- Remove all clothing to avoid missing injuries but also avoid excessive heat loss (infants – warming blankets, overhead heaters).
- Do not neglect to monitor vital signs while examining for injuries.
- Analgesia – paracetamol, tilidine (Valeron®) for axial injuries. Morphine (0.2 mg/kg in 20 ml 5% Dextrose) by slow infusion for trunk injuries or post-surgery.

Head and neck

- Primary injury – irreversible. Secondary injury (brain swelling, cerebral oedema) is common – prevent by early, adequate resuscitation, oxygenation, and hyperventilation ($PaCO_2$: 3.5–4.0 kPa).
- Raised intracranial pressure – watch for SIADH (low Na^+, high urinary specific gravity).
- Intra-cranial haematomas – clinical signs are subtle compared with adults – watch carefully for changes in level of consciousness, abnormal behaviour.
- Basilar skull fractures involving anterior cranial fossa – there is a small but clinically significant risk of bacterial meningitis. Use of prophylactic antibiotics is controversial. Perform CSF culture early if signs of meningeal irritation develop.
- CT scan – indicated as for adults.
- Non-penetrating C-spine injuries are uncommon, mostly at C1/C2. If there is doubt – X-ray in flexion. Significant cord injury can occur without fractures ('SCIWORA'). Be familiar with anatomic variants in children.

Thorax

- Majority of injuries are minor – rib fractures, small pulmonary contusions.

- Most pleural collections are small effusions – drain only if clinically indicated (splinting, dyspnoea, underlying atelectasis).
- Ruptured diaphragm, cardiac contusion – less common, but life-threatening. Diagnose clinically, and X-ray on high index of suspicion.
- Give supplemental oxygen whether symptomatic or not.
- IV morphine (see above) for rib fractures.

Abdomen

- Ensure that the stomach is deflated before physical examination.
- Intra-peritoneal haemorrhage (liver, spleen, kidney) – usually self-limiting. Watch vital signs, circulatory shock will precede abdominal distension. Surgery is indicated for massive or ongoing haemorrhage.
- Ruptured viscus and peritonitis – surgery based primarily on clinical impression/deterioration in signs (free air on initial X-ray in only 10%).
- IVP is necessary for all children with macroscopic haematuria or loin mass/tenderness suggesting significant renal injury.
- CT scan is seldom indicated in acute phase as the need for surgery is a clinical decision.
- Diagnostic peritoneal lavage – not indicated in vast majority and compromises subsequent clinical examination.
- Laparoscopy in case of a possible intra-abdominal (old) injury: Fibrin and/or pus? In selected cases laparoscopic (assisted) repairs.

Musculo-skeletal

- Epiphysis (cartilaginous growth plate) is the weakest part of musculo-skeletal system – growth plate fractures are common; sprains and ligament injuries are rare before adolescence.
- Beware of compartment syndrome following reduction of supra-condylar fractures of the humerus or fractures around the knee joint (pain on passive extension of wrist, or dorsiflexion of the foot). Early (open) fasciotomy of all compartments if suspected.
- Compound fractures – early debridement and systemic antibiotics are the cornerstones of preventing bone and soft-tissue sepsis.
- Possible vascular injury – on-table angiography followed by exploration and repair if indicated.

Non-accidental injury

Suspect non-accidental injury where:
- There is a delay in seeking medical care.
- History is unforthcoming, vague, or inconsistent with type or degree of injury.

- Multiple hospital attendances for minor complaints.
- Obvious injuries – cigarette burns, bruising away from bony prominences, perianal or genital injury.
- Multiple injuries in various stages of healing or incidentally diagnosed (skeletal survey).
- Diagnostic features such as bucket-handle fractures.
- Consult with social worker, Child Protection Unit, or childcare agency before confronting parent(s).
- Complete the necessary documentation in order to contribute optimally to the judicial process.

Pitfalls

- Not following APLS® principles.
- Not undressing and examining the whole patient.
- Underestimating shock due to compensatory mechanisms.
- Missing concurrent multiple injuries.
- Contributing circulatory shock to head injury (although this is possible in a small child with a relatively large head, it is unusual, and a cause for the shock always has to be searched for).
- Not communicating adequately with parents and child caretakers.

Recommended reading

Sanchez, J., Paidas, C. N. 1999. Childhood trauma now and in the new millennium. *Surgical Clinics of North America,* 79:1503–1540.

Stylianos, S. 1998. Late sequelae of major trauma in children. *Pediatric Clinics of North America,* 45:853–860.

34

Trauma in pregnancy

Jones Omoshoro-Jones

Trauma is the leading cause of non-obstetric maternal death in South Africa. It involves 3% of females admitted to a trauma unit, and accounts for 6% of the complications seen in pregnancy. Nearly 70% of cases seen are victims of non-accidental injury, and interpersonal violence during pregnancy is a significant cause of maternal and foetal morbidity and mortality. Foetal outcome is very dismal, with a 61% mortality rate.

General principles

The initial treatment priorities are similar to those for non-pregnant women. Specific management principles pertaining to the pregnant woman are given below.

Identification of the circumstances surrounding the event

Repetitive injuries account for 60% of trauma related to domestic violence. As with child abuse, this information must be identified, documented, and reported as appropriate.

Awareness of incidental pregnancy

Pregnancy unsuspected by the woman or trauma physicians occurs in 8%–11% of cases. Early recognition of pregnancy by use of an emergency-room urine screening pregnancy test (pregnosticon) in all women admitted to hospital, followed by pelvic ultrasonography if positive, is therefore imperative.

Impact of changes in pregnancy

The associated anatomic and physiologic changes (Table 34.1) impact significantly on the management of the patient as signs and symptoms of injury, responses to resuscitation, as well as the result of diagnostic tests, are altered. Maternal resuscitation impacts on foetal outcome. An aggressive and active management policy should be instituted early. Injured pregnant women should be managed in a facility with advanced trauma care and obstetrics capabilities.

Table 34.1 Physiological changes in pregnancy

Uterine:
- Progressive enlargement; at symphysis pubis by 12 weeks, umbilicus by 20 weeks, costal margin by 36 weeks.
- Initially protective, foetus vulnerable as wall thins with stretching and amniotic fluid decreases.

Musculoskeletal:
- Decreased elasticity of ligaments, joints and muscles: pubic symphysis and sacro-iliac joints widen.

Gastro-intestinal:
- Cephalad displacement of bowels by growing uterus.
- Decreased gastric volume and generalized gut hypomotility predispose to reflux, early satiety and vomiting with increased risk of aspiration.

Haematological:
- Relative anaemia. Absolute leucocytosis.
- Hypercoagulability state predisposes to disseminated intravascular coagulopathy and thrombotic events.

Cardiovascular system:
- Increased intravascular volume. Relative anaemia.
- Progressive tachycardia: heart rate – 20 beats faster than pre-pregnancy state. Hence decreased sensitivity of pulse rate as sign of shock.
- Cardiac output increased by > 1.5 litre/min at 10 weeks. BP drops by – 15 mmHg in second trimester. Hence relative hypotension.
- Supine hypotension common due to above and compression of IVC by gravid uterus.

Respiratory system:
- Mild tachypnoea, elevated tidal volume, relative hypocapnea by third trimester.
- Increased O_2 consumption, splinting of diaphragm, with above, impact on respiratory drive and reserve.

Renal system:
- Glomerular filtration rate and renal blood flow increased, with serum urea and creatinine levels halved compared to pre-pregnancy levels.

Management

See Figure 34.1 on page 365.

Resuscitation

Specifics of note here are:
- Hypovolaemic shock may be masked by changes in pregnancy. As a result of the increased blood volume associated with pregnancy, hypotension is a late feature of shock. Look at peripheral perfusion, urine output, and the haemoglobin level. Central venous pressure measurements with fluid boluses may be indicated to establish an adequate intravascular volume.

Figure 34.1 Clinical evaluation of the injured pregnant patient

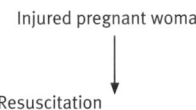

Injured pregnant woman

↓

Resuscitation

- A, B, C, D, E
- Resuscitation same as for non-pregnant woman
- Essential X-rays (C-spine, chest, pelvis, as required)

↓

Secondary survey (full clinical examination)

- Abdomen: Palpate size of uterus
            Estimate foetal age
            Presence of contractions
            Uterine irritability
            Auscultate foetal heart rate
- Pelvis   – palpate
- Vaginal   – ruptured membranes
             Bleeding
- Urine test, β HCG, ultrasound
- Completion of radiological investigations

↓

Definitive management

- After excluding a spinal cord injury, prevent supine hypotension by applying a tilt to the right side of the mother's pelvis with a towel. This shifts the side of the gravid uterus off the IVC, ensuring reasonable venous return for optimal cardiac function.
- Prevent hypothermia: transfuse or infuse warm fluids, blood or products. Avoid over-exposure. Cover-up patient warmly using space blankets or warming blankets.
- Use type-specific blood to avoid Rhesus iso-immunization.

Medications

- Intubation: Short-acting benzodiazepine such as midazolam (Dormicum®) recommended. Foetal depression is minimized or avoided (especially if in third trimester and emergency delivery may be required).
- Analgesia: Small doses (1–2 mg/kg) of morphine intravenously.
- Antibiotics/anti-tetanus prophylaxis: Administer as appropriate. Avoid aminoglycosides in first and second trimester. Third generation

cephalosporins (e.g. cefuroxime 750 mg) in combination with metronidazole or co-amoxiclavulinate (Augmentin® 1.2 g) provide good coverage.

- Avoid vasopressors: A shocked patient needs fluids not adrenaline, dopamine, or phenylephrine! Injudicious use of these agents in an injured pregnant woman may result in a calamitous decrease in uterine blood flow with decreased placental perfusion and consequent foetal loss from hypoxia.

Blood tests:
- ABG, U & E estimation
- ß-HCG analysis (if urine pregnancy test is equivocal)
- Blood grouping, typing and cross-match, Coomb's test DIC screen is very important as placental abruption predisposes to DIC in severe trauma.

Radiology: Pregnancy does not preclude acquisition of important films such as cervical spine, chest, and pelvic X-rays in a severely injured woman. Lead shields are available to prevent undue foetal X-irradiation.

Secondary survey and further management

- Haemodynamically unstable patients require resuscitative surgery.
- Stable patients are treated as per outcome of the secondary survey and special investigations ordered. Further treatment is tailored towards the over-riding clinical problem, i.e. trauma surgical or obstetrics.

Intra-abdominal injuries: Acute abdominal signs are notoriously marred in pregnancy. Suspect an intra-abdominal injury in the setting of:
- Polytrauma
- Any penetrating trauma
- Shock refractory to resuscitation
- Decreasing Hb despite blood transfusion

Uterine rupture: Clinical features consist of:
- Abdominal pain (provided normal level of consciousness)
- Inability to palpate fundal height
- Easy palpation of foetal parts

Abruptio placentae: Clinical features are:
- Abdominal pain
- Irritable uterus
- Vaginal bleeding

Pelvic examination: Pre-requisites: sterile condition. Note any perineal wound, laceration, contusion, or bleeding. Liquor may be detected with use of nitrazine dipstix analysis (liquor has pH of 7, vaginal fluid pH 5). A positive nitrazine test suggests ruptured membranes.

Specialized treatment

The indications for laparotomy are outlined in the box below.

Indications for laparotomy
- Evidence of intra-peritoneal haemorrhage: haemodynamic instability
- Acute abdomen
- Unexplained or refractory shock
- Spinal cord injury with an inability to assess the abdomen clinically as a result
- Penetrating trauma
- Failed non-operative management

Obstetrics and foetal considerations

Confirmation of the pregnancy using pelvic ultrasonography
- Determination of gestational age (GA)
- Assessment and estimation of foetal viability

Foetal viability. GA of 24 weeks may be compatible with life with appropriate management. Generally, however, a GA of 28 weeks or a birth weight of 1 000 g and above are considered as most compatible with life.

Assessment of viability
- Clinically: history of movements and determine fundal height
- U/S: assessment of GA, lie, presentation of foetus, placental position, amniotic fluid volume, and the presence of retro-placental clot.

Cardiotocography. This monitors foetal condition. Foetal distress is characterized by abnormally frequent uterine contractions (about 10 per 10 minutes) resulting in late decelerations and foetal tachycardia with reduced variability or the characteristic sine-wave pattern. Foetal distress may signify placenta abruptio. In the absence of foetal distress, delivery may be expedited in a severely injured mother with the use of steroids to promote foetal lungs maturity. In the presence of foetal distress, delivery should promptly follow aggressive maternal resuscitation and stabilization. Table 34.2 outlines the predictors of foetal mortality.

Table 34.2 Predictors of foetal mortality in pregnant trauma patients

Foetal factors:	Maternal factors:
• Gestational age (50% at 26 weeks)	• Hypotension/haemorrhage
• Gestational weight (< 750 gm, 90%; > 750 gm, 40%)	• Injury severity score > 25
• Foetal heart rate < 110 beats/min	• Acidosis
• Abruption placenta	• DIC

Conclusion

Trauma in pregnancy is a significant event. Optimal management remains difficult and challenging, as well as fraught with many pitfalls.

Early recognition of the pregnant state in all injured women of child-bearing age, knowledge of the changes in pregnancy, the peculiar responses of the pregnant woman to shock, the mechanism of injury, and early institution of aggressive resuscitation efforts, coupled with early involvement of a qualified trauma surgeon and obstetrician, are the requisites to guarantee the best possible outcome for the injured mother and her foetus.

Pitfalls

• Not realizing that a female trauma patient is pregnant. All females admitted to an emergency unit between the ages of 12 to 45 must be screened for pregnancy.

References reading

Daponte, A., Khan, N., Smith, M. D., Degiannis, E. 2003. Trauma in pregnancy. *SAJS*, 41: 51–56.

35

Emergency care of the sexual assault survivor

Lorna Martin

The annual reported incidence of sexual assault is around 50 000 cases per year, although this may be a vast underestimation of the true numbers.

The immediate management of the sexual assault survivor involves medical treatment, as well as obtaining specimens for medico-legal requirements. If the patient has reported the assault to the police or has intentions to do so, careful attention needs to be paid to the collection of forensic evidence. This includes the detection, documentation, and interpretation of all injuries, as well as the collection of biological trace evidence.

Responsibilities of the trauma team towards the patient

- Maintain an empathetic and supportive approach to these severely traumatized patients.
- Present a clear explanation of the medical procedures and interventions involved, including anti-retroviral treatment.
- Perform a very thorough examination and recording of findings.
- Allow a patient to start the process of re-empowerment immediately, by involving him/her throughout the process.

Responsibilities of the trauma team towards the police and justice system

- The doctor and assisting nurse act as the 'medical detectives', and optimally utilize the opportunity to gather as much forensic evidence as possible, keeping in mind that they may have to testify in court.
- Documentation must be complete, legible, and safely archived.

Consent

- Written consent is mandatory for examining these patients and obtaining forensic specimens.

- Patients who are 14 years or older can give assent.
- For patients who are 13 years or younger, consent must be given by the parent or legal guardian. If no parent or guardian is available, consent must be obtained from the Superintendent of the health care facility.
- Alternatively, if a charge has been laid with the police, consent for minors may be obtained from the Magistrate.
- Consent must be fully informed, given freely and without coercion.

Life-threatening injuries

Examine all patients for life- and limb-threatening injuries, utilizing the ABC principles, while stabilizing the cervical spine as indicated. Treat these injuries and stabilize the patient accordingly. Stable patients: note that the collection of forensic evidence must occur simultaneously with the examination to ensure that no evidence is lost and to minimize contamination. This should take place in suitable premises with adequate lighting, all equipment must be on hand, a nurse should be present, and if requested by the patient, a relative or friend. Refer also to the discussion of collection of forensic evidence under the heading Examination.

History

A detailed and appropriate history must be obtained for the presenting complaint. Other important aspects are:
- Making definitive statements on behalf of the patient must be avoided: use phrases 'as the patient remembers' and 'alleges'.
- The patient may remember more detail at a subsequent interview by a police officer or prosecutor that may differ from what she/he has told you. This is understandable, but may be misinterpreted by the court.
- A complete detailed history directs the examination, collection of forensic evidence, and management.

General history

The patient's name, age, and sex must be obtained, as well as details of medication, allergies, and other relevant previous medical history.

Details of incident

The following must be established:
- Date and time
- Loss of consciousness
- Assailants – number and identity if known
- Where it happened; on what surface it took place

- What clothing was removed, if any, by whom, how
- Relative position of both parties during the attack; any steps taken to resist; any possible injuries to assailant
- What type of threats – verbal, physical, whether weapons were used
- Type of sexual or indecent activity that occurred, attempted or actual penetration of external genitalia, vagina, oral, anal, or other; any type of oral activity – licking, sucking, kissing; use of any foreign objects including hands; ejaculation by assailant; use of condom.

Details of circumstances after the incident

Ask whether patient has urinated, defaecated, bathed, showered or washed; establish whether there is any pain, discharge, or bleeding; or whether there has been any change of clothing.

Gynaecological history

- Parity
- LMP
- Menstrual cycle history
- Pregnancy details
- Contraceptive use

Collection of biological evidence in the stable patient

The goal of collecting forensic evidence is to obtain a sample of the perpetrator's DNA (Crime Sample), and reference samples from the patient (Control Sample).

- The evidence must be properly collected, preserved, and packaged with no contamination from other sites.
- Use the Sexual Assault Evidence Collection Kit provided by the police. The SAECK comprises a box with the necessary equipment for the collection and preservation of all body evidence in a step-wise manner. It includes Dacron swabs with swab drying racks, sterile water, catch paper, combs, self-adhesive evidence seals, and blood collecting equipment.
- Change gloves frequently during collection to minimize contamination of evidence. Explain this to the patient.

Oral specimen. In the event of oro-genital contact, use the package labelled oral samples. Use the swab to carefully swab under the tongue, along the gum line, cheeks, and palate. Place the swab into a perforation of the drying rack of the swab guard box, and seal with evidence seal.

Sanitary towel and panties. If present, collect and place into the bag provided, seal with the evidence seal.

Evidence on patient's body. Two sealed packages are provided to collect and preserve any biological evidence on the patient's hair, skin, fingernails, and any foreign debris. Solicit the patient's help for possible location of such material.

Material under fingernails. Use swabs provided for fingernails, moisten with sterile water provided, and swab under fingernails of each hand, using one swab per hand. Place swabs into drying rack of swab guard box labelled 'Evidence' on the patient's body.

Dried secretions on skin. Use Dacron swab to swab areas of body where possible saliva or semen is deposited. Ask the patient for possible location if assailant licked, kissed, or bit him/her. Place swab into drying rack of swab guard box labelled 'Evidence' on the patient's body – as above, then close and seal with evidence seal.

Head hair. Use the comb provided to comb the patient's hair over the catch paper labelled 'Head Hair Combing'.
- Put the comb into paper and refold, seal catch paper with evidence seal provided.
- With the patient's consent, pull five reference head hairs from the sides, top, and front. Place into catch paper labelled 'Pulled Reference Head Hair', refold and seal.
- Matted hair – any matting of the head or body hair should be carefully cut away over the catch paper labelled 'Debris A'. Refold and seal with evidence seal.

Foreign debris. Any foreign debris on the patient's body should be scraped away over catch paper labelled 'Debris B', e.g. soil, leaves, sand, fibres, hair. Refold paper and seal with evidence seal.

Pubic hair. Combing of the pubic hair with the comb provided is done to obtain any loose hair or debris that may be useful for identification of the assailant.
- Place catch paper marked 'Pubic Hair Combing' under the patient's buttocks and with downward strokes comb the pubic hair region.
- Look for any matting, carefully cut away, and place onto catch paper.
- Place comb onto catch paper, refold, and seal with evidence seal. With the patient's consent, pull reference pubic hairs, place onto catch paper labelled 'Pulled Reference Pubic Hair', refold and seal.

Ano-rectal specimens. Collect specimens in the event of ano-rectal assault. Remember the patient may not verbalize this event. Always collect before genital specimens to prevent contamination of that area.

External anal swab. Moisten swab provided, carefully swab the anus extending slightly into the anal canal. Place the swab into perforation A of the drying rack of the swab guard box labelled 'Ano-rectal specimen'.

Rectal swab. Apply gentle traction to the buttocks to dilate the sphincter, and then carefully swab the anal canal and rectum. Place the swab into perforation B of the drying rack of the Ano-rectal specimen swab guard box. Close and seal with the evidence seal.

Genital specimens. Three swabs are provided for this step to be collected in order.

External genital swab. Moisten one swab with sterile water provided. Swab external and internal labia majora and minora, clitoris, peri-urethral area, and fossa navicularis, applying gentle pressure.

Place swab into perforation A of drying rack of swab guard box labelled 'Genital Specimen'.

Tampon. If present, collect and place into box labelled 'Tampon'.

Vaginal swab. This swab is necessary before any medical examination to ensure that the original condition of the vagina is maintained and to curb inadvertent loss of foreign body fluids induced by the medical examiner. Insert a sterile, warmed, unlubricated speculum.

Swab the anterior and posterior vaginal fornices. Place swab into perforation B of drying rack of swab guard box labelled 'Genital Specimen'.

Cervical swab. Swab the cervical os, place swab into perforation C of swab guard box labelled 'Genital Specimen'. Close and seal with evidence seal.

Reference DNA specimen. This specimen is to obtain a control reference sample of blood from the patient by venepuncture and deposition of blood into storage device 'Marshal' cassette.

After collection of blood into an EDTA tube, place blood-dispensing device into the top of tube and invert, depositing one drop into each well of the Marshal cassette. Place cassette into padded envelope provided and seal with evidence seal.

All evidence packages and swab guard boxes are placed back into the SAECK box with the completed accompanying form. Ensure that all details on the box are correctly filled in, and then seal the box with the tamper-proof evidence seal.

Examination

If life-threatening conditions have been assessed and managed, proceed with general examination in a compassionate way, with a nurse and relative or friend of the patient present if requested.

General examination

The examination should take place as soon as possible to minimize the degradation of biological evidence. The new SAECK allows for the collection of forensic evidence for up to five days after a sexual assault.

- Ask patient to change into clinic gown, undressing over a large catch sheet, which must be folded and placed into evidence box. If clothing is the same as that worn at time of attack, examine carefully for trace evidence and collect, also for damage/signs of struggle, etc.
- Note patient's general appearance and demeanour, emotional and mental status, look for signs of distress or discomfort, and whether under influence of alcohol or drugs.
- Note all details on examination form.
- Perform a full general physical examination recording vital signs and height, weight, and physique/body build.
- A pregnancy test must be performed.

Detailed general examination

- Careful inspection of the whole body for injuries must be performed.
- Eyes – look for petechial haemorrhages, which may be an indication of throttling.
- Inner aspects of lips and mouth – look for petechial haemorrhages from rough kissing, hand over the mouth, slaps to face, oral penetration.
- Inspect finger imprint contusions and fingernails.
- Examine all abrasions, especially around neck and inner aspects of thighs.
- Look for 'love bites' – tiny petechial haemorrhages and bites which may show pattern of dentition of perpetrator, especially over neck, breasts, and thighs.
- Look at the surface of the body that was in apposition to the surface on which the patient was forced during the attack, e.g. the back, buttocks, and calves if attacked lying on back. Remember that this is not the only position in which sexual attacks occur.

- Examine abrasions for the piling up of the epithelial layers to indicate the direction of the applying force.
- Look at the hands and forearms for 'defence' wounds.
- Describe all injuries and wounds correctly as abrasion or graze, laceration or tear, contusion or bruise, incised wound or cut, penetrating incised wound or stab, or gunshot wound.
- Describe each injury in terms of size (measure if possible), shape, area on body relative to known landmark, and age.
- Make an attempt to correlate the injury with the possible mechanism of infliction, and to history.
- Avoid contamination by the examining finger or hands. Remember that injuries to the genitalia are caused by the use of fingers, foreign objects, and weapons, as well as the penis.
- For both male and female patients, begin with examination of the anus, to avoid contamination with the genitalia when taking swabs.
- Carefully examine the anal margin for any bruising, abrasion, or laceration. Forceful penetration of the anus often leads to mucosal peri-anal and rectal tears.
- Injuries to the vulva may comprise fingernail scratches, especially of the inner aspects, and friction between the penetrating organ and unlubricated labia causes abrasion as the labia are forced inwards.
- Commonly the hymen is deficient anteriorly, and more pronounced posteriorly, therefore damage to the hymen occurs almost invariably to the posterior quadrant. Tears of the hymen may extend into the vaginal wall or the perineum. There is often contusion and abrasion of the hymenal orifice either with or without tears. This finding is consistent with forced penetration, but it is difficult to distinguish between penile and digital penetration. Also note that full penetration of the penis and even repeated sexual intercourse may not lacerate the hymen. The hymen is quite capable of stretching and therefore rupture or tearing does not necessarily occur on first penetration. The cause of a lacerated hymen is not always a penis. A torn hymen may extend and cause slight tearing of the vaginal wall, and in cases of forceful penetration or large organ disparity deeper and more serious tears of the vagina will occur.
- Vaginal contusions are seen as areas of darker red against the overall redness of the vaginal mucosa. Bruising tends to occur on the anterior wall in its lower third, and on the posterior wall in its upper third. The posterior fourchette is the most common site of injury. Posterior tears of the hymen, fossa navicularis, or of the posterior fourchette may extend into the perineum.

Remember that in many cases, naked-eye injuries may be absent and this cannot be interpreted as lack of forced sexual intercourse.

Management

- Look for life- and limb-threatening injuries and manage appropriately.
- Do baseline blood tests for HIV, RPR and TPHA for syphillis, hepatitis B and C.
- Additional tests may be required if antiretroviral treatment is to be commenced (see below).
- Check for known allergies to any of the suggested treatment regimes before prescribing.
- Do tetanus toxoid vaccination 0.5 ml imi for any wounds, unless vaccinated in past 10 years.

Prevention of pregnancy

Give Ovral® 2 tablets immediately and 2 tablets 12 hours later. Give an antiemetic as nausea is a common side-effect. Repeat pregnancy test after one month.

Prevention of sexually transmitted diseases

Non-pregnant patient
- Ciprofloxacin 250 mg stat
- Metronidazole 2 g stat (warn against any use of alcohol)
- Doxycycline 100 mg 12 hourly, for a week.

Pregnant patient
- Ceftriaxone 125 mg imi stat
- Erythromycin 500 mg qid for 7 days
- Metronidazole 2 g stat

Hepatitis B status

- If Hepatitis B surface antibody level is greater than 10 international units per litre (ideally more than 100 IU/litre), the person is immune. If less than 100 IU/litre, give hepatitis B immunoglobulin *within* 48 hours. Repeat in 28 days.
  Dose: Less than 5 years of age: 200 IU imi (intra-muscular injection)
                  5–9 years: 300 IU imi
                  over 10 years: 500 IU imi
- If the core antibody is positive, the patient is acutely or chronically infected (IgM antibody is positive if acutely infected).

HIV prophylaxis

- The option to prophylaxis should be offered to patients who present within 72 hours of the assault.
- Complete information should be given to patients about their risk of infection, and the fact that treatment assumptions are based on occupational exposure and mother-to-child transmission (evidence on prophylaxis for sexual assault is currently unavailable).
- Baseline HIV testing should be discussed and offered.
- The patient should be fully counselled, before this is done. Side-effects of medication must be explained.
- One of the suggested treatment options is AZT 300 mg 12 hourly and 3TC 100 mg 8 hourly, or Combivir® one tablet twice daily for 28 days.
- Laboratory monitoring (full blood count, renal, and liver profiles, and repeat HIV testing) and follow-up must be ensured. Blood tests should ideally be repeated at three weeks, six weeks, and six months.
- Patients who are HIV positive at the time of sexual assault should not be offered prophylaxis, but referred to appropriate service for management of their disease.

Counselling

Counselling and follow-up visits must be offered to all patients and each patient must be regularly assessed in terms of physical and emotional healing.

Treatment regimens, their side-effects, and the results of blood tests require close monitoring.

Pitfalls

- Not ensuring adequate space, trained staff, and the availability of required forensic collection kits in your unit.
- Not paying immediate attention to life-threatening injuries.
- Not re-examining the patient as injuries to the genitalia are often very small and bruising often only shows up after 24 to 48 hours.
- Not providing counselling for HIV testing and rape survivors.
- Ignorance of forensic evidence gathering.
- Not giving the correct prophylaxis for pregnancy, hepatitis B and HIV *within the correct time.*
- Inadequate and illegible documentation.
- Not organizing follow-up of the whole patient and monitoring for drug side-effects.
- Not consulting with the prosecutor before the court case, and not keeping a copy of the documentation.

References

Martin, L. Provincial Administration of the Western Cape Training Manual on Management of the Sexual Assault Survivor.

SAECK (Sexual Assault Evidence Collection Kit) provided by the SA Police Services.

SAPSwebsite:http://www.saps.gov.za/8crimeinfo/bulletin/942000/rape-.html

36 Respiratory failure

Lance Michell

Acute respiratory failure may occur in the trauma patient either directly as a result of the trauma to the lungs or thorax, or as a secondary and often preventable event. The early recognition of injuries that can lead to respiratory failure and prompt intervention with respiratory support are the key aspects of managing this problem.

Causes of respiratory failure in trauma

Airway obstruction (partial or complete)

Airway obstruction may be divided into direct and indirect causes.

Upper airway obstruction (larynx and above)

Direct	*Indirect*
Decreased consciousness	External compression
Injury to face/tongue/	(haematoma)
mandible/larynx	Oedema (inhalation
Foreign body	hot/toxic gases)
Vomitus	Oesophageal intubation
	Post-extubation laryngeal
	oedema

Lower airway obstruction (trachea and bronchi)

Direct	*Indirect*
Foreign body	Oedema from toxic gases
Blood	Bronchial secretions
Vomitus	Blocked/kinked endotracheal
Ruptured trachea/bronchus	tube

Neurological

Direct	*Indirect*
Brainstem injury	Opiate suppression (brainstem)
Cervical cord injury above C4	Neuromuscular junction
Phrenic nerve damage	blockade

Disturbance of the mechanics of ventilation

Direct	*Indirect*
Pneumothorax	Iatrogenic causes
Haemothorax	(hydrothorax or
Open chest	pneumothorax from
Multiple rib fractures	a central line)
Ruptured diaphragm	
Abdominal compartment syndrome	

Acute lung injury (ARDS)

Direct	*Indirect*
Lung contusion	Shock
Toxic gas	Trauma
Near drowning	DIC
Aspiration acid gastric contents	Massive blood transfusion
Pulmonary infection (diffuse)	Sepsis
	Fat embolism syndrome

Pneumonia

Direct	*Indirect*
Aspiration	Inadequate cough
	Intubation
	Atelectasis

Other causes of respiratory failure include:
- Pulmonary embolism
- Cardiogenic pulmonary oedema

Mechanisms of respiratory failure

Acute respiratory failure can be divided into two broad types, ventilation-perfusion mismatch (type I) and ventilation failure (type II), as described below.

Ventilation-perfusion mismatch (type I)

- Overall ventilation is adequate but blood passing through the lungs is not fully oxygenated.
- Caused by parenchymal lung disease:
  - lung contusion
  - pneumonia

- – pulmonary oedema (cardiogenic/fluid overload)
- – ARDS
- – atelectasis/lobar collapse
- – pulmonary embolism
- *Blood gases are:* $PCO_2\downarrow PO_2\downarrow$ (Compensatory hyperventilation reduces or maintains PCO_2 but is less effective at increasing PO_2.)
- *Management:* Increase inspired O_2, continuous positive airway pressure (CPAP), or mechanical ventilation with positive end expiratory pressure (PEEP).

Ventilation failure (type II)

- The lungs are normal but not enough air is moving in and out. CO_2 accumulates and O_2 decreases in alveoli but there is normal gas exchange across alveolar capillary interface.
- Caused by an interference with respiratory mechanics; partial airway obstruction; depression of respiratory centre; abdominal distension.
- *Blood gases:* $PCO_2\uparrow$, $PO_2\downarrow$.
- *Management:* Remove the cause or mechanical ventilation (only increasing the inspired O_2 may mask rising PCO_2).

Common causes of respiratory failure in the trauma patient

Acute respiratory distress syndrome (ARDS)

Acute respiratory distress syndrome frequently develops in critically injured patients and is not a single disease but a clinical syndrome, which results from a common response of the lungs to a variety of insults.

Definition
ARDS consists of:

- Acute onset
- Bilateral pulmonary infiltrates on chest X-ray
- $PaO_2/FiO_2 < 200$ mmHg (27 kPa);
  for less severe acute lung injury < 300 mmHg (40 kPa)
- No evidence of left ventricular failure

Aetiology
Direct lung injury:

- Pulmonary contusion
- Aspiration of gastric content
- Smoke inhalation

- Pneumonia
- Near drowning
- Negative pressure from obstructed airway

Indirect lung injury:
- Prolonged shock
- Severe sepsis
- Massive blood transfusion
- Fat embolism syndrome
- Pancreatitis

Pathogenesis
- Inflammatory response
- Increased pulmonary capillary permeability to albumin
- Alveolar flooding with albumin-rich fluid
- Inactivation of surfactant
- Dependent areas of lung collapse and are perfused but not ventilated
- Decreased lung compliance (decreased 'stiffness')
- Neutrophils invade and damage lung parenchyma
- Late fibrosis

Treatment of ARDS
- Treat the underlying cause (e.g. control sepsis, fixate fractures)
- Support respiratory system with intubation and mechanical ventilation (see below)
- Avoid fluid overload
- Consider steroids in the late, fibrotic phase.

Figure 36.1 CXR showing the typical 'snowstorm' appearance of ARDS

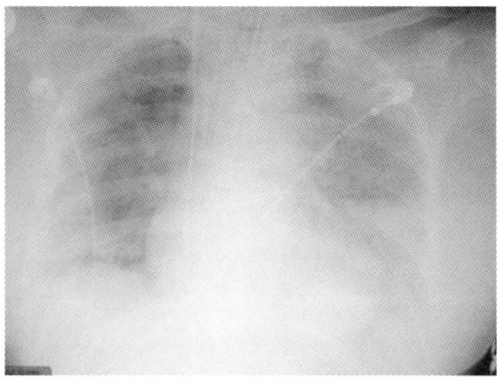

Figure 36.2 The pathogenesis of blunt chest trauma resulting in type I respiratory failure

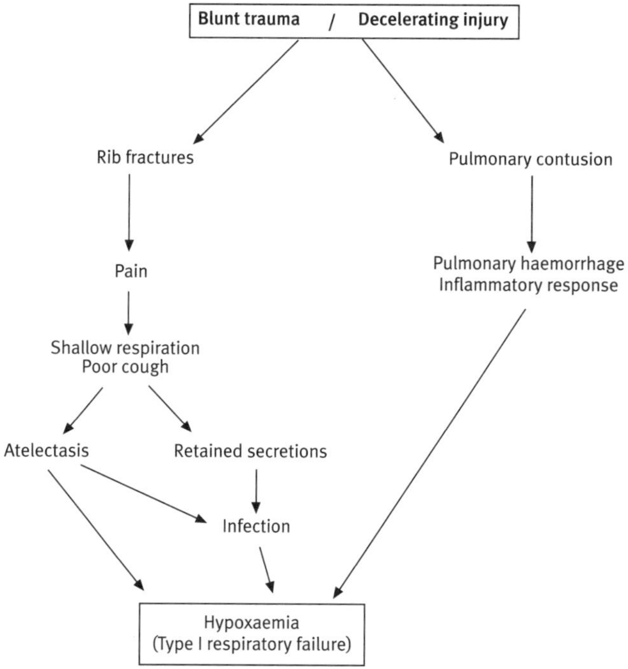

Blunt chest injury

Blunt chest injury is common and easily underestimated. A flail chest occurs when an unstable segment of chest wall moves paradoxically with respiration (chest wall depression on inspiration). The flail worsens as the pulmonary contusion decreases lung compliance. Only a gross flail interferes with the mechanics of ventilation sufficiently to cause a degree of type II respiratory failure.

Management
Good pain control is essential. The options are:
- Non-steroidal anti-inflammatory agents
- Systemic opiates
- Intercostal catheter for unilateral local analgesia
- Epidural catheter for opiate/local anaesthesia

Chest physiotherapy and mobilization is an essential component of management.

An oxygen mask or CPAP (continuous positive airway pressure) by mask can be used for:

- Less severe injury
- Awake, cooperative patient
- No other serious injuries

Intubation and ventilation (early) for the more severe injury:

- Unable to oxygenate on CPAP
- Uncooperative patient
- Multiple trauma

Conservative management using epidural analgesia and CPAP reduces intensive care unit (ICU) time as a pneumonia frequently complicates intubation and ventilation.

NB: Look for common associated injuries: aortic tear, cardiac contusion, liver and spleen injury, and diaphragm rupture.

Aspiration of gastric contents

- Massive aspiration causes asphyxia.
- Acid aspiration can cause a severe ARDS.
- Food particle aspiration causes bronchial obstruction, lobar collapse, and pneumonia with abscess formation.

Prevention

- Intubate at-risk patients with a cuffed endotracheal tube.
- Intubate using rapid sequence induction for skilled intubators.
- Use naso-gastric tube.

Management

- Immediate: Intubate and suction trachea. (There is no role for lavage, steroids, or early antibiotics.)
- Provide respiratory support as for ARDS.
- Perform bronchoscopy for lobar collapse and removal of large particles.
- Treat later (almost inevitable) infection with broad-spectrum antibiotics, including anaerobic cover.

Fat embolism syndrome

This relatively rare condition occurs in 2–5% of patients with fractures, especially long-bone or pelvic fractures.

Aetiology

Micro-emboli of fat, usually derived from bone marrow, lodge in capillaries and under certain conditions trigger a local inflammatory response.

Clinical features

The main features, which typically develop 24–72 hours after injury, consist of:

- *Petechiae.* Classically on the axillae, chest, and conjunctiva, and occurs in 55% of patients. If present with one of the other two conditions below this confirms the diagnosis.
- *Respiratory distress.* An ARDS-like response that can cause severe hypoxia but usually has a good prognosis with correct management.
- *Cerebral involvement.* Includes confusion, headache, and decreased level of consciousness. Often the first sign and often missed.
- In addition, a systemic inflammatory response syndrome (SIRS) is usually present.

Predisposing factors

- Inadequate fracture stabilization
- Prolonged shock

Treatment

Respiratory support in an ICU is required. The prognosis is generally good.

Nosocomial pneumonia

Nosocomial pneumonia frequently occurs in trauma patients because of:

- Intubation
- Aspiration
- Immune suppression due to inflammatory response and blood transfusion
- Poor cough and shallow breathing

Prompt antibiotic therapy, chosen empirically from local microbiology data, is essential.

Management of respiratory failure

Clinical presentation

The patient:

- Complains of difficulty with breathing but more commonly is too breathless to talk
- Has rapid respiratory rate (> 30 breaths/min in an adult)
- Has rapid shallow breathing pattern

- Uses accessory muscles
- Is unable to talk in full sentences
- Shows onset of mental confusion

NB: Clinical diagnosis of severe respiratory failure requires immediate intervention without waiting for confirmatory blood gases. Exclude non-pulmonary causes of apparent respiratory failure, e.g. gastric dilatation, abdominal compartment syndrome, severe metabolic acidosis, and panic attack.

Special investigations

- *Pulse oximetry:* An essential monitor for all patients with or at risk for respiratory failure.
  $SaO_2 < 90\%$ requires confirmation and intervention.
- *Blood gases:*
  $PaO_2 < 8$ kpa (60 mmHg) on 40% facemask.
  $PaCO_2 > 6.5$ kpa (50 mmHg).
- *Chest X-ray:*
  Assists with diagnosis rather than severity.
  Always check for easily reversible causes, e.g. pneumo-/haemothorax.
- *Pulmonary function tests:*
  Vital capacity < 15 ml/kg correlates with inability to clear secretion – intubation often required.

Management

Remove the cause if possible by:

- Draining pneumo-/haemothorax
- Reversing muscle relaxants with neostigmine
- Reversing opiates with naloxone
- Administering a diuretic if in pulmonary oedema
- Providing respiratory support

Types of respiratory support

Oxygen therapy

- Ensure the patient is able to ventilate adequately.
- Use 40% facemask.
- Monitor closely with pulse oximeter.

CPAP facemask

When using the CPAP facemask, ensure the following:

- The patient must be able to ventilate adequately.

- The facemask must be applied with CPAP machine and tight-fitting mask and harness.
- It requires an awake, cooperative patient.

Mechanical ventilation

Non-invasive ventilation:
- Ventilation with special ventilator and face or nasal mask
- Avoids disadvantages of intubation
- Currently little or no role in trauma

Invasive ventilation:
- Requires intubation and ICU ventilator
- Requires admission to ICU
- Current standard of care for acute respiratory failure

Extracorporeal membrane oxygenation (heart-lung machine)

Consider in severe hypothermia or where oxygenation cannot be achieved with conventional ventilation and there is a reversible condition. No benefit has been shown in clinical trials of acute respiratory failure.

Managing a ventilated patient

Airway

- A securely tied, cuffed endotracheal tube (ETT) is essential.
- Oral ETT: Usually easier to insert but uncomfortable and requires more sedation.
- Nasal ETT: More comfortable but there is a risk of sinusitis.
- Tracheostomy: Indicated where the intubation period is > 7–10 days. It reduces laryngeal damage and aids weaning.
- Suction ETT to remove secretions using sterile technique.
- Maintain ETT cuff pressure of 30 cmsH$_2$O to prevent tracheal stenosis.

Ventilator settings

Mode of ventilation
- Volume control modes allow setting of tidal volume.
- Pressure control modes limit inspiratory pressure but tidal volume varies with lung compliance.

- Pressure support mode allows good synchrony with patient breathing.
- Synchronous intermittent mandatory ventilation (SIMV) is the easiest mode to use, allows patient synchrony, and has better acid-base control.

Settings

- Set minute volume using tidal volume or inspiratory pressure level and rate. Tidal volume should be 6 ml/kg.
- Rate 15–20/min to control PCO_2.
- Inspiratory time is 30–50% of respiratory cycle.
- FiO_2 (inspired O_2 concentration) of between 0.4–1.0 (40%–100% O_2) to control PaO_2. Use the lowest FiO_2 to maintain a $PaO_2 > 8$ kPa or $SaO_2 > 90\%$.
- PEEP (positive end-expiratory pressure) improves oxygenation and keeps the alveoli open for gas exchange. Set at between 0 to 20 cmsH$_2$O. Use low values (5cmsH$_2$O if patient hypovolaemic or has raised intra-cranial pressure). Higher levels of PEEP protect lungs in ARDS.
- Alarms: Set alarms for low minute volume and high airway pressure (airway pressures > 40 cmsH$_2$O). Ventilation-induced lung injury is caused by overdistention of normal alveoli using excessive tidal volumes. This can worsen ARDS and cause multiple organ failure.
- Severe ARDS may require additional measures:
  - Recruitment manoeuvres
  - Prone ventilation
  - Permissive hypercapnoea

Sedation

- Opiates (e.g. morphine infusion) if pain present
- Benzodiazepines are the mainstay of sedation
- Avoid muscle relaxants

Nutrition

Begin enteral feeding early once the patient is haemodynamically stable.

Weaning from the ventilation

Test for weaning as soon as:
- The patient is haemodynamically stable
- FiO_2 is down to 40% and PEEP < 6 cmsH$_2$O
- The patient is able to breathe spontaneously
- The patient is able to maintain own airway

The best predictor of successful extubation is ability to breath comfortably with rate < 30 breaths per minute for two hours on CPAP or a T-piece.

Conclusion

A wide variety of conditions cause respiratory failure in the trauma patient and many of these are preventable. Close observation and monitoring must be used to detect patients who require respiratory support. Mechanical ventilation is a high-risk activity and only meticulous attention to detail can prevent iatrogenic complications.

Recommended reading

The acute respiratory distress syndrome network. 2000. Ventilation with lower tidal volumes as compared with traditional volumes for acute lung injury and the acute respiratory distress syndrome. *New England Journal of Medicine*, 342:1301–8.

Marik, P. E. 2001. Aspiration pneumonitis and aspiration pneumonia. *New England Journal of Medicine*, 344:665–71.

Tobin, M. J. 2002. Advances in mechanical ventilation. *New England Journal of Medicine*, 344:1986–1996.

Ware, R. M, Matthay, M. A. 2000. The acute respiratory distress syndrome. *New England Journal of Medicine*, 342:1334–49.

Accidental hypothermia

Pradeep H Navsaria

Accidental hypothermia is defined as an unintentional decline in core body temperature (35 °C).

Classification

Hypothermia is classified as:
- Mild: 35 to 32 °C
- Moderate:< 32 to 28 °C
- Severe: < 28 °C

Risk factors

The following are the main risk factors for hypothermia:
- Extremes of age (especially the elderly)
- Ethanol abuse
- Malnutrition
- Poverty
- Mental disease
- Neuroleptic drugs
- Hypothyroidism
- Cold-water immersion
- Winter-sports players

Physiology of thermoregulation

- Thermoregulation is coordinated in the pre-optic anterior hypothalamus.
- The thermal conductivity of water is 20–30 times greater than air. Therefore, immersion in water results in rapid onset hypothermia.
- Heat is lost from the body by four mechanisms:
  1 Radiation (55%)
  2 Evaporation (airway – 5%, skin – 25%)
  3 Conduction (10%)
  4 Convection (5%)

Figure 37.1 Scheme of thermoregulation

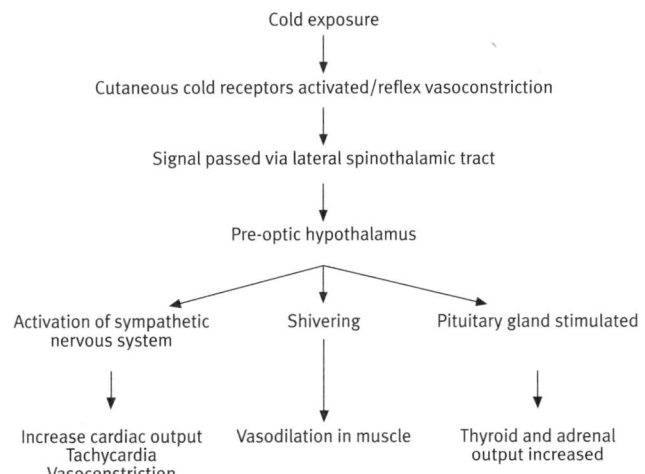

Effects on organ systems

The effects of hypothermia depend on the severity of hypothermia, the cause, and the premorbid state of the patient.

Effect on cardiac system

The cardiac response to hypothermia is variable and depends on the degree of hypothermia.

- Initially: tachycardia, increased cardiac output, peripheral vasoconstriction, increased peripheral vascular resistance
- Below 32 °C: conduction impaired, heart rate and cardiac output decreases
- Sinus bradycardia and the J or Osborne wave, which is a positive-negative deflection immediately after the QRS complex seen on electrocardiogram, are hallmarks and are seen in 30% of cases.
- Any arrhythmia or block can occur:
  - atrial fibrillation common below 32 °C
  - ventricular fibrillation may occur below 28 °C.
- Cardiac output is virtually nil below 25 °C

Effect on respiratory system

- Bronchorrhea and bronchospasm

- Early tachypnoea followed by hypoventilation
- Oxy-haemoglobin curve shifted to left (further aggravated by hypocapnia and alkalosis)

Effect on renal system

- Cold diuresis: shunting of blood from periphery to central circulation – lowers intravascular volume
- Oxidative tubular activity depressed – decreased sodium and water resorption
- Can render patient hypovolaemic

Haematological changes

- Volume depletion results in haemoconcentration and increased blood viscosity predisposing to thrombosis
- Clotting impaired
- DIC (disseminated intravascular coagulation)

Effect on endocrine system

- Hyperglycaemia initially – insulin release inhibited, peripheral use of glucose diminished
- ACTH (adrenocorticotropic hormone) and TSH (thyroid-stimulating hormone) increased
- Catecholamines and cortisol also elevated

Effect on acid-base balance

- Lactic acidosis due to decreased peripheral perfusion – compensatory respiratory alkalosis
- Severe hypothermia – respiratory depression occurs – respiratory acidosis

Diagnosis

Diagnosis is made on rectal or oesophageal measurement of core temperature using a low-reading thermometer.

History

Take history of pre-existing medical condition, trauma, and alcohol.

Examination

Perform ABCD examination:

A – establish a patent airway, administer warm, humidified oxygen

B – breathing (exclude pneumothorax, pneumonia, fractured ribs, lung contusion)

C – circulation (establish venous access, commence warm fluid infusion)
D – disability + 'degree of temperature'

Perform a complete head-to-toe examination.

Laboratory evaluation

A laboratory evaluation includes:
- Full blood count and coagulation profile
- Serum electrolytes
- Renal function
- Blood glucose
- Arterial blood gases (correct for temperature of patient)
- Blood cultures
- Thyroid function tests (if indicated)

Special investigations and procedures

Special investigations include:
- Chest radiograph
- Electrocardiogram
- Foley catheter
- Central venous catheter
- Computerized tomography of brain if any concern of a head injury

Continuous monitoring of the following is necessary:
- Vital signs
- Central venous pressure
- Urine output
- Serial electrolytes
- Arterial blood gases
- Blood glucose levels

Administer warm humidified oxygen and warm intravenous fluids to all patients. Give thiamine intravenously if alcohol abuse is suspected. Do not correct bradycardia with atropine until the patient is normothermic. Commence broad-spectrum antibiotics if sepsis is suspected.

Rewarming strategies

These strategies may be:
- Passive (no added heat), or
- Active (added heat)
  Active rewarming may be: external (surface) or internal (core)

Passive external warming

- Maintain a warm environment – ambient temperature > 25 °C.
- Remove all clothing, blanket insulation.
- Keep head covered – 30% of body heat can be lost via the head.

Active external warming

Use heat sources – immersion in warm water, hot water bottles, and heaters.

Beware of 'afterdrop', a phenomenon of decrease of core temperature after the start of external warming – supposedly initiated by peripheral vasodilation and shunting of cold, acidotic blood full of metabolic waste to the core tissues.

Active internal warming

Humidified heated oxygen:
- Face mask or endotracheal intubation
- Inspired air should not exceed 40 °C

Warmed intravenous fluids:
- Warmed intravenous fluids or blood
- Warm to 40 °C – can use microwave oven

Peritoneal lavage:
- Use standard diagnostic peritoneal lavage kits or open method using a Foley catheter.
- Infuse 1 litre of warmed balanced salt solution into peritoneal cavity for a minute and then drain.
- Fluid rates of up to 10–12 litre/hr are possible.

Pleural lavage:
- Use standard tube thoracostomy – preferably the left side.
- Infuse 1 litre warm normal saline into pleural cavity for a minute and then drain.
- Repeat until temperature is > 32 °C.

Extracorporeal blood warming:
- Femoro-femoral bypass – requires full heparinization and not a modality for trauma patients
- Veno-venous bypass – heparinless pumps available, can be used in non-arrested trauma patient

Diathermy:
- Restores body heat by ultrasonic waves, microwaves, or shortwaves.
- Delivers heat to core tissues without an invasive procedure.
- Haemorrhage is a contraindication.

Warming strategy for hypothermic patient

Aim to warm patient by 1–2 °C per hour.

Mild hypothermia: Passive external warming; warm intravenous fluids and inspired gases

Moderate hypothermia: Above + pleural lavage

Severe hypothermia: All of above. Consider shortwave heating. With temperature < 25 °C consider bypass heating methods

Mortality

The prognosis is poor in the following circumstances:
- When associated with trauma
- When patient is elderly
- With severe hypothermia
- With attempts at rapidly rewarming patients

Frostbite

Treatment for frostbite is as follows:
- Admit patient.
- If < 24 hours – rewarm in a water bath at 40 °C.
- If > 24 hours – do not re-warm.
- Administer tetanus prophylaxis.
- Administer opiates and non-steroidal anti-inflammatory drugs for analgesia.
- Remove all blisters.
- Elevate affected limb.
- Administer antibiotics – penicillin 1 000 000 units six hourly.
- Refer to a plastic/hand surgeon for assessment.

Pitfalls

- High index of suspicion – use low-reading thermometer.
- Determine the cause of the depressed level of consciousness (head injury, stroke, hypothermia, drugs, substance abuse).
- Beware of afterdrop.
- Hypoglycaemia often occurs during rewarming.
- Cold diuresis and fluid deficit increases as rewarming occurs.

- Apnoea, asystole, and absence of brain activity; usual signs of death can be present in severe hypothermia.
- Treatment for each case should be individualized.

Recommended reading

Danzl, D. F., Pozos, R. S. 2002. Accidental hypothermia. (Review article) *NEJM*, 331(26):1756–1760.

Juricovich, G. J. Greiser, W. B., Luterman, A., Curreri, P. W. 1987. Hypothermia in trauma victims: An ominous predictor of survival. *J Trauma*, 27(a):1019–1024.

38 Acute renal failure

Lance Michell and Andrew Nicol

Acute renal failure (ARF) in the trauma patient is associated with a mortality of 20% if this is the only failed system, increasing up to 80% mortality in multiple organ failure.

One of the most important goals of resuscitation from shock is to re-establish urine flow, as this not only indicates that the kidneys are receiving an adequate blood supply but that the rest of the organs are also being adequately perfused.

Definitions

Renal failure is defined as follows:
- *Acute:* (Hours to days) deterioration in renal function, resulting in a compromise of fluid and electrolyte homeostasis
- *Oliguria:* Urine output of < 0.5 ml/kg/hour for four hours
- *Anuria:* Urine output of < 50 ml per day

Aetiology

The aetiology of renal failure is as follows:

Pre-renal:
Hypovolaemia
Blood loss
Burns
Pump failure (CCF, tamponade, myocardial infarct)
Abdominal compartment syndrome

Renal:
Acute tubular necrosis
Ischaemia
Aminoglycosides
Intravenous contrast
Myoglobin
Glomerulonephritis
Interstitial nephritis

Post-renal:
Ureteric disruption
Urethral trauma
Blocked Foley catheter
Prostatic obstruction

Table 38.1 Biochemical distinction between pre-renal and renal causes of ARF (only valid in oliguric patient with previously normal kidneys and when no diuretic has been administered)

	Pre-renal	Renal
Urine osmolality	> 500 mOsm/l	< 350 mOsm/l
Urine specific gravity	> 1.020	< 1.010
Urinary sodium (Na)	> 10 mEq/l	> 20 mEq/l
Urinary: Plasma urea ratio	> 20	< 10
Fractional excretion of Na	< 1%	> 3%

$$\text{Fractional excretion of Na (FENa)} = \frac{\text{Urinary Na x Plasma creatinine}}{\text{Plasma Na x Urinary creatinine}}$$

Management approach to the 'oliguric patient'

The management of the 'oliguric patient' is set out in Figure 38.1.

- A diuretic in established renal failure should only be administered when the preload is adequate. The aim is to convert oliguric acute renal failure to polyuric renal failure, which is easier to manage.
- Dialyse if indicated.

Indications for haemodialysis

- Serum potassium > 7 mmol/litre
- Fluid overload with pulmonary oedema
- Serum urea > 50 mmol/litre
- Serum creatinine > 500 μmol/litre
- Base excess > −10 meq/litre

Pitfalls

- Administering furosemide to an oliguric patient in order to increase urine output without determining the adequacy of the preload and the underlying cause.
- Administering potassium containing intravenous fluids to anuric patients.

Figure 38.1 Management approach to the 'oliguric patient'

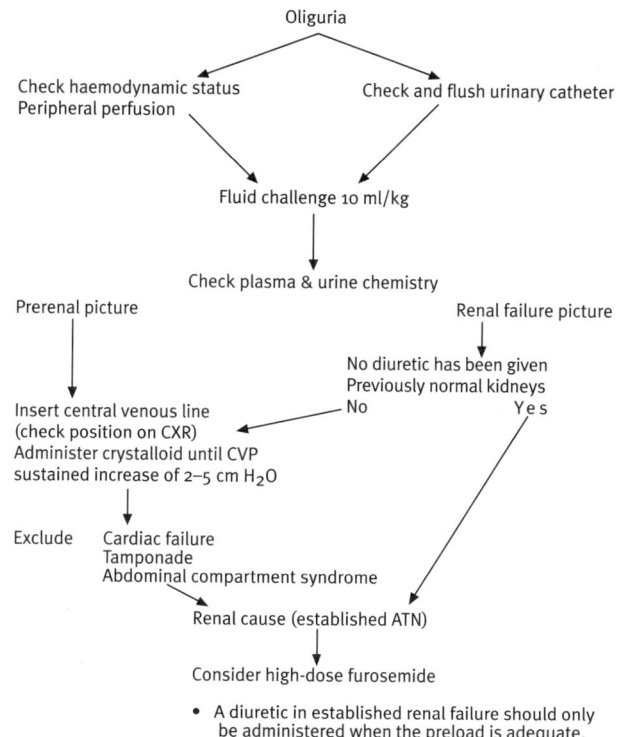

- A diuretic in established renal failure should only be administered when the preload is adequate. The aim is to convert oliguric acute renal failure to polyuric renal failure, which is easier to manage.
- Dialyse if indicated

Recommended reading

Oh, T. E. (ed.) 1997. Intensive care manual. Fourth edition. London: Butterworth-Heinemann Medical.

PART 4

Specific injuries

Elbie van der Merwe

The prevalence of burns in developing countries is significantly higher than in developed countries. Factors contributing to this are poor socio-economic conditions resulting in informal housing, paraffin flame devices used for cooking, and limited education. Researchers from Africa found that despite the increased availability of electricity in areas where infrastructure is developed, increased use and (often careless) handling of flammable (kerosene) and explosive agents for domestic purposes can contribute to the incidence of burns.

Although highly specialized burn units are located in the main centres, most burn victims are initially treated in peripheral hospitals and emergency units, where early, efficient, and appropriate emergency management will significantly influence the patient's eventual outcome.

Emergency management of the burns victim

The following are the main priorities in the initial treatment of burns:

- Airway maintenance and protection
- Breathing assessment and support
- Circulation: vascular access and initial fluid management
- Pain control
- Exposure, assessment of extent of burns
- History and head-to-toe examination
- Documentation
- Wound care
- Treatment plan, fluids, oral intake, drugs, monitoring
- Admission or transfer
- Prevention of early complications and secondary insult

Primary survey

A: Airway

The airway may be already compromised at the time of arrival or may become compromised during the resuscitation period. Swelling may increase over 24–36 hours.

The airway may be damaged directly by inhalation of the heat from the fire, toxic inhalants or smoke, causing mucosal damage and subsequent oedema. It may be indirectly compromised by the neurological status of the patient. Disorientation and coma indicate a significant exposure to carbon monoxide (CO) or the presence of associated closed head injury.

Signs of airway compromise or imminent compromise
- Hoarseness and stridor
- History of closed space smoke exposure
- Burns to the face, neck, and chest
- Singed nasal hair and/or mucous membranes
- Altered level of consciousness
- Oedema of oropharynx or epiglottis

Management of the airway
- The swelling may progress extremely rapidly and if there are any indications of risk, the patient should be intubated before obstruction occurs.
- Oro-tracheal intubation is the most convenient, safe route.
- If intubation via an oral or nasal route is not possible, consider cricothyroidotomy or tracheostomy.
- If the possibility of cervical spine injury exists (explosion, vehicular collision, fall from a height), the head and neck should be manually immobilized during intubation, and then protected with a hard collar and head blocks until radiologically cleared.
- Use a high-volume, low-pressure cuffed endotracheal tube.
- Use a safe, standardized intubation technique, with low-dose sedation, pre-oxygenation, cricoid pressure, and constant reassuring communication with the patient.

Inhalation injury

The pathophysiology of inhalation injury remains poorly understood and over the past years, few improvements in treatment have occurred.

Inhalation injuries are classified into three types:

1. Upper airway injury (supraglottic) is due to the heat of the burn and results in swelling of the upper airway. This causes airway problems within 24 hours.
2. Large airway injury includes the trachea and bronchi. It is due to the large particles from the fire and causes respiratory problems in the first 48 hours.
3. Alveolar injury occurs due to small particles: this is seen particularly when synthetic materials were involved. The respiratory problems may develop over 72 hours after the injury and usually cause hypoxia, V/Q mismatching, increased airway resistance, decreased pulmonary

compliance and increased pulmonary vascular resistance. Infectious complications may present as tracheobronchitis or pneumonia.

B: Breathing

Pulmonary function and inhalation injury

- Assess rate of breathing, air entry, and breath sounds, to identify associated injuries, haemo- or pneumothorax, underlying lung disease, or early signs of inhalation injury.
- Treat chest injuries appropriately.
- Obtain a chest X-ray, arterial blood gas, and serum carboxyhaemoglobin levels.
- Administer humidified oxygen by mask with a reservoir bag (at 12 to 15 ℓ/min, to achieve a FiO_2 of 1.0) or use Continuous Positive Airways Pressure (CPAP) to prevent or help to reopen collapsed alveoli and atelectatic lung zones.
- Inhalation of toxic gases such as cyanide, hydrogen sulphide, or hydrogen chloride results in severe injury of the lower respiratory mucosa. Smoke from 'clean' combustion causes less damage, while hot air inhalation usually causes upper airway injury.
- Suspect pulmonary damage due to smoke inhalation when there is a history of fire in an enclosed space, confusion, or depressed level of consciousness, tachypnoea, cough, wheeze, rhonchi, crepitations, or where there are peri-oral or intra-pharyngeal burns and carbon in the sputum.
- Inhalation injury is strongly suspected when the face, neck, and chest are burnt, but may be present without these burns.
- Carbon monoxide (CO) inhalation results in the formation of carboxyhaemoglobin, which has a high affinity to oxygen and consequently reduces oxygen delivery to the cells. Look for cherry red mucous membranes and wounds.
- The constricting effects of a circumferential or extensive truncal burn may mechanically restrict breathing unless escharotomies are performed.
- Assisted ventilation (IPPV) with PEEP (positive end-expiratory pressure) is indicated for early respiratory decompensation ($PaO_2 < 10$ kPa), taking care to prevent barotrauma.
- Fibre-optic bronchoscopy may be required and repeated to assess the extent of airway injury.
- Nebulizing with heparin (as a free radical scavenger and to prevent fibrin plugs), bronchodilators, or mucolitic agents may be helpful.
- Antibiotic is prescribed only after sputum is cultured and the sensitivity to the antibiotic has been obtained.

C: Circulation

Patients with significant burns have a large insensible loss of fluid from their wounds. The amount of loss is proportional to the surface area of the burn, the depth, and the time elapsed. Effective fluid resuscitation is important but warnings regarding the sequelae of over-resuscitation are increasingly prevalent. Effusions, iatrogenic intra-abdominal hypertension and compartment syndromes may develop.

- Assess blood pressure, peripheral pulses, and circulation, especially the distal perfusion of a circumferentially burnt extremity. Consider the possibility of underlying injuries causing haemorrhagic shock.
- Fluids may be given orally or intravenously. The oral route can be used in smaller burns of < 20% TBSA (total body surface area) in adults and children with even more extensive wounds. There is a growing trend to utilize the enteral route for fluid resuscitation. This should be started as soon as possible to maintain gut motility.

Figure 39.1 Rule of Nines in adults and children

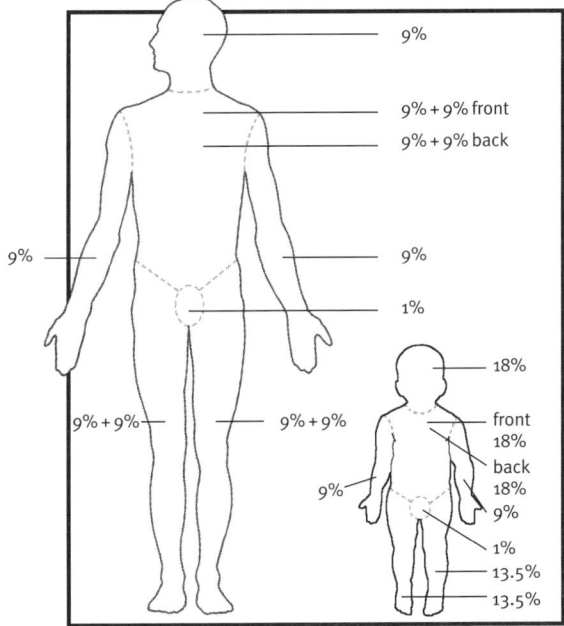

- Access is preferable via a central venous pressure (CVP) line or 2 peripheral lines with a large-bore cannula (14–16 gauge) through unburnt skin. If necessary a venous cut down may be used through damaged skin. A CVP line should not be kept for longer than five days. On removal the tip can be sent for microbiology culture and sensitivity to identify possible secondary infection from the line.
- Draw blood for urea, electrolytes, carboxyhaemoglobin levels, glucose, drug, and alcohol screen.
- For significant burns, place two large-bore peripheral lines and commence fluid resuscitation with Ringer's lactate solution at 2–4 ml/kg/% total body surface area (TBSA).
- Place urinary catheter for patients with burns of > 20% TBSA, to monitor output (0.5–1 ml/kg/h). Check urine for blood, protein, and myoglobin.
- Monitor ECG, pulse rate, blood pressure – invasive (IBP) or non-invasive (NIBP) – and oxygen saturation. An arterial line is strongly recommended in monitoring the blood pressure which can fluctuate over the whole resuscitation period of 24–48 hours.

Determine the fluid requirements
- Use the Rule of Nines to assess the extent of the wounds (adapt for children).
- Weigh the patient if possible (kilogram).
- Use the Parkland Formula (or any other formula) for the first 24 hours: 2–4 ml/kg/% TBSA burn. The 24-hour period starts from the time of injury. Half of the calculated amount is given over the first eight hours, the rest is given over the subsequent 16 hours. Allow for change in the treatment regime at any time required.
- The maintenance fluid requirements of small children must be taken into account as well. Allow for oral feeding when possible.
- Assess the need for blood in the first 24 hours and postpone infusion to day two or three if possible. A low Hb (8–10 mg/dl) in previously healthy young patients can be accepted.
- Maintain hourly urine volume of 0.5–1 ml/kg as the minimum goal.
- Trends are more important observations than single readings.
- Keep in mind that compromised patients with underlying disease, inhalation injury, or high-voltage electrical burns, or patients with low reserves may be very unstable during the fluid resuscitation phase. Constant evaluation and adjustment of the regime may be necessary.

D: Disability and analgaesia
- Altered levels of consciousness may be due to hypoxia, circulatory compromise, or an additional injury.

Do a basic neurological assessment, including pupils, level of consciousness (GCS), and peripheral motor and sensory function.

- The importance of pain-relieving drugs cannot be overemphasized. Pain leads to anxiety, increases the metabolic response to trauma and increases oxygen consumption.

- *Paediatric patients:*
  Morphine (0.05 mg/kg/hr diluted as a slow constant infusion)
  Midazolam (0.1 mg/kg increments) potentiates the effect of opiates
  Tilidine hydrochloride sublingually
  Ketamine (1–4 mg/kg IV or IM)

- *Adults:*
  Opioids: morphine 0.1–0.2 mg/kg in incremental doses of 1–2 mg IV until pain is under control
  Fentanyl (2–4 μg/kg) for procedures at the bedside
  Propofol, ketamine, and Entonox® may be useful

- A combination of analgesics and sedatives can be administered, providing the patient remains cooperative. Careful monitoring is advised.

Figure 39.2 Escharotomy incisions

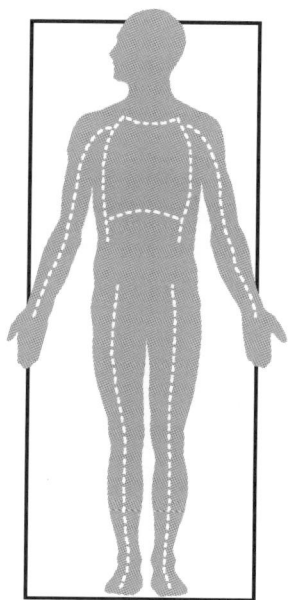

E: Exposure

- During transport, the patient's burns should be covered with sterile dry, non-adherent dressing, or with a sterile hydrogel.
- Once in the emergency unit, all clothing is removed to fully assess the depth and extent of the wounds, but the patient must be protected from hypothermia.
- Log-roll to inspect the back, if this has not already been done.
- After the removal of all loose skin and blisters, the wounds and surrounding areas are scrubbed and cleaned.

Burn evaluation

- Extent: % TBSA: see Rule of Nines.
- Establish depth:
  Superficial: epidermal, superficial dermal
  Deep: deep dermal, sub-dermal (full thickness)
- Superficial wounds are red, wet, painful, blanche with pressure, then show rapid capillary refill, develop little swelling.
- Deep dermal wounds are red with mottled white or grey, dry and less painful, with more swelling. It is easier to determine exact depth after the first 48 hours.
- Full thickness burns are pale white to dark brown or black, leathery, with no sensation and profound swelling in the subcutaneous tissue.
- Assess location: involvement of face, hands, joints, etc. is an indication for referral to a specialist centre.
- At the end of the primary survey, reassess the airway breathing and circulation.

Secondary survey

History

Obtain important information from the scene of the accident:

- Cause of the fire
  - stove sets clothing alight: always deep wounds
  - house on fire: think about inhalation injury
  - explosion: possibility of other injuries
- Nature of the burning material
- Enclosed space
- Period exposed to the fire or smoke
- Time elapsed since the incident
- Condition of the patient – intoxicated or unconscious

Additional information that is required:

- Previous medical history
- Last meal
- Allergies
- Medications

Head-to-toe examination

- Look for other injuries.
- Re-assess airway and breathing.
- Assess response to fluid therapy.
- Check for contact lenses, constricting jewelry, dentures, hearing aids.
- Examine corneas.
- Examine ears, mouth, throat.
- Request appropriate X-rays.
- Consider the need for escharotomies for deep circumferential burns of trunk or limbs.
- Document all findings, treatment, and results, including detailed drawings of the extent and depth of various burnt areas.
- Tetanus prophylaxis should be given, unless the patient has had a booster within the previous five years.

Wound care

- Ensure that escharotomies have been done where required, before wounds are covered. (See Figure 39.2.)
- Topical antibacterial agents are usually not necessary in the first 48 hours and may alter the appearance of the wounds.
- Apply sterile hydrogel dressings until the receiving doctor has inspected the wounds (if patient is to be transferred to a burns centre or specialist).
- Elevate swollen hands and feet.
- Formal burns dressings are usually instituted by the staff of the burns ward.
- The dressing should be non-adherent, exudate absorbent, protecting the wound from bacterial colonization, and keeping the patient comfortable.
- Suitable antibacterial agents are silver sulfadiazine for large areas which is still used in 79% of cases, and chlorhexidine or povidone-iodine for cleaning smaller wounds (< 15% TBSA). Novel antimicrobial agents and old-fashioned treatments are resurfacing. Both sugar and honey have been used with good effects as dressings for wounds. Carica papaya fruit has been shown to be excellent at debriding wounds and

cleaning infected wounds. Aromatherapy using essential oils is a fast growing area of interest as well. Topical antibiotics should never be used, as the emergence of resistant bacterial strains are encouraged and agents such as neomycin are absorbed through the wound, leading to deafness in children.

- Vacuum assisted closure (VAC dressing) can be used with acute or chronic wounds. Negative pressure applied to a wound facilitates granulation tissue while maintaining a clean wound bed and eradicating infection.

Monitoring

Check the following regularly:

- Airway obstruction
- Heart rate (ECG)
- Blood pressure
- Urine output
- Central venous pressure (if a central line has been inserted)
- Oxygen saturation (O_2 Sats)
- Respiratory rate if not on ventilatory support
- Perfusion of fingers and toes, rather than peripheral pulses
- Need for additional fluid or decrease of infusion

Classification of burn injuries

Burn injuries are classified as follows:

- Flame burns
- Scald burns: boiling water, cooking oil, hot food, steam
- Electrical injury
- Chemical burns
- Contact burns
- Others: friction burns and 'cold' burn injury (liquid nitrogen)

Typically, children sustain scald burns and adults are burnt by flames from cooking devices (paraffin stoves), house fires, and assaults. The patients may have associated blunt or penetrating injuries due to collapsing buildings or explosions. Always look out for signs of non-accidental injury and abuse.

Electrical burns

Special problems to look out for are deep contact and hidden exit wounds, severe muscle injury with development of compartment syndrome, rhabdomyolysis with myoglobinuria, arrythmias, additional injuries, and the risk of development of renal failure.

Admit all electric burns patients for at least 24 hours for limb elevation and ECG monitoring.

Check urine for myoglobins, if present institute a saline diuresis, consider mannitol and alkanization.

Chemical burns

Alkaline burns damage tissue progressively and relentlessly until all the chemicals have been removed from the wound bed. This may require copious lavage or scrubbing of the wound, starting as soon as possible (on scene).

Acid burns cause tissue necrosis due to protein denaturation, and this may act as a barrier to deeper penetration of the acid. Wounds need to be washed copiously as well.

Treatment plan

Aims of burns patient management

Scarring is minimized and optimal functional and cosmetic outcomes are achieved by adhering to the following principles:

- Effective resuscitation
- Aggressive wound management
- Early excision and grafting. Surgical techniques vary from scraping, brushing, sharp dissection, bulk tissue removal and amputations. Blood-saving techniques include: warm saline-soaked pads, compressive dressings or tourniquets, subcutaneous injection of vasopressors or using the tumescent technique
- Wound coverage after necrotectomy is essential. Allografting deep dermal wounds and autografting full thickness wounds remain the golden standard
- Maintain sufficient nutritional support – orally
- Prevent infection by anticipating problems:
    - remove intravenous lines (five days) and catheters as soon as possible
    - mobilize the patient early to prevent respiratory infections and muscle wasting
    - aggressively maintain an optimal immune status by supporting the patient not only physically but also emotionally
    - isolate patients with resistant organisms to prevent spread
    - avoid prophylactic or unnecessary antibiotic use
    - minimize blood transfusion by tumescent operating techniques to decrease blood loss and by accepting low serum haemoglobin levels (Hb < 10 mg/dl in the ward, and Hb = 10 mg/dl intra-operatively)

- Physiotherapy and exercises to maintain range and function
- Early rehabilitation and scar control
- Constant emotional support and effective stress management

Nutritional support

After calculation of nutritional needs, oral alimentation is started within 24 hours after injury.

- Protein requirement = 3 gm x % TBSA burn + 1 gm x patient mass (kg)
  Paediatric protein requirement = 1 gm x % TBSA burn + 3 gm x patient mass
  Protein requirements divided by 6.25 = nitrogen (N) requirements
- Calorie requirements = 1 500 kcal/m^2 BSA + 1 500 kcal/m^2 TBSAB
  1–12 months: 2 100 kcal/m^2 BSA + 1 000 kcal/m^2 TBSAB
  1–11 years: 1 800 kcal/m^2 BSA + 1 300 kcal/m^2 TBSAB
  $\times 630$ = Kilojoule (non-protein Kj) requirements)
  1 Kcal = 4.18 Kj
- Fat should provide < 2 % total calorie intake as energy is required to metabolize fat and some fats are immunosuppressive
- Commercially available high protein drinks, 250 ml 4–6 hourly provide much of the total protein and energy requirements
- Micronutrients: vitamins, minerals, and trace element supplementation
  Daily requirements:

Vit A:	10 000–250 000 IU
Vit B1:	3 mg
Vit B2:	2.4 mg
Vit B6:	2 mg
Vit B12:	5 µg
Vit D:	400 IU
Nicotinic acid:	20 mg
Vit C:	1 000 mg,
Vit E:	100 mg
Folic acid:	5 mg,
Zn:	220 mg
Glutamine:	20 mg

  Calcium, magnesium, and phosphate levels should be monitored
- Anabolic stimulants may be considered
- Careful use of beta-blocking agents to reduce energy expenditure
- Semi-elemental feeds may be considered if burn is > 30% BSA

Table 39.1 Dressings

Biological dressing		
Allograft	Fresh donor skin Cryopreserved donor skin Glycerol preserved skin Amniotic membrane	Relatively inexpensive, carries the risk of disease transmission, CMV, HepB, HIV, All temporary
Xenograft	EZ-Derm™	Temporary
Cultured skin	Epithelial autograft Epithelial allograft TransCyte™	All temporary
Synthetic skin	Biobrane Alloderm™	Temporary
Skin substitute Synthetic composite dermal analogue	Integra™	Expensive, used instead of allograft Permanent

Surgical wound management – a guideline

- Remove blisters.
- Treat superficial wounds with antibacterial creams, transparent polyurethane film, or biological dressings.
- Alternatively, cover smaller wounds with hydrocolloid dressings.
- Mobilize hands with small wounds and protect them inside a plastic bag.
- Re-assess deep dermal wounds 2–5 days after the injury. The majority will then be reclassified as either full thickness or superficial burns. If at five days post-injury, it looks as though the wound will not be healed in 14 days, it should be treated as full thickness burn.
- Full thickness wounds require early excision and an immediate cover with the patient's own skin (autograft), cadaver skin (allograft), or if small enough but tendon, bone cartilage, and joints are exposed, a flap procedure may be considered.

Skin substitutes

When donor sites are scarce, coverage in this circumstance can be obtained by skin substitutes. These materials may be biologic, synthetic or a combination of both.

Pitfalls

- Black singed areas in the wound bed may look like normal skin in pigmented people. In reality these are very deep wounds.
- The first six hours after facial burns are the 'golden hours' to place an endotracheal tube. Swelling of mucous membranes is a life-threatening complication.
- If a patient is to be transferred, elective intubation may be considered prior to transfer if the patient has facial burns.
- There is a tendency to underestimate the depth of the wound but overestimate the wound size.
- The visible burn in electrical burns underestimates the degree of tissue damage.
- Referral to a plastic surgeon should be considered early for burns to the eyes, ears, or hands.
- CVP lines should not be kept for routine infusion. Line infection with gram-negative septicaemia may be fatal.
- NSAI drugs are extremely dangerous during the resuscitation phase. Acute tubular necrosis is imminent.
- Oral feeding is the rule. Parenteral nutrition is contraindicated in the burn patient.
- Hypothermia is a serious complication. Do not apply wet drapes during resuscitation or leave the patient uncovered while operating.

Recommended reading

Baxter, C. R. 1974. Fluid volume and electrolyte changes in the early post-burn period. *Clinical Plastic Surgery,* 1:693–703.

Boswick, J. A. (ed.) 1987. *The art and science of burn care.* Rockville, MD: Aspen Publishers.

Brown, T. L. H., Muller, M. 2003. Parimony, simplicity and survival in burn care. *Burns,* 29:197–198.

Clark, W. R., Nieman, G. F. 1988. Smoke inhalation. *Burns,* 14:472.

Clark, W. R., Bonaventural, M., Meyers, W. 1989. Smoke inhalation and airway management at a regional burn unit: 1974–1983. Part I: Diagnosis and consequences of smoke inhalation. *Journal Burn Rehabilitation,* 10:52–62.

Demarest, G. B., Hudson, L. D., Altman, L. C. 1979. Impaired alveolar macrophage chemotaxis in patients with acute smoke inhalation. *Am Rev Respi. Dis,* 119:279–86.

Edwards-Jones, V., Greenwood, J. E. 2003. What's new in burn microbiology? James Laing Memorial Prize Essay 2003. *Burns,* 29:15–24.

Fitzpatrick, J. C., Cioffi, W. G. 1996. Diagnosis and treatment of inhalation injury. In D. N. Herndon (ed.) *Total burn care.* Philadelphia: WB Saunders Company Ltd, p 184.

Gomez, M., Logsetty, S., Fish, J. S. 2001. Reduced blood loss during burn surgery. *Journal of Burn Care Rehabilitation,* 22:111–117.

Herndon, D. N., Barrow, R. E., Linares, H. A., et al. 1988. Inhalation injury in burned patients: Effects and treatment. *Burns Incl Therm Inj,* 14:349–56.

Latarjet, J., Choinere, M. 1995. Pain in burn patients. *Burns,* 21:344–346.

Mullner, T., Mrkonjic, L., Kwasny, O., Vecsei, V. 1997. The use of negative pressure to promote the healing of tissue defects: A clinical trial using the vacuum sealing technique. *British Journal of Plastic Surgery,* 50:194–199.

Muller, M. J., Gilpin, D. A., Herndon, D. N. 1996. Modulation of wound healing and the postburn response. In D. N. Herndon (ed.) *Total burn care.* Philadelphia: WB Saunders Company Ltd, p. 231.

Nebraska Burn Institute. Advanced Burn Life Support Providers Manual, Lincoln, NE: Nebraska Burn Institute, 1987.

Olabanji, J. K., Oginni, F. O., Bankole, J. O., Olasinde, A. A. 2003. A ten-year review of burn cases seen in a Nigerian teaching hospital. *Journal of Burns & Surgical Wound Care,* 2(1):1, Available from www.journalof-burns.com

Pruitt, B. A. 1997. The evolutionary development of biologic dressings and skin substitutes. *Journal of Burn Care Rehabilitation,* 18:S2–5.

Rode, H., Millar, A.J.W. 1999. Burns. In V.C. Harrison (ed.) *Handbook of Paediatrics.* Cape Town: Oxford University Press.

Simko, S. 1981. Reflections on the organization of mass burns treatment. *Acta Chir Plast,* 23(3):197–200.

Smailes, S. T. 2002. Noninvasive positive pressure ventilation in burns. *Burns,* 28:795–801.

Steenkamp, W. C., Van der Merwe, A. E., De Lange, R. 2002. Burn injuries caused by paraffin stoves. *South African Medical Journal,* 92:445.

Warden, G. D. 1992. Burn shock resuscitation. *World J Surg,* 16:16–23.

Barotrauma and decompression sickness

Jonathan Rosenthal

Diving has become a very popular sport in southern Africa with tens of thousands of dives being done annually, often in remote areas. Unfortunately, obeying all the 'rules' does not exclude diving injury. It is essential that these cases be recognized immediately and appropriately treated to minimize the chances of permanent disability or even death.

Pathophysiology of barotrauma, air embolism, and decompression sickness

Over-pressure of air-containing spaces occurs on ascent from depth, with resultant barotrauma to lungs, sinuses, and ears. This is due to expansion of the gas in these spaces as ambient pressure decreases. At worst, severe overpressure with systemic arterial gas embolism can be fatal, even from shallow depths.

Decompression sickness occurs when ascent is too rapid to allow enough time for gas dissolved in tissue fluids to equilibrate and to be removed through ventilation. Dissolved gas (especially nitrogen) then enters a gaseous phase in the tissues or in the circulation. These bubbles cause injury (e.g. neurological or musculoskeletal) via embolic effect, but importantly also via an endothelial injury that can progress over days.

Decompression sickness may be precipitated by too rapid ascent from the depth, by exercise, or by altitude, such as travel by air or over mountain passes shortly after a dive. Inexperienced divers, and older or obese divers, are at greater risk. Symptoms are more likely to occur in previously injured areas. However, it is important to note that even when all the 'rules' of diving are followed; decompression sickness can still occur.

Clinical presentation: Decompression sickness

Cases can present up to one week after diving, but the majority present within the first six hours after diving. Denial of symptoms is common.

- *Musculoskeletal cases* may present with severe joint pain, usually of the large joints, with minimal clinical findings (the term 'the Bends' derives from the fact that the affected joints are usually less painful when held in flexion).

- *Neurological deficit* may be present in 25% of musculoskeletal cases, involving the spinal cord or central nervous system. Obstruction of epidural veins of the spinal cord may present with back pain, paresthesiae or paralysis.
- *Cerebral symptoms* include headache, confusion, hallucinations, visual disturbance, convulsions, and cranial nerve VIII involvement with nausea and vomiting, nystagmus, vertigo, and tinnitus – referred to as 'staggers'.
- *Cutaneous involvement* causes skin rash, mottling, pruritis.
- *Pulmonary involvement* presents with dyspnoea, haemoptysis, cough, pleuritic pain (known in diving tradition as 'chokes').
- *Other systems* that can be affected include the coronary vessels leading to myocardial ischaemia and lymphatic obstruction with resultant oedema.
- Severe decompression illness may lead to circulatory collapse and death.

Clinical presentation: Air embolism

- Loss of consciousness or focal neurological deficit occurs immediately or shortly after ascent, due to occlusion of cerebral arterial vasculature.
- Acute myocardial infarction or cardiac arrest may occur due to embolic occlusion of coronary arteries.
- Subcutaneous emphysema, pneumothorax, or mediastinal emphysema may be present.
- Cerebral air embolism may lead to permanent disability or death.

Management

Treatment with recompression and circulatory support clears retained gas, oxygenates ischaemic tissues, and reduces endothelial injury – therefore essential, even with delayed presentation. Failure to treat with recompression, even if symptoms seem to have resolved, can lead to delayed neurological sequelae and dysbaric osteonecrosis.

- Assess ABCs and protect C-spine if indicated.
- If air embolism is suspected, the patient may be best kept in the left lateral decubitus Trendelenburg position.
- Administer 100% high-flow oxygen by rebreathing mask (mask with reservoir).
- Check blood pressure, pulse rate, and blood glucose.
- Monitor continuous ECG and oxygen saturation.

- Infuse intravenous crystalloid such as Ringer's lactate at 500 ml (i.e. maximal tolerated rates) per hour (patients can take fluids orally if able), and treat dysrhythmias and seizures as indicated.
- Obtain dive history: number of dives, time up, bottom time, depth, buoyancy problems, etc.
- Establish history of symptoms: onset and location of pain, treatment to date, previous medical history.
- Do clinical and neurological examination: level of consciousness, motor, sensor, and cerebellar systems, respiratory exam, musculoskeletal examination, skin inspection.
- Do special investigations: all patients require emergency unit chest X-ray, urea, and electrolytes (but do not let this delay recompression in severe cases).
- Suspect and treat hypothermia.
- Contact diving physician as early as possible.
- Discuss drug treatment with diving physician, e.g. the role of aspirin or lignocaine.
- The best diagnostic tool is often a trial of pressure in the decompression chamber.
- Contact a diving specialist:
  Divers Alert Network duty doctor: sharecall 0860 242 242
  National Hyperbarics Cape Town: 021 671 8655

Pitfalls

- Patients with rapid ascent may have pulmonary overpressure injury (including pneumothorax) and arterial gas embolism.
- Delayed onset suggests decompression sickness (i.e. nitrogen bubbles coming out of solution into gaseous phase).
- Obeying the 'rules' does not exclude decompression illness or embolism.
- Maintain vigilance for pneumothorax.
- Diving accidents often present with central or peripheral neurology.
- Remember pressure care!
- History is vital – keep witnesses for questioning by diving physician.
- Keep dive computers and equipment (they may be required for forensic evaluation).

Recommended reading

Bennett, P., Elliott, D. (eds.) 1993. *Physiology and medicine of diving*. Fourth edition. London: WB Saunders.

Bove, A. A., Davis, J. C. (eds.) 1990. *Diving medicine*. Philadelphia: WB Saunders.

41 Non-accidental trauma

Roux Martinez

Non-accidental injury occurs inside and outside the family unit, as well as in institutions, even hospitals. Worldwide, this problem is prevalent at all socio-economic levels and it has major social, health, and financial implications. This phenomenon occurs in our country as well, although true incidence is unknown and probably much higher than suspected. The so-called battered woman and abused child are familiar to most trauma centres. Husband abuse, however, as well as abuse of the elderly, infirm, imprisoned, and institutionalized, also occur and are often misdiagnosed. Abuse and domestic violence are commonly associated with the socio-economic stress caused by poverty, alcoholism, unemployment, and limited parental education.

Contributing factors

Much research has been done to identify the profiles of both abuser and victim, their motives, the patterns of injury, and the emotional cycles in which abuse tends to occur.

The afflicted are usually vulnerable to some extent, for reasons of their physique, sex, age, or financial and emotional dependence.

Most victims are repeatedly abused before they finally seek medical or social help. Some victims never seek help until it is too late.

Abuse happens by commission (assault) or omission (neglect).

Abuse can be verbal, sexual, physical, emotional, or even by psychological manipulation or threatening behaviour.

By not recognizing a patient's call for help, the very trauma staff may continue the chain of abuse.

Role of the trauma team

The trauma team plays a crucial role in identifying, treating, and reporting abuse in a sensitive and objective manner.

Reluctance to report suspected abuse is often due to:

- Inadequate staff training or lack of confidence
- Fear of making possible false accusations
- Reluctance to be involved in the legislative process
- Personal views and attitudes of the caregiver, which can cloud objectivity.

Recognizing non-accidental trauma

Patients presenting to the emergency unit do not always give a true history as to the origin of the abuse. It behoves the clinician to have a high index of suspicion and look out for subtle indications that abuse has taken place. At the same time, caution should be exercised as unfounded accusations could lead to litigation and emotional distress.

The abused woman

- Is usually abused by the man with whom she has a primary relationship
- Often presents with psychiatric labels and psychosomatic complaints
- Is often young and married early
- Is often from a very traditional or conservative belief system
- Often is or becomes socially isolated, but may also be in the social limelight
- Often comes from a family where abuse occurred
- Often has an increased incidence of para-suicide, alcoholism, and drug abuse
- Will often deny the abuse when questioned by staff
- Starts being abused during pregnancy, but existing abuse patterns can also increase or decrease during this time
- Has a fourfold increase in the incidence of low birthweight infants
- Blames herself or external factors for the abuse
- Hopes that someday her abuser will change
- Hopes that the medical staff will realize what is happening to her, without having to tell them

The abuser

- Is often an underachiever, insecure, with poor self-esteem
- Often abuses alcohol and drugs
- May suffer from personality disorders or other psychiatric problems
- Sees himself as head over her and the household
- Is often very jealous and manipulative
- Blames her for being deserving of or looking for his abuse
- Goes through cycles of aggression and remorse
- Is often financially or emotionally stressed
- Reacts at times of maximal personal interaction, such as holidays and weekends
- Is often from a family where abuse occurred
- Will often override your history-taking and attempts to examine the patient, and will hover around you and the patient
- May pretend to be extremely interested, loving, and supportive

The abused child

- Is most often abused by his/her own parents, especially the mother or primary caregiver
- Comes from families in all socio-economic strata, but often comes from a highly stressed environment due to financial problems, chronic illness, behavioral problems, retardation, or physical handicaps
- Is often in the age group under four years
- Often has parents with alcohol or drug problems
- Often has parents who were abused as children
- Is often an unwanted child or of an unwanted sex

Child abuse in South Africa

According to the April 2002–March 2003 SAPS statistics regarding crimes against children, 55% of reported crimes were rape, 7% were assault, 11% were abandonment, 1% child exploitation, 5% were child stealing, 9% child abuse, 18% indecent assault. 83.5% of all crimes aginst children are committed by persons known to the child, often at home.

The abused child can present with:
- Unexplained injuries
- Delayed presentation of injuries, or repeated visits to the emergency unit
- A history that does not match the clinical findings or age
- Withdrawn and disinterested in their environment, or may actually tell you that an adult caused the injuries
- Long-bone fractures in different stages of healing, Salter-Harris fractures, or metaphyseal tears (bucket handle appearance)
- Retinal haemorrhages or petechiae
- Burns (cigarette, circumferential with defined edges if submerged in hot water, iron, heater, or stove marks)
- Bruises, which can be imprints of the objects used in the assault
- Strangulation marks
- Perforated eardrums
- Sexually transmitted diseases
- Nervousness or being withdrawn
- Signs of forced feeding (bruising of mouth, lips, frenulum)
- Nutritional and educational neglect

Differential diagnosis of suspected child abuse

It is extremely important to identify and appropriately deal with cases of child abuse. At the same time, it should be kept in mind that many conditions can mimic child abuse, and an incorrect diagnosis and wrongful accusation may cause infinite harm.

- Accidental trauma: differentiate by careful history, injury patterns, recurrences
- Birth trauma: obtain birth history. Can present with bruising, retinal bleeds up to a month later. May have skull, clavicle, femur, and humerus fractures
- Osteogenesis imperfecta: multiple fractures, osteopaenia, blue sclerae, dental abnormalities
- Rickets: Vitamin D deficiency, renal disease, bowing of long bones. Reduced serum phosphates and increased serum alkaline phosphatase
- Scurvy: calcified subperiosteal haemorrhages, poor wound healing, bleeding gums, petechial haemorrhages
- Congenital syphilis: metaphyseal widening, chronic periostitis, positive serology
- Copper deficiency: osteoporosis and pathological fractures
- Infantile cortical hyperostosis: hyperplasia of subperiosteal bone with no metaphyseal involvement. Mandible and clavicles often affected
- Bleeding disorders: haemophilia, Von Willebrand's disease, Henoch-Schönlein purpura, meningococcal purpura. Abuse can co-exist!
- Cultural scarification: usually typical patterns for different tribes. Cauterization marks and acupuncture in certain cultures
- Mongolian spots: first two to three years of life
- Blistering skin conditions: may mimic burns (Erythema multiforme, impetigo, staphylococcal scalded skin syndrome, chicken pox)
- SIDS (sudden infant death syndrome) may mimic non-accidental suffocation
- Cardio-pulmonary resuscitation: can cause rib fractures and retinal haemorrhages

The abused institutionalized and geriatric patient

Some or all of the following may be present:
- Unexplainted falls, e.g. 'accident prone'
- Restraints used
- Branded as difficult patient or trouble maker
- Over- or under-medicating
- Pinch marks
- Defensive type injuries
- Retinal detachment
- Dehydration or malnourishment
- Decubitus ulcers

- Poor hygiene
- Extreme fearfulness, depression, theft of their belongings
- Signs of physical torture, beatings, dehydration, malnourishment, restraint injuries, depression, and suicide attempts in prisoners

Management

Managing an abuse victim is a specialized team effort that involves medical, social, legal, psychological, forensic, and police experts. The emergency unit is often the first step in this long and often frustrating journey.

- Be sensitive and empathetic and patient.
- Do not be judgemental or accusatory.
- Observe patient/partner or parent attitudes and interactions carefully.
- Ensure safety and confidentiality.
- Ask all superfluous relatives and caregivers to leave the examining room.
- Take a very thorough history.
- Access previous medical records if available.
- Fully undress the patient and then cover.
- Perform a thorough, but minimal required examination for the distressed child.
- Note that sexual assault examination in a child must be performed by a specialized team.
- Carefully examine inner aspects of limbs, pelvic examination in adults, throat and neck, inside of the mouth, palms, soles of feet, and between fingers and toes.
- Perform toxicology screen and test for therapeutic drug levels where indicated.
- Do a very thorough clinical documentation as your notes may be used in a court of law.
- Explain that injuries appear unusual and that investigations may be indicated to rule out other medical causes that can mimic abuse.
- Allow the patient to be part of the decision-making process.
- Never blame the patient for 'accepting' abuse.
- Assess for suicidal intention.
- Assess safety situation for children at home if the mother is the victim.
- Perform radiology: X-rays for under 5-year children should include at least skull, chest, pelvis, spine, and long-bone views. About 20% of abused children will present with bony injury.
- Make liberal use of CT scanning and bone scanning for healing fractures and head and abdominal injury. Radionucleide bone scanning will detect abnormalities 24–48 hours after injury and stay positive for months thereafter, with a low (12%) false-negative rate.

- Re-examine the patient with subtle signs after 24 to 48 hours, as some bruises may only then become evident.
- Maintain a low threshold for admission as this will also allow access to specialized staff for further counselling and intervention.
- Provide adult patients who refuse admission or further investigations with contact numbers for future reference.
- Ensure early involvement of the rest of the multi-disciplinary team.
- Make an effort to know and liaise with the anti-abuse organizations and professionals in your community (see addendum for list of contact numbers and resources).

Reporting child abuse and the procedure that follows

- Report your suspicions to the South African Police Service, and in particular the Family Violence, Child Protection and Sexual Offences Units (FCS).
- Do a thorough examination with good documentation of findings, and photographs of all injuries if possible.
- The investigating team will start with taking a statement from the person accompanying the child.
- Hereafter the child will be interviewed at home or in a place where the child is comfortable.
- Statements from witnesses will be taken and evidence collected.
- A completed docket will be sent to the prosecutor, who will interview the child with closed circuit television.
- The child will be sent for counselling and therapy.

Pitfalls

- Lack of knowledge and understanding of abuse and its symptoms.
- Not wanting to be involved.
- Allowing personal bias and accusational attitudes to influence decisions.
- Poor history-taking and inadequate case documentation.
- Not looking for occult injuries.
- Not reporting suspected abuse.
- Not involving multi-disciplinary team early on.

References and recommended reading

Jaudes, P. K. 1984. Comparison of radiology and radionucleide bone scanning in the detection of child abuse. *Paediatrics*, 73:166.

Mc Farlane, J. 1989. Battering during pregnancy: Tip of an iceberg revealed. *Women Health,* 15(3):69.

Meadow, R. 1989. ABC of child abuse, epidemiology. *British Medical Journal,* 298:727.

Tercier, A. 1992. Child abuse. In P. Rosen, R. M. Barkin (eds.) *Emergency medicine: Concepts and clinical practice.* Third edition. St Louis: Mosby Year Book.

http://www.n/m.nih.gov/medlineplus/domesticviolence.html

Gunshot wounds and blast injury

Herman du Plessis

Gunshot wounds in South Africa are unfortunately extremely common, especially in areas with high levels of criminal activity, gangsterism and lawlessness. Innocent bystanders are frequently injured in gangster shootouts, especially in areas where unemployment, drug and alcohol abuse are rife. Violent interpersonal disagreements, previously perpetrated with knives, sticks (knopkieries) or fists, are now settled with firearms, often unlicensed and easily obtainable.

Principles of wound ballistics

Ballistics is the study of the flight of missiles. Wound ballistics is a special type of terminal ballistics, and is concerned with the action of missiles in human tissue.

The potential energy of a missile or bullet is predicted by the formula: $E = \frac{1}{2}MC^2$ (M = mass, C = velocity). The kinetic energy that is eventually dissipated into the tissues, is proportional to tissue injury. By increasing the mass of the missile, energy is increased, but by increasing the velocity, energy is quadrupled, potentially causing much greater damage. When a missile traverses the body, a smaller amount of energy is deposited in the tissue than when the bullet lodges in the body, as all the potential energy is then transferred to the tissues. Low-velocity missiles ($< 1\,000$ feet per second) are associated with 'civilian' weapons, which produce considerably less tissue damage on impact than high-velocity missiles ($> 3\,000$ feet per second), which are usually from hunting or military weapons.

Permanent and temporary cavitation

The permanent cavity is a physical deficit caused by tissue lost in the actual path of the missile, and will vary in size depending on the size, shape, velocity, and deforming characteristics of the bullet.

The temporary cavity is the temporary displacement of tissue, beyond the actual path of the missile, as the missile travels through. The size of the temporary cavity is proportional to the kinetic energy lost (dissipated into tissue) by the missile. At a velocity of over 800 m sec^{-1} ($\pm 2\,500$ ft sec^{-1}) a substantial temporary cavity is created around the tract, where tissue is disrupted by the shock wave (energy dissipation) of the missile. The tissue in this zone is significantly injured by stretch and compression, and disruption of tissue architecture takes place on a cellular level.

Ammunition

Hunting ammunition mostly consists of soft-nosed lead points, designed to mushroom open on impact. This ensures that a big permanent cavity is created through massive energy loss, killing the animal.

Military ammunition, on the contrary, must be full metal jacketed, according to the Geneva Convention. This metal shell is then filled with lead. This missile will often traverse the victim intact, unless it hits bone, which will cause it to break up, and lead to significantly more tissue damage. The aim in warfare is not to kill, but only to injure the enemy, necessitating a major commitment of medical and strategic resources to the treatment of the injured.

Clinical presentation of gunshot wounds

Entrance wounds are usually smaller than exit wounds, but may contain fibres of clothing or foreign material.

Entrance wounds of close-range gunshot wounds may be surrounded by punctate tattoo marks, caused by burning gunpowder travelling with the missile.

Entrance wounds may be identified by the circumferential abrasion around the wound, caused by the spinning motion of the bullet.

Exit wounds are generally irregular in shape and do not have gunpowder tattoo marks or the circular abrasion marks on the edges of the wound. The bullet tract may not always follow a linear route between entrance and exit wounds.

Management

The management of the severely injured remains according to the principles of A, B, C.

- When airway and breathing problems have been controlled, and external bleeding stopped as far as possible, the patient usually requires further surgical management in the operating room.
- Vascular and organ injuries are all managed on their own merit (see relevant chapters).
- Most chest injuries can be managed by intercostal drainage and volume replacement.
- Low-energy transfer wounds sometimes need no treatment at all, or very limited drainage or local debridement.

- High-energy transfer injuries need aggressive and radical debridement of wounds, removal of foreign bodies, fragments and dead tissue, and thorough rinsing. Wounds are then left open (unsutured, but bandaged) to drain properly. Wound inspection is done 3–5 days later, and the wounds can then be closed by suture if clean.
- In the presence of bowel injury, especially large bowel, the debridement and irrigation must be meticulous and extensive to remove all bowel content and organisms from injured muscle, to prevent infection. Broad-spectrum antibiotics have a definite place as adjunct in these cases, and wound inspection needs to be performed within 48 hours.
- Pencillin is still the antibiotic of choice for the treatment and prophylaxis of clostridia.

Pitfalls

Care needs to be taken to avoid the following pitfalls:
- Not recognizing the extent of the damage caused by high-energy transfer missiles and bullets.
- Inadequate debridement of wounds, especially those contaminated by bowel content.
- Discarding removed bullets, as this may be of forensic importance.

Blast injuries

Mechanism of an explosion

An explosion can be defined as the chemical reaction that takes place when a small volume of solid or liquid matter is detonated and converted to a large volume of warm gas. Compressed air around the sphere of expanding gas creates a shock wave that moves rapidly away from the centre of the explosion.

The shock wave consists of a high-pressure phase (over pressure) of extremely short duration, followed by a low-pressure phase, lasting 5–10 times longer. This wave is the cause of injury to the victim and damage to the surrounds. The energy of the shock wave diminishes with distance.

The shock wave causes injury by:
- Spalling (breaking the interface between different densities, like an underwater explosion)
- Implosion (compression and release of internal gas areas – small explosions)
- Inertia (different reactions in tissue of different densities, causing tearing of ligaments)

Table 42.1 Blast effects on the human body

Over pressure	Organ	Effect
10–15 psi	Ear	Drum perforation
30–50 psi	Lung	Alveolar injury, oedema, haemorrhage
80–100 psi	Lung	Pneumothorax, air embolism
150 psi	Brain Viscera	Haemorrhage, rupture
200 psi	Limbs	Traumatic amputations

(psi = pounds per square inch)

Blast effects on the human body

Injuries

Primary injuries

These are caused by the shock wave that subjects the body to devastating pressure changes. Eardrums, airways and hollow organs may rupture or perforate, liver and spleen are torn and lacerated. Near the origin of the explosion, limbs are disrupted and amputated, or total and fatal disintegration of the body may occur.

Secondary injuries

These injuries are caused by missiles, such as fragments of casing, rocks, glass, and masonry, propelled at high velocities by the explosion. This leads mainly to lacerations and penetrating foreign body wounds, but also to fractures and tattoos from sand and soot.

Tertiary injuries

These injuries occur when the body is lifted and flung against inert objects.

Miscellaneous

Burns are often present due to heat or fire generated by the explosion. Inhalation injury is caused by hot gas and smoke.

Management

Management is as follows:

- Follow the standard Airway, Breathing, Circulation, Disability approach.
- Protect the spine until injuries are excluded radiologically.
- After establishing an airway, assess for pneumothorax or haemothorax and treat by drainage.
- Ventilation may be necessary because of pulmonary contusion and/or inhalation injury.
- Small-volume (pressure control) ventilation is recommended to reduce the risk of air embolism.
- Bleeding is controlled, and high-flow IV lines are established. Draw blood for arterial blood gas, carboxyhaemoglobin levels and cross-match.
- Assess disability and document all findings.
- Emergency surgery such as laparotomy or limb amputation may be required to control bleeding.
- Frequent reassessment is essential, especially of the ventilated patients, in case of later development of tension pneumothorax.
- Liberally X-ray spine, chest and abdomen in two planes, small wounds may be due to foreign bodies that have penetrated the gastro-intestinal tract, requiring surgery.
- Absent distal pulses in the presence of multiple blunt and penetrating injuries may need formal angiography to determine the level of vascular injury.
- Wounds often need scrubbing, debridement and suture in the operating room, as many are deeper than first suspected, or contain foreign material.
- All patients involved in any explosion need to have their ears examined for tympanic rupture, and have a high risk of long-term partial deafness.

Pitfalls

Care needs to be taken not to miss any of the following:

- The seemingly dazed and uninjured walking wounded, who need careful assessment. They often have blast lung and tympanic rupture – they cannot hear commands, only a ringing in the ears and may become hypoxic.
- Minor eardrum perforations.
- Major internal injuries when confronted by extensive superficial injuries.
- Inhalation injuries and hypoxia.

Further reading

Du Plessis, H. J. C. 1991. Management of gunshot wounds. *Journal of Trauma and Emergency Medicine (SA)*, 8:375–376.

Du Plessis, H. J. C. 1994. Missile injuries. *Journal of Trauma and Emergency Medicine (SA)*, 11:1019–1022.

Explosive blast injuries. In M. S. Owen Smith. 1981. *High velocity missile wounds*. London: Edward Arnold.

Explosions and explosive device related injuries. In S. L. Wiener, J. Barrett. *Trauma Management*. 1986. Philadelphia: WB Saunders.

Frykberg, E. R., Tepas, J. J. 1988. Terrorist bombing. *Annals of Surgery*, 208:569–576.

Owen Smith, M. S. 1981. *High velocity missile wounds*. London: Edward Arnold.

Patterns of injury. In D. V. Feliciano, E. E. Moore, K. L. Mattox. 1996. *Journal of Trauma*. Stamford: Appleton and Lange.

Scharf, G. M., du Plessis, H. J. C. 1990. Management of injuries due to explosive devices. *Journal of Trauma and Emergency Medicine (SA)*, 7:242–251.

Wound ballistics. In S. C. Wiener, J. Barrett. 1986. *Trauma Management*. Philadelphia: WB Saunders.

43 Bites and toxic stings

Curt Minnie

Although bites and stings occur frequently and many seem unimportant, for example, a dog bite, occasionally these seemingly innocuous wounds can lead to major complications, or the patients present with serious consequences that need urgent, active management, such as snake bites.

The African perspective is that we occasionally see injuries by wild animals which are lethal, or which may be disfiguring. Extensive knowledge of every type of bite or sting may not be possible for all practitioners, but the principles of management should be known to all, and resources for detailed information should be available in all emergency units.

Mammalian bites

Mammalian bites are common presenting problems of which the true incidence is unknown.

The four main issues of concern are:
1. Threat to life (uncommon)
2. Amount of soft tissue damage
3. Risk of infection and sepsis
4. Possible transmission of disease (see Table 43.1)

Pathophysiology

Most mammalian bites are not life threatening, but the following aspects are important:

Table 43.1 Potential disease transmission by mammalian bites

Animal bites	Human bites
Rabies	Hepatitis B & C virus
Bubonic plague	Tuberculosis
Tularaemia	Actinomycosis
Leptospirosis	Scarlet fever
Rat bite fever	Syphilis
Erysiplothrix	Gonorrhoea
Tetanus	HIV
Cat scratch fever	

- Larger animals may exert tremendous closing pressures (15–30 kg/cm^2).
- Dog bites are a combination of crush and tearing injuries.
- Soft tissue damage with necrotic tissue offers an ideal nidus for infection.
- Cat bites usually are a combination of scratches and deep puncture wounds.
- Larger herbivores (e.g. hippo) may cause severe crush and closed degloving injuries.
- Bites by large carnivores, although rare, cause massive soft tissue injury and loss of life.
- Human bites have a reputation for infection, but this may be because of the increased risk in closed fist injuries.

Management principles

The principles for management are:
- Thorough history documenting circumstances of injury
- Meticulous examination with documentation of findings including diagrams
- Seeking advice from a surgeon whenever any doubts arise
- Applying ATLS® principles

Wound management

- Most wounds can be managed in the Emergency Department.
- Well anaesthetized wounds facilitate examination.
- Digitally explore the lateral margins and base of the wound.
- Exclude the following common complications in all cases:
  - distal neurovascular injury
  - bony injury
  - tendon injury
  - retained foreign body
  - joint injury or penetration.
- Scrub or irrigate wounds with saline or dilute iodine solution.
- Debride compromised tissue and edges.
- Avoid agents toxic to tissues (e.g. peroxide, concentrated iodine or alcohol) in wounds.
- Once adequately debrided and irrigated, most wounds can be closed primarily.
- High-risk wounds (Table 43.2) or wounds with established infection should not be sutured.

- High-risk wounds require follow-up wound inspections and consideration for delayed closure.
- Routine culture of uninfected wounds is not required.

Prophylaxis

Antibiotic prophylaxis remains controversial and is indicated in the following circumstances:
- High-risk wounds
- Cat bites
- Deep puncture wounds
- Significant co-morbid disease, e.g. diabetes
- Immune-compromised patients
- Closed-fist injuries

Other treatment includes:
- Amoxicillin-clavulanic acid for 5–7 days could be used unless the patient is allergic to penicillin.
- Cefuroxime, doxycycline, erythromycin, co-trimoxazole, or ciprofloxacin may be used.
- Follow-up examinations for signs of infection should be routine at 48 hours.
- Consider the need for tetanus prophylaxis, as well as rabies prophylaxis, in endemic areas.
- HIV prophylaxis must be considered for all human bites.

Table 43.2 Bite wound infection risk and causative factors

Infection risk	Wound factors	Victim factors
Cat (40–50%)	More than 12 hours old	Age < 5, > 50 years
Human (15%)	Peripheral location	Substance abuse
Dog (2–5%)	Closed-fist injury	Diabetes
	Puncture wound	Malignancy
		Immune compromise:
		Transplant
		Radiotherapy
		Chemotherapy
		Medication
		Asplenism

Admission criteria

Patients showing the following should be admitted to a hospital:
- Tenosinovitis
- High risk for infection
- Obvious severe infection or cellulitis
- Closed-fist injuries
- Any complicated hand wounds

Closed-fist injuries

Consider all wounds in the metacarpo-phalangeal region to be closed-fist injuries. These wounds often present late and already infected, having been assumed to be minor injuries.
- Always examine these wounds through a full range of motion.
- Always examine radiologically, as 60–70% are positive for fractures, foreign bodies, or air in the joints.
- There should be a low threshold for admission, elevation, and intravenous antibiotics, as sepsis of the hand may have devastating long-term consequences.

Snake bite

Only some 10% of South African snakes are venomous. Not all bites will result in envenomation.

Snake venom can be categorized as neurotoxic, cytotoxic, or haemotoxic, although overlap does occur.
- Neurotoxic snakes include mambas and neurotoxic cobras.
- Cytotoxic snakes include the puff adder, gaboon adder, horned adder, and the cytotoxic (spitting) cobras.
- Some of the smaller adders, such as the berg adder, have both cyto- and neurotoxic effects.
- Haemotoxic snakes are the boom slang and vine snake (also known as the bird or twig snake).
- Consult with local experts regarding the venomous species in your area.

Management principles

- Provide immediate resuscitation if required (respiratory support).
- Determine the degree and severity of envenomation.
- Decide whether antivenom is indicated.
- Prevent complications.

Emergency management

- Identify snake if possible.
- Clean away excess venom if present and rinse out eyes if contaminated.
- Place patient in a well-monitored area and secure venous access.
- Remove any bandages and keep limb immobilized.
- Provide analgesia if required (beware of agents that may decrease respiratory effort).
- Monitor vital signs regularly, including vital capacity/peak expiratory flow.
- Clean and debride wounds.
- Provide tetanus prophylaxis.
- Be prepared to intervene rapidly should respiratory support be required.
- Be prepared to treat anaphylaxis.
- Admit all patients for at least 24 hours as delayed symptoms may occur.
- Assess for signs of significant envenomation.

Features of envenomation

- Cytotoxic features including pain, swelling, numbness, and paraesthesia occur almost immediately.
- Systemic features include weakness, nausea, vomiting, dysphagia, diplopia.
- Respiratory distress or cranial nerve palsy may occur within minutes to hours, indicating neurotoxicity.
- Haemotoxic complications may develop in hours to days.
- Never ascribe any symptom or complaint to hysteria.

Use of polyvalent antivenom

- The antivenom must be indicated.
- There is a risk of anaphylaxis because of the equine immunoglobulin components.
- The antivenom is manufactured by the SAIMR (South African Institute of Medical Research) and is supplied in 10 ml ampoules.
- The package insert contains additional important information and should be carefully studied.

Indications

The following are indications for treatment:
- Progressive painful swelling of a hand or foot
- Swelling extending to or involving a proximal joint

- Swelling of the head, neck, or chest
- Respiratory distress with deteriorating vital capacity/peak expiratory flow rates
- Neurological dysfunction such as diplopia, dysphagia, slurred speech, and muscle weakness
- Bites by mambas, large puff adders, or gaboon adders, before signs of toxicity
- If foetal distress becomes apparent in a pregnant victim
- In children with any signs of envenomation (see Recommended reading)

Neurotoxic effects may not be immediately reversed by administration of polyvalent antivenom, but recovery will be hastened. The symptomatic patient will therefore still require respiratory support.

Cytotoxic tissue damage is likely to be limited by timeous administration of polyvalent antivenom.

Boomslang antivenom, however, will rapidly reverse all haemotoxic effects at any stage of the process.

Contraindications to polyvalent anti-venom treatment

- Bites of small adders, sea and bird snakes
- Peripheral bites with mild non-progressive swelling in adults
- Boomslang bites (this type of bite requires specific antivenom available from the SAIMR)

Dosage

- Use 80–120 ml in 200 ml 5% dextrose water intravenously.
- Larger doses may be required to reverse respiratory neuromuscular dysfunction.
- Boomslang antivenom is given as 20 ml intravenously, occasionally with a second dose of 10 ml.

Patients should be in an ICU environment and managed by a specialist. Consider transferring patient to a larger centre if required.

Scorpion stings

Toxic scorpions in South Africa belong to the Buthidae group (small pincers and big stings), notably *Parabuthus granulatus* and *P. transvaalicus*. Although most scorpions are harmless, stings from the Buthids can be neurotoxic and are potentially lethal.

They may be found in Mpumalanga, the North and North-West Provinces, and the Western Cape.

All scorpion stings are painful.

Features of envenomation

- There may be severe local pain.
- This will be followed by myalgia, paresthaesia, and hyperesthaesia.
- There may be fever, hyperreflexia, dysphagia, sweating, and increased adrenergic activity.
- Children may become very agitated, restless, and may convulse.
- Airway compromise and complete respiratory failure may follow.

Emergency management

- Patients should be closely monitored in an appropriate area.
- Be prepared to manage ensuing airway obstruction and support ventilation.
- Consider scorpion antivenom in cases of severe envenomation.
- Dose: 10 ml intravenously, with 5 ml follow-up dose occasionally required.
- Antivenom reaches its peak effect after 4–8 hours.
- The wound should be cleaned and dressed.
- Tetanus prophylaxis must be provided.
- All bites are very painful and analgesia must be provided.
- Avoid any opiates as they may potentiate respiratory failure.
- Injecting local anaesthetic around the wound works very well.
- Calcium gluconate intravenously may reduce symptoms.
- Patients should be managed in an ICU environment.
- Consider transfer to a larger centre if required.

Spider bites

Most South African spiders are non-toxic.

Neurotoxic spiders belong to the Latrodectus species, e.g. button (widow) spiders. Violin, crab, and sac spiders are cytotoxic.

Features of neurotoxic envenomation

- Intense burning at the site of the bite with associated lymphadenopathy is experienced.
- Severe myalgia, hyperreflexia, tremor, and abdominal rigidity may follow.

- Marked sympathetic arousal may be present with hypertension and tachycardia.
- Fever, nausea, and vomiting may also be present.

Emergency management

- All patients with symptoms should be hospitalized and closely monitored in an appropriate area.
- Any wounds should be cleaned and debrided.
- Tetanus prophylaxis should be considered.
- Severe neurotoxic envenomation may require Latrodectus antivenom.
- Dosage: 10 ml IV, occasionally with a follow-up dose of 5 ml if required.
- Response is usually within 10–30 minutes.
- Be prepared to treat severe anaphylaxis.
- Calcium gluconate intravenously may reduce painful spasms.

Hymenoptera stings (bees and wasps)

These occur throughout South Africa. Allergy to Hymenoptera venom is common and repeat exposure may be life threatening.

Clinical features of envenomation

- There may be intense burning at the site with pruritis and rapid swelling.
- In patients with a known allergy to the venom, varying degrees of allergic reaction may follow.
- Severe anaphylaxis may follow even a second exposure.
- Massive envenomation (100–300 stings) may lead to a syndrome characterized by rhabdomyolysis and progressive multiple organ failure.

Management of minor exposures

- Remove sting carefully.
- Clean wound.
- Local therapy with ice, antihistamines, and topical steroid may provide relief.
- Consider tetanus toxoid if indicated.

Exposures in patients with known allergy or patients with previous multiple stings

- Remove sting carefully.
- Clean wound.

- Consider tetanus toxoid if indicated.
- Admit patient to observation area.
- Monitor vital signs for 4–6 hours.
- Consider intravenous steroids and antihistamines early.
- Be prepared to treat anaphylaxis.

Management of massive envenomation

- Remove all stings.
- Resuscitate aggressively.
- Be prepared to treat severe anaphylaxis, massive swelling, and airway obstruction.
- Give intravenous steroids and antihistamines early.
- Monitor haemodynamic status very carefully.
- Refer to Specialist for further therapy in ICU.
- Consider transfer to a major centre.

Pitfalls

- Seemingly insignificant human or animal bites can have severe septic complications if not managed correctly from the start.
- The early signs of neurotoxic snake bite are subtle and should be carefully elicited.
- A photo atlas or reference manual should be available to identify the snake/spider/scorpion involved.
- The benefits of appropriate antivenom administration, when indicated, in the Intensive Care environment, far exceed the risks.

Recommended reading

Muller, G. J. 1993. Black and brown spider bites in South Africa. A series of 45 cases. *South African Medical Journal*, 83:399–405.

Muller, G. J. 1993. Scorpionism in South Africa. *South African Medical Journal*. 83:405–411.

Schrire, L. Muller, G. J., Pantanowitz, L. 1996. The diagnosis and treatment of envenomation in South Africa. *South African Institute for Medical Research*.

http://www.n/m.nih.gov/medlineplus/bitesandstings.html

Psychological trauma

Gerrit van Wyk

Physical trauma is almost always accompanied by emotional trauma, which may have far-reaching effects on the patient's long-term functioning. For example, motor vehicle accident survivors frequently experience incapacitating anxiety and inability to deal with traffic. Emergency medical care providers are not always aware of the extent and gravity of the late psychological consequences of crime, natural disasters, and interpersonal violence.

Post-traumatic stress disorder (PTSD), the long-term effect of unresolved emotional trauma, is potentially debilitating and long-lasting. Intensive specialist treatment is usually required, while an appropriate response soon after the traumatic incident could have avoided these complications.

There is no doubt that children are particularly susceptible to the long-term effects of injury and the emotional distress that accompanies pain and hospitalization. Various specialized techniques of assessment and treatment are available to assist young survivors of trauma.

Causes of psychological trauma

Psychological trauma (emotional shock), may be caused by:

- An event outside the usual range of human experience, distressing to almost anyone.
- Witnessing or learning of the trauma, death, or serious injury of a family member or close associate.
- The subjective experience of an event, not so much the objective content of the event itself.
- An experience associated with intense threat and/or horror.

Where one person may be severely traumatized by a certain experience, another person would seem to be largely unaffected.

The psychology of trauma

The critical traumatic incident is usually experienced as:

- A breakdown of coherence, meaning, predictability, and understanding of how the world is
- An intense loss of control over environment and destiny
- An intense experience of powerlessness and helplessness
- An experience of extreme vulnerability and insecurity

Understanding and empathy are essential for an appropriate response to the victim's distress.

Typical reactions following trauma

- Emotional fluctuation from numbness and unreality to fear, anger, sadness, and even guilt and self-recrimination
- Difficulty sleeping, bad dreams
- Difficulty concentrating
- Low energy, fatigue, loss of drive
- Tension and nervousness, easily startled, easily panicked
- Pre-occupation with what has happened and what could have happened
- Repeatedly reliving aspects of the traumatic event, flash-backs
- Physical symptoms of stress, such as headache, indigestion, hypertension, hyperventilation, muscle tension, dizziness, tremors
- Intense reactions of fear and discomfort when confronted with objects, situations, people, smells, sounds, anything that reminds of the incident
- Tendency to avoid people, places, feelings, memories, anything associated with the traumatic incident
- Overwhelming fear of repetition of the event, pre-occupation with security and safety

Phases of recovery

The phases of recovery from a traumatic incident are set out in Figure 44.1.

Should significant symptoms persist after four weeks, specialized treatment is indicated.

Determinants of recovery

Various factors can increase vulnerability to trauma and delay recovery.

Figure 44.1 Phases of recovery

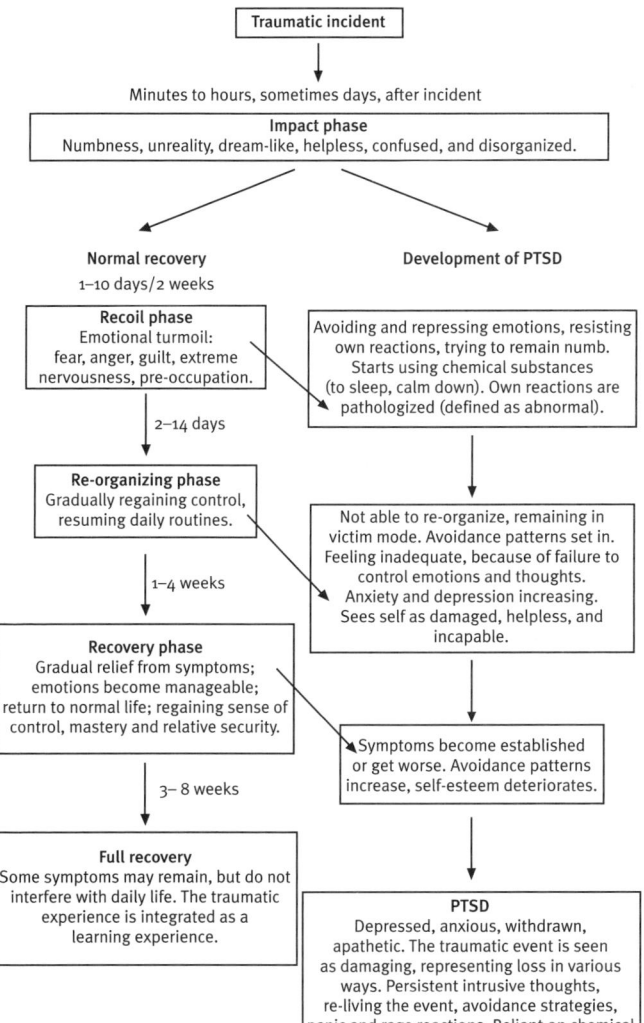

An alternative approach to the recovery process is also in three phases:
1. *Victim phase:* experienced as being a helpless victim
2. *Survivor phase:* grateful for survival, realizing it could have been worse
3. *Full recovery phase:* trauma is seen as a growth, albeit a painful experience. Once some form of benefit is recognized, strength or wisdom gained from the bad experience, the trauma is resolved.

Factors relating to the traumatic incident

- Natural disasters have a greater impact than man-made disasters.
- Incidents involving darkness, fire, noise, injury, blood, or death are more difficult to resolve.
- Rape and intense military combat have the highest incidence of PTSD.
- The trauma seems to be worse if the person was alone.
- Away from home, or in a foreign situation, the impact is greater.
- Motor vehicle accidents and criminal violence are the most common causes of post-traumatic stress in South Africa.

Factors relating to the person

- Persons with a history of previous trauma or a psychiatric history are at risk of complications.
- Single persons, divorced persons, persons living alone are more vulnerable.
- Pre-existing stress such as familial, occupational, or financial stress make recovery more difficult.
- Children under the age of eight and adults over the age of 50 are more vulnerable.

Factors relating to the aftermath of the trauma

- Hospitalization and sick leave often cause a delay in recovery.
- Social support structures are an important aid to recovery.
- Validation/recognition that the experience was real, significant and distressing, and that the victim is blameless, is essential.
- Counselling can speed up recovery and diminish the incidence of PTSD.
- Counselling is more effective if commenced soon after the trauma (preferably the same day) and if the victim is counselled in situ.
- Development of avoidance patterns makes PTSD more likely.
- Anxiolytics do not aid the recovery process due to the risk of habituation and pathologizing (turning the normal trauma reaction into an illness).

- Expectations of the victims concerning their own reactions to the trauma are crucial to the recovery. Victims need to be reassured that their reactions are normal and appropriate.

Post-traumatic stress disorder

- PTSD is an extension and exacerbation of the typical early reactions and symptoms following psychological trauma, i.e. reliving, hyper-arousal, numbing and avoidance.
- Symptoms persisting longer than a month can be regarded as PTSD. Prior to this they are regarded as normal and appropriate responses.
- PTSD usually resolves spontaneously within six months after the traumatic incident. If symptoms persist after six months the condition is regarded as chronic and the prognosis is diminished drastically.
- The condition is commonly associated with alcohol and drug abuse, rage reactions, and depression, and often causes major social and occupational dysfunction.
- Treatment of PTSD is essentially psychotherapeutic. Psychotropic medication, specifically adrenergic and SSRI anti-depressants are palliative at best.
- The most effective treatment is cognitive-behavioural therapy, a specialized, but cost-effective form of psychotherapy. Various other approaches are used with varying success.

Head injury and trauma

- Concussive head injury is often associated with post-traumatic amnesia, even in mild cases of concussion. This will distinguish concussion from psychological trauma.
- Emotional trauma leads to amnesia for aspects of the traumatic event, where concussive amnesia is more of a 'blanket' type.
- The expected reliving and avoiding reactions following emotional trauma are absent after concussion, but other signs, such as fatigue, headache, absent-mindedness, difficulty concentrating, and emotional lability, are shared.
- Concussion may cause adjustment difficulties (post-concussion syndrome), but is not usually the cause of PTSD.

Advice to victims of trauma

- Give yourself time to recover; you will not be your usual self for a while. Your reactions and feelings are a normal part of recovery which takes about three weeks.

- Do not hesitate to ask for support and understanding from those close to you.
- Communicate your experience to others close to you as often as you can and in as many ways as you can – talking, discussing, drawing, writing.
- Avoid alcohol, drugs, tranquillizers, and sleeping tablets.
- Re-establish your regular routines as soon as possible.
- Do not put off going back to work.
- Do not try to be 'strong': do not avoid crying or feeling afraid, or any other feelings you may have. The feelings will diminish by themselves – fighting against your feelings will only complicate your recovery process.

Pitfalls

- Guard against labelling these reactions as unreasonable, unnecessary, or in any way abnormal, disordered, or sick. Pathologizing these reactions will feed feelings of inadequacy and add to their already overwhelming sense of disempowerment, often the start of PTSD.
- Benzodiazepines and other sedatives should be administered with circumspection because of a high risk of habituation in traumatized persons.
- The response of family members, friends, and work colleagues is significant for the recovery of the victim. Their responses could either aid or obstruct normal recovery. It is useful to give some guidance to them on how to react.
- The psychological impact of trauma is all too often disregarded in the rush of the emergency room, while the after-effects can be potentially disastrous. These complications are avoidable by responding empathetically to the patient's distress and by appropriate early counselling.

Recommended reading

Hodgkinson, P. E., Stewart, M. 1998. *Coping with disaster: Handbook of post-disaster psychosocial aftercare.* London: Routledge.

Resick, P. A. 2001. *Stress and trauma.* East Sussex: Psychology Press.

Van Wyk, G. C. B. 2001. *Trauma in the Workplace: The new way of managing trauma: Turning a bad experience into good.* Cape Town: Traumaclinic.

PART 5

Specific issues

For many things in medicine, one can say that if there is more than one system, it is because there isn't a single system that works well. Certainly, one could make that argument about scoring systems. It is the purpose of this chapter to summarize what is wanted from a scoring system and to review the attempts made in that direction.

Scoring systems were first used by the Egyptians, who divided injuries into three groups – treatable, contentious, and untreatable. The fundamental principles remain unchanged.

A scoring system may be defined as 'a system of quantifying the total impact of individual injuries'. It is not the same as an audit. An audit is 'a retrospective review of available data that allows evaluation of activities within a unit'. A scoring system may help audit a unit but can also provide prospective information about the prognosis of an individual trauma victim.

Scoring systems can be divided into three types: physiological, anatomical, and outcome analysis.

Physiological scoring systems

These scoring systems include the simplest ones used on a day-to-day basis.

The **Revised Trauma Score** measures BP (blood pressure), GCS (Glasgow Coma Scale), and RR (respiratory rate). This simple scoring system is used for prehospital assessment.

The **APACHE** (Acute Physiology Score and Chronic Health Evaluation) system is a more complex system that is widely used in intensive care units.

Anatomical scoring systems

These systems classify injuries on the basis of their anatomical location and severity.

- The original system known as **AIS** (Abbreviated Injury Scale) was devised in 1971 and divided the body into six regions and graded injuries from 1–5.
- A more detailed version, **CRIS** (Comprehensive Research Injury Scale), has not gained general acceptance.

- The AIS has been modified into the **ISS** (Injury Severity Score), which uses the sum of the square of the highest scores for each region.
- This has been changed again into the **NISS** (New Injury Severity Score), which is the sum of the three highest scores.
- More recently, a scoring system utilizing the ICD–10 diagnostic coding system has been devised.

Outcome analysis systems

Ideally, a scoring system would give us information about a patient's prognosis before resuscitation was started. This would allow more efficient utilization of resources and one would theoretically avoid the emotionally and financially unsatisfactory situation of spending time and resources on patients with injuries incompatible with life. Both the simple GCS and the more complicated ISS were found to correlate with mortality, but neither were able to predict the probability of an individual surviving. One of the major prognostic variants is age: neither of these systems takes age into account. The aim of outcome analysis systems is to provide this information.

The **TRISS** (Trauma Score and Injury Severity Score Analysis) methodology is a mixture of the ISS and the trauma score and can be used to predict the probability of survival.

TRISS:

$P(s) = 1/(1+e^{-b})$:

$b = b_o + b_1 (RTS) + b_2 (ISS) + b_3 (age factor)$

Application of scoring systems

The problem with all the anatomical systems and particularly the outcome analysis systems is that they are cumbersome and require either dedicated personnel or computer systems. This makes them relatively expensive to use. Clearly, the decision not to continue with treatment is a major decision and would have to be based on absolute confidence with the scoring system and could only be implemented if the probability of mortality was 100%. There are few times the outcome analysis system would in fact change management.

The ideal system: Can it exist?

The more complicated the system, the more accurate it is when used to compare the performance of one centre with another centre.

Having looked at the problems with existing systems, what would the ideal system be? It would be accurate, simple, repeatable, cheap, give reliable prognostic information, utilize the existing coding system used by a hospital and internationally. No such system exists.

Conclusion

Scoring systems are used to quantify injuries. All involved with trauma management would agree that it would be better to prevent trauma than treat the victims. Society needs information in order to implement changes that may prevent accidents occurring. The medical profession needs to supply the governing bodies with information so that appropriate policy may be drafted. For that, accurate statistics regarding the aetiology of trauma are required. Thus, any scoring system should ideally provide demographic information to prevent duplication of resources.

Scoring systems have different roles to play, depending on what stage in the management of a patient they are utilized. In the prehospital stage, they allow formalization of the decision of which is the nearest appropriate facility and most appropriate mode of transport. At all levels, they allow comparison between units, auditing, research, and planning of facilities.

There is no doubt that scoring systems have a role to play in the management of trauma victims and in the planning of facilities. The structure of trauma facilities varies widely nationally and internationally. Rural areas may have very different facilities from the large urban centres. There is no 'one system fits all' available and there never will be such a system, but standardization among scoring systems used internationally is nevertheless vital.

Recommended reading

Conrad, M. H., Nwariaku, F. Trauma scoring. In F. Nwariaku, E. Thal (eds.) 1999. Second edition. *Parkland Trauma Handbook.* London: Mosby.

Muckart, D. J., Bhagwanjee, S., Gouws, E. 1997. Validation of an outcome prediction model for critically ill trauma patients without head injury. *Journal of Trauma,* Dec, 43(6):934–8, discussion 938–9.

Organ Injury Scale of the American Association for the Surgery of Trauma (OIS–AAST). 2000, http://www.aast.org.

Medicolegal aspects of trauma

Johan W van der Spuy

The key considerations of the medicolegal aspects of trauma are:
- Clinical assumptions are shortcuts to disaster.
- No notes may mean no defence.
- Derogatory criticism should be avoided.
- You should be clear and yet concise in what you say and in what you write.

Medicolegal topics are arranged alphabetically:
- Affidavits
- Alcohol and drugs
- Amputations
- Blood transfusion
- Certificates
- Communication
- Consent
- Documentation
- Emergencies away from your hospital or rooms
- Evidence in court
- HIV testing
- Missed injuries
- Mistaken identity
- Professional insurance
- Rape cases
- Referrals
- Statements in unguarded moments
- Subpoenas

Affidavits

Affidavits are formal documents to be used by lawyers and courts. The better one's affidavit, the less likely it is that one will be called to give evidence in court.
- Do not use abbreviations; if you must do so define your abbreviation (e.g. 'RBB means right bundle bunch block').

- Avoid using technical jargon.
- Sign or initial all amendments.
- Sign or initial each page; the last page must be signed and dated.
- Provide your first names, surname, and contact data.
- Be clear, concise, and objective.
- Clarify what you found, what you did, when you stopped caring for the patient, what his/her condition was when last seen, and who was to be in charge of the patient thereafter.

Alcohol and drugs

Alcohol intake is common in the hours before injury. Common errors and pitfalls are:

- Assuming that the smell of liquor on the breath indicates that a considerable amount had been taken and that the patient's clinical state of consciousness is due to that.
- Forgetting that intoxicated patients are prone to head injury, as well as to other injuries.
- Overlooking the possibility of drugs, hypoglycaemia, diabetic ketosis, hypoxia, hypothermia, etc. being the cause or part of the equation.
- Discharging patients too soon, before they had regained their faculties, before they can look after themselves properly, and before they had been re-examined when sober.
- It is good practice to give such patients advice sheets in regard to important injuries, which may manifest over the next day or two (head, neck, abdomen, chest, and limbs).

Amputations

- Always get valid consent.
- Explain and record the reasons for amputation and the level at which amputation is to be made.
- X-rays and photographs are invaluable and say more than words.
- Primary stump closure in amputations for trauma carries considerable risk of complications; delayed formal closure is advisable.
- Tetanus prophylaxis and prophylactic antibiotic cover are essential.
- Check that it is the correct side – particularly when the opposite limb is also injured.
- Do not cover the stump with a cage and/or blankets post-operatively; when stump haemorrhage occurs, it must be readily visible.

Blood transfusion

Avoid identification errors at all cost! The doctor is responsible for ensuring that:

- The specimens going to Blood Bank are correctly labelled.
- The blood to be transfused is correctly identified as being for the particular patient (not the folder!).
- The blood is fit for transfusion.
- Reactions are reported to the Blood Bank.

Remember:

- The blood container and tubing must be kept for 24 hours after infusion to allow proper investigation in the event of transfusion reactions.
- Adult Jehovah's Witnesses should *not* be given blood against their expressed wishes. However, South African law dictates that lifesaving blood transfusion may not be withheld from minor children of Jehovah's Witnesses – parental refusal is then invalid by law. Always liaise such situations with your medical superintendent and with your senior doctor or a peer.

Certificates

- False statements may lead to professional censure, if not criminal prosecution.
- Only certify facts based on personal observation.
- If asked to certify a fact which you cannot verify, qualify the situation by adding, 'as I am informed', 'in my opinion', or something similar.
- Date your certificate and make all dates safe against fraud: 02.02.2002.

Communication

- Communication errors and misunderstandings are at the root of many clinical tragedies and most litigation or professional disciplinary disasters.
- Hand-overs to colleagues and instructions to nursing staff are classic situations favouring communication foul-ups. Writing it and saying it is much safer than just saying it.
- Telephonic instructions also often lead to errors – ask for 'play-back' to verify that the message had been received correctly; it is also prudent to make brief notes about what such messages were.
- Patients and relatives must be reasonably informed about what is happening and what is to happen. Establish rapport; understand that they are stressed and allow for that. Do not make false promises like 'everything will be fine' in critical cases; give a somewhat guarded prognosis

and assure them that you are doing your best. When they understand and are kept informed, patients and relatives are also more lenient on us for our inevitable shortcomings and little mistakes.

Consent

- Consent is necessary for all procedures under general or regional anaesthesia. Strictly speaking, it is also necessary for procedures under local anaesthetic (e.g. suturing of simple lacerations) but in conscious patients implied consent is usually adequate. When in doubt, play safe.
- Informed consent is necessary – the patient must understand the why, the what, and the foreseeable consequences.
- Only majors may sign consent, i.e. those aged 21 years, those aged 18 and who are self-supporting, and those who are legally married (regardless of age).
- A mother may sign for a child, even when she is still a minor herself.
- One spouse cannot sign consent for the other while the latter is of sound mind and capable of giving consent.
- A parent or legal guardian must sign consent for procedures on a minor. However, when parents or legal guardians unreasonably deny consent for essential procedures on a child, the law charges the doctor with the responsibility of getting a magisterial order to proceed in the best interests of the child.
- Telephonic consent may be taken in emergencies but then one must:
  - ensure the identity of the consentee and the exact relationship to the patient
  - get a second person to take the consent directly from the consentee
  - get both persons taking the consent to sign the consent form
  - ensure that the consentee is the nearest contactable next-of-kin to the patient
  - get the consentee to endorse the telephonic consent with written consent as soon as possible afterwards.
- It is extremely unwise to perform procedures against the declared wishes of a major person and without legal consent, e.g. when the person refuses permission on religious or other grounds.
- At times the surgeon may be confronted with unusual emergency situations: the patient may not be able to sign consent and no next-of-kin may be contactable (e.g. with an unidentified unconscious patient). If delay will endanger life or limb, the surgeon and one other doctor must sign consent jointly. Notwithstanding any of the above, emergency situations may arise when the doctor has to act without the requisite consent in order to save the patient (for instance, when emergency

front-room thoracotomy is necessary). In such cases, be sure to record the circumstances in writing as soon as possible and to liaise with a senior colleague (e.g. a medical superintendent) before or very soon after the procedure.

Documentation

This is your most important commitment beyond being competent. Court procedures often occur several years later when memory of details is impossible. Courts grant written notes great credence, as opposed to vague memories and statements regarding what you will have done in such a situation.

Illegible writing is a major source of misunderstanding and consequent error, as well as one's own personal and legal embarrassment.

Be sure to record:
- Date and time of first and subsequent examinations. Record day, month, *and year* and use 24-hour time readings
- In traffic trauma it is becoming increasingly important to record whether or not alcohol and/or drugs had been involved and whether injured occupants had used their seatbelts or had been ejected from the vehicle
- Vital signs
- Wounds and external marks or lesions (site, size, and appearance)
- Appearance of clothes (so often omitted; so important later)
- Fractures
- Examination findings
- Results of special investigations
- Operative procedures and findings
- Medication prescribed (drugs and intravenous fluids)
- Treatment orders, particularly those for removing drains, catheters, etc.
- Sign and write your name adequately and *legibly*.

Never write derogatory remarks about the patient, relatives, nursing staff, the referring doctor, or colleagues in the notes, no matter how irritated you feel at the time. These have a habit of rebounding!

Never alter the original notes or add to the records at a later date in order to 'whitewash' your part in the patient's care. Quite frequently copies of the original notes had already been made before you make your amendments or additions. Even though you are not guilty of misconduct, such actions are regarded very seriously by assessors, disciplinary enquiries, and courts – it implies that you have something to hide and are trying to cover it up.

Emergencies away from your hospital or rooms

These emergencies are mostly at the roadside following traffic accidents. It is one's ethical and medicolegal duty to render assistance if an emergency is defined and one may then not refuse to help.

Once the emergency situation has been solved, care can be transferred to any person competent to deal with the case. Points to remember at the accident site are:

- Safeguard yourself and the patient.
- Prevent secondary collisions.
- Take reasonable action to save life and protect limbs (attend to airway, stop bleeding, splint fractures as best possible).
- Move the patient only if the environment is hostile.
- Point out dangerous situations to first-aiders and ambulance personnel.
- Do what is within your capabilities.
- Remember that others on the scene (e.g. a trained paramedic) may have more expertise and experience in prehospital care than you have.
- You are not obliged to accompany the patient to hospital if the ambulance crew can handle the situation.
- Do not abandon the patient until the situation appears safe.
- Record drugs and treatment given.
- Provide a note to go with the patient.

Evidence in court

- A doctor giving evidence about a patient whom he/she treated is an expert witness in court – a situation different to that of a person being a witness to the fact only (as, for instance, a person who saw an accident occur and merely relates in court what he/she saw). An expert witness is entitled not only to relate the facts concerned but also to present the logical sequelae and deductions arising from such observations.
- Court will judge. Give evidence only. Do not slant your evidence according to your sympathies or feelings.
- Speak clearly, say exactly what you mean, and say it as simply as possible.
- Do not answer questions which are unclear or ambiguous; if necessary, request more clarity.
- Distinguish very clearly between fact and opinion.
- Distinguish very clearly between certainty, probability, and possibility.
- Do not appear to be expert when you are not. When you do not have the answer or cannot express an opinion, say so.
- Do not be pushed into giving yes-or-no answers on complex matters unless you are comfortable to do so.

- Do not say things that you are not prepared to defend.
- If you omitted to examine a specific clinical aspect, say so. Do not make it up on the spur of the moment.
- Answer the question and do not over-elaborate or sidetrack – the opposition thrives on this.
- Do not get annoyed during cross-examination. It is the right and the duty of the opposing side to test the validity of your evidence. They love getting you cross because then you are distracted and more easily tripped up.

HIV testing

In elective situations it is internationally agreed that, except for anonymous surveys, informed consent should be obtained before testing for HIV antibodies in living patients.

Emergency situations raise other considerations and the doctor should use discretion in the interests of both the patient and the members of the health-care team:

- Until HIV status of the patient is known, precautions should be taken as if the person is HIV-positive.
- A need-to-know situation arises in cases of needle-stick injuries to staff. It is fairest to then take the test and advise the patient afterwards if it is positive.
- If HIV-positivity and consequent immunocompromise are suspected in a patient, special care and management may be necessary and then testing of an unconscious patient becomes acceptable as part of patient management.
- It is your duty to pass on information of HIV-positivity to other health-care workers and sexual partners of the patient who may be affected.
- Warn staff not to pass from one patient to another when there is any possibility of blood on their hands or gloves.
- Consult with colleagues when uncertain and in unusual situations.

Missed injuries

Classic situations for missing injuries are:
- Unconscious, drunk, or drugged patients
- Not undressing the patient adequately (or fully in the case of unconscious patients or those with multiple injuries)
- Not assessing the patient oneself and relying on the findings of nurses, students, or colleagues
- Unconscious, inebriated, or spinal cord-injured patients
- Being sidetracked by externally obvious injuries

- Inadequate subsequent reassessment
- Assuming that referral letters and hand-over information represent the full and unquestionable truth
- Not listening to the patient, the relatives, the nursing staff, and juniors

Lesions that are prone to be missed are:
- Rib-cage fractures
- Injuries to posterior parts of the body
- Perineal injuries
- Mandibular and facial bone fractures
- Closed degloving lesions
- Pulse inequalities or deficits
- Spinal cord lesions in unconscious or polytrauma patients
- Peripheral nerve and brachial plexus injuries
- Foreign bodies (particularly glass) in wounds

Mistaken identity

This is a common medicolegal issue because the sequelae vary from unpleasant to catastrophic. It is best avoided by:
- Checking patient names!
- Checking the names and dates on X-rays and other special investigations before acting thereon.
- Check sides; left-right confusion can be disastrous.
- Be particularly careful in labelling and identifying individual fingers and toes correctly.
- Never handle the records or films of more than one patient at the same time.
- Do not put X-rays back on the bed after viewing – put them back into the packet of the appropriate patient.
- Check identity against the patient – *not* against the folder.
- Be doubly careful about patient identification with blood transfusion.

Professional insurance

Anyone in medical practice is strongly advised to have such cover – even in non-clinical situations litigation or disputes may arise regarding contracts or remuneration.

It is strongly advised that cover is obtained from a reputable organization with established international standing, like the Medical Protection Society. Be particularly wary of competitive schemes, usually offered at very attractive lower premiums. Scrutinize the cover provided by such schemes very carefully. They often do not cover your legal costs and do not always offer legal representation in regard to Health Professions Council disciplinary enquiries into your practice or conduct. They also tend not to provide legal representation in contractual disputes with your partner/s or employer.

When you stand accused, be strongly advised not to make admissions or statements, nor to provide explanations of your actions, before you have liaised with the legal advisers of your medical insurers.

Do not assume that your employer (e.g. state, province, or private concern) will accept the responsibility for clinical complications arising from work done while in their service. They may but they may not!

Do not wait for lightning to strike – every doctor is vulnerable and litigation is increasing.

Rape cases

- Identify, note, and treat all non-gynaecological injuries.
- Make a specific record of the mental and psychological state of the patient.
- Keep clothes and do not wash it, otherwise valuable evidence may be destroyed.
- The patient should not be washed until fully assessed medicolegally in order not to lose vital evidence (blood stains, semen, assailant's hair, scratched skin under victim's nails).
- Vaginal and speculum examination should preferably only be done as part of the procedure when specimens are taken. A preliminary examination tends to destroy evidence.
- Blood for VDRL and HIV testing should be taken to establish the victim's status at the time of rape.
- It is considerate to have a woman doctor treating/investigating the patient whenever this is feasible; otherwise have a female nurse in attendance. Rape victims have just had an unpleasant experience with a male or males.
- Psychiatric and Social Work support should be offered.
- The choice of whether or not to lay a charge rests with the patient. If a charge is to be laid, it must be done as soon as possible and is best lodged with the police station nearest to where the offence had been committed.
- If the patient is fully conscious and declines to lay a charge the doctor need not take forensic specimens but it should be emphasized to the patient that the evidence becomes less reliable with the passage of time, should she change her mind later. Documentation should nevertheless be meticulous as a charge may eventually be laid.
- When rape is suspected in an unconscious patient one should proceed with the forensic examination and the collection of specimens.

- Slide specimens are to be fixed and handed to the police in a sealed, signed envelope.

Referrals

The rules for staying out of trouble are:

- Always come when you are called out. Mistakes of judgement are often condoned; those from lack of commitment to patients or juniors are not accepted as readily.
- When handing over a patient, ensure that your own records are up to date and clear. Also ensure that the person taking over understands *all* the relevant facts and issues, and preferably record that you have done so.
- When receiving a patient, do not assume that all the relevant facts and perspectives have been given to you. If the case is in any way complicated or complex, spend some time going over it afresh. Where necessary, make your own investigations. Do not be afraid to ask questions about previous findings or management. Record the time when you took over the patient's care and sign such recording.

Pitfalls

- Be very careful not to make adverse or derogatory statements. Count to 1 000 – the walls have ears!
- Do not make statements when you are upset or angry. More particularly, do not write such statements into the medical records.
- Be careful of what you say when you think patients are still asleep, cannot hear, are still sedated, or have not yet recovered from anaesthetic.
- Guard against derogatory criticism of colleagues or their actions.
- Statements aimed at concealing your own possible negligence can be incriminating.

Subpoenas

Good affidavits often prevent subpoenas to testify in court.

Upon receiving a subpoena, it is advisable to contact the relevant Public Prosecutor (in criminal cases) or the instructing attorney (in civil matters) and establish whether your evidence will indeed be necessary. Often there is merely some lack of clarity about terminology in your affidavit, which can be cleared up telephonically. Even if you are needed in court, it can often be arranged that you are contacted when really necessary, rather than to be present from the start, provided that you can guarantee availability at short notice.

Recommended reading

Claasen, N. J. B., Verschoor, T. 1992 . Medical negligence in South Africa. *Digma*.

Strauss, S. A. 1991. *Doctor, patient and the Law*. Third edition. Pretoria: J L van Schaik.

47 Brain death and organ donation

Alexia Michaelides

The majority of potential organ donors arise from lethal head injuries. At any given time, all over the world, there is always a tremendous shortage of donor organs and an oversupply of patients in end-stage organ failure awaiting life-saving transplants. It is the ethical responsibility of all medical professionals who work in the trauma environment to identify and refer potential organ donors. Donors and donor families should ideally be managed by trained professionals such as Transplant Coordinators. However, should a Transplant Coordinator not be immediately available, the following guidelines are almost universally applicable:

- Identify the potential organ donor
- Establish the cause of death
- Ascertain that donor criteria are met
- Establish brainstem death
- Obtain consent from the family
- Institute appropriate medical management
- Refer to the transplant team

Identifying the potential donor

The potential donor may be recognized by certain mechanisms or cause of death, but should be thoroughly assessed for the presence of exclusion criteria.

Cause of death

The potential organ donor is a patient who has sustained irreversible brain injury due to:

- Direct head trauma
- Intracerebral haemorrhage
- Cerebral ischaemia (e.g. drowning)
- Drug overdose
- Primary brain tumour (i.e. no metastases)

Exclusion criteria

The potential donor should be under the age of 70, although age is not considered an absolute reason for exclusion.

The potential donor should have no history of:
- Malignancy, other than primary brain tumour
- Systemic sepsis
- Tuberculosis
- Sexually transmitted diseases
- Viral infections such as hepatitis B & C, HIV, systemic herpes, and acute viral illnesses such as encephalitis, meningitis, or malaria
- Insulin-dependent diabetes mellitus
- Long-standing hypertension
- A history of IV drug abuse
- A history of recent tattooing and body piercing

If a patient fails to meet the criteria for solid organ donation, consideration should be given for tissue donation (e.g. corneas, bone, skin). If there is uncertainty regarding the eligibility of the potential donor, obtain advice from a Transplant Coordinator.

Establish brainstem death

Brainstem death is the irreversible cessation of all functions of the brain. A patient who is declared brainstem dead is considered to be legally dead.

Criteria for establishing brain death

- The cause of death must be defined.
- Toxicology screen may be required to exclude presence of central nervous system (CNS) depressants and toxins.
- Correct metabolic disturbances prior to testing, e.g. hypoglycaemia, hyponatraemia.
- Correct hypothermia ($< 35\,°C$) and ensure adequate oxygenation and circulatory support.
- Ensure arterial blood gas PCO_2 is within normal range (4.5–6.1 kPa).
- Two doctors must make the diagnosis of brainstem death.
- The doctors must be registered with the SA Medical and Dental Council. One must be registered for more than five years, the other may not be an intern.
- Neither doctor may be a member of the transplant team.
- The tests do not have to be done separately or within any specified time.
- The certification of brainstem death is a clinical diagnosis.

Testing for brainstem death

- Pupillary reflex: pupils show no response to light (i.e. fixed), although not necessarily dilated
- Corneal reflex: no response to light touch with cotton wool
- Gag and cough reflexes: absent with suction or movement of endotracheal tube
- Pain response in facial distribution: supra-orbital pressure must not elicit any facial movement (spinal and tendon reflexes elsewhere may be present)
- Oculo-cephalic reflex: absence of eye movement relative to rapid head turning
- Oculo-vestibular reflex: absence of eye moment relative to iced water injection onto tympanic membrane
- Apnoea test: this is to be done last and in the following sequence:
  1 Pre-oxygenate the patient for 10 minutes with 100% oxygen
  2 Ensure the PCO_2 is within normal range (4.5–6.1 kPa or 35–45 mmHg) before disconnecting the ventilator
  3 Disconnect ventilator and administer oxygen via endotracheal tube at 10–12 ℓ/min with a catheter
  4 Observe the patient for 10 minutes for any signs of spontaneous respiration
  5 Do a blood gas at 10 minutes and reconnect the ventilator
- If the patient becomes hypoxic and unstable on testing, repeat the blood gas every three minutes.
- As soon as the PCO_2 rises above 6.5 kPa or 50 mmHg, and the patient shows no attempt at spontaneous respiration, the ventilator can be reconnected and the patient declared apnoeic.
- Provided no spontaneous respiration occurs within 10 minutes and the PCO_2 is > 6.6 kPa or 50 mmHg, there is no brainstem function.

Additional tests that can be performed but are not necessary to establish legal brain death, are cerebral angiography, cerebral blood flow scans, EEG, and atropine administration.

Consent for donation

Obtaining consent is a complex process which should be dealt with in a sensitive manner.

Approaching the next-of-kin

As soon as both doctors have completed the tests and have confirmed brainstem death, this is the time of death. Organ donation should only be discussed with the family once the diagnosis of brainstem death has been made. Transplant Coordinators are frequently more successful than physicians in obtaining consent.

Legal aspects

The Human Tissue Act allows adults to donate all or parts of their body for research or transplantation. In South Africa, organ donation is by required consent, which means that telephonic or written consent is required from the next-of-kin. Consent can legally be given by the following relatives:

- Spouse
- Son or daughter older than 18 years
- Either parent
- Legal guardian
- Sibling
- Other authorized person (e.g. common-law spouse)

Should a discrepancy exist between the wishes of the donor and that of his/her family, this can often be resolved with help from the transplant social worker/psychologist or Transplant Coordinator. In reality, the family's wishes are frequently honoured over the donor's.

If the donor has died as a result of unnatural causes, the State Pathologist or District Surgeon of the area must give permission for the removal of the organs.

Permission for the surgical procedure for removal of organs must be obtained from the Medical Superintendent of the hospital or Manager of a private hospital.

Supporting the family

It is important to be able to answer any questions that the family may have regarding funeral proceedings, costs, and procedures. Many families take solace by realizing that their loved one has helped save the lives of others.

The Transplant Coordinator is responsible for ensuring that the correct procedure is followed. To assist the family, a psychologist or social worker, or other person with counselling experience in organ procurement matters, should be present.

Medical management of the organ donor

The principle of donor management is to maintain tissue oxygen delivery by supporting oxygenation and ventilation, and optimizing haemodynamics.

Oxygenation and ventilation

- Maintain adequate ventilation and oxygenation by monitoring blood gases.
- Perform regular endotracheal suctioning to minimize pulmonary complications.
- Maintain adequate haemoglobin for optimal oxygen-carrying capacity: transfuse packed cells if required.

Haemodynamics

- Maintain systolic BP > 90 mmHg, and CVP 10–12cm H_2O by means of fluid administrations of colloid and crystalloid. This may require 3–4 litres rapidly.
- If the BP fails to respond and only if adequately hydrated, commence a dopamine infusion at 3–5 µg/kg/min and titrate according to BP. Avoid the use of adrenalin and only use dobutamine if the patient is showing signs of cardiac failure or has a diagnosed cardiac contusion.
- Utilize TNT or phentolamine for hypertension (not for hypertensive episode during coning process) if necessary.
- Maintain normothermia.
- Replace previous hour's urine output plus 100 ml and replace potassium as required.
- If diabetes insipidus develops, desmopressin or DDAVP can be administered, but with caution and in very small doses. DDAVP is preferable, with two puffs down the endotracheal tube usually being sufficient.
- Bradycardias are common and will not respond to atropine, but may respond to low-dose dopamine.
- If CVP is adequate, but urine output is low, furosemide can be administered up to 120 mg maximum.
- Monitor serum electrolytes and replace potassium accordingly.
- Monitor glucose and treat with insulin if necessary.

Pitfalls

- Unnecessary weaning of oxygen.
- Inadequate fluid resuscitation leading to circulatory collapse.
- Unnecessary use of inotropic support.
- Incorrect diagnosis of diabetes insipidus resulting in unnecessary administration of desmopressin or DDAVP.
- Administration of pentothal or midazolam resulting in excessive delays in diagnosing brain death.

Recommended reading

Organ Donor Fact Finder. Everything You Need To Know. (Fact-file on donor management) Organ Donor Foundation of South Africa. Available at most Transplant and Intensive Care Units in SA.

Addendum: Resources for health care workers and trauma victims

ALCOHOLISM:

Alcoholics Anonymous (General office)	Johannesburg	011-452-9907
	Cape Town	021-592-5047
	East Rand	011-421-1534
	Pretoria	012-322-6047
	Van der Bijl Park	016-455-2986
	Durban	031-301-4959
	Port Elizabeth	041-367-3637
	East London	043-741-3865
Alcoholics Victorious (men)	Cape Town	021-786-1981 (24hr)
Alcoholics Victorious (women)	Cape Town	021-797-1270 (a/h)
Avalon Treatment Centre	Cape Town	021-637-9100
Alateen	Cape Town	021-592-3970 (24 hrs)
Al-Anon	Cape Town	021-592-3970 (24 hrs)
Detoxification services		
Karl Bremer Hospital	Cape Town	021-918-1511
GF Jooste Hospital	Cape Town	021-690-1000
Bridges	Cape Town	021-852-6065
Sanca	Cape Town	021-945-4080 (a/h)
CMR	Cape Town	021-945-1064
AA LONERS	Johannesburg	011-615-8207

ALLERGY AND ASTHMA

Allergy and Asthma Network		www.aanma.org
Allergy Society of SA	Cape Town	021-447-9019

ANXIETY DISORDERS

		www.anxiety.org
Depression and Anxiety Support Group		080-011-8392

BAROTRAUMA

National Hyperbarics	Cape Town	021- 671-8655
Duty doctor		086-024-2242

BURNS UNITS

Tygerberg Hospital Burns Unit	Cape Town	021-938-4911
Red Cross Children's Hospital Burns Unit	Cape Town	021-658-5111

Chris Hani Baragwanath Hospital	Johannesburg	011-933-8000
Nkosi Albert Luthuli Hospital	Durban	031-240-1000
Milpark Hospital	Johannesburg	011-480-5923
Sunninghill Hospital	Johannesburg	011-806-1826
SA Burns Society, Prof A Madaree	KwaZulu-Natal	031-240-1171

CHILD ABUSE

Childline National Number		086-132-2322
Child Emergency		080-012-3321
		080-005-5555
Childline	Cape Town	021-461-1114
	Johannesburg	011-484-0771
	Potchefstroom	018-293-0045
	Bloemfontein	051-430-3311
	Port Elizabeth	041-453-0441
	Durban	031-312-0904
	Pietermaritzburg	033-394-5177
Child Protection Unit of South African Police	Cape Town	021-376-3030
		021-592-2601
	Durban	031-307-7000
		080-011-1213
Kuilsrivier Support Group for Abused Children and Women	Cape Town	021-483-3880
		021-903-3333
Bathuthuzele Youth Stress Clinic	Cape Town	021-959-2283
		080-060-0411
Ilitha Labantu	Cape Town	021-633-2383
Tygerberg Social Work Unit for Traumatised Children	Cape Town	021-938-4164

DOMESTIC VIOLENCE

List of shelters:	www.npa.gov.za/SOCA/SOCAShelters.asp	
Nicro	Cape Town	021-422-1690
Women's Help Line		080-015-0150
St Annes	Cape Town	021-448-6792
Western Cape Network on Violence Against Women	Cape Town	021-633-5287
United Sanctuary for Battered Women	Cape Town	021-572-1811
	Cape Town	021-572-5459
Women in Need	Cape Town	021-425-2095
FAMSA	Cape Town	021-447-7951
Embizweni Workshop for Men with Violent Tendencies	Cape Town	021-364-1195
POWA (People Opposing Women Abuse)	Johannesburg	011-642-4345
	Johannesburg	011-933-2333
Stop Women Abuse		080-015-0150

	Pretoria	012-460-0733
Salvation Army Shelter for Battered Women	Pretoria	012-327-3005
Masimanyane Shelter	East London	043-743-9169
Mother of Hope (shelter)	Port Elizabeth	041-585-4265
Salvation Army Haven of Hope	Port Elizabeth	041-585-5363

DRUG ADDICTION

Cape Town Drug Counselling Centre	Cape Town	021-447-8026
Crescent Clinic	Cape Town	021-762-7680
Denovo Treatment Centre	Cape Town	021-988-1138
Hottentots Holland Drug Counselling Centre	Cape Town	021-852-4820
Ramot Treatment Centre	Cape Town	021-939-2033
Stepping Stones Treatment Centre	Cape Town	021-783-4230
Kenilworth Manor	Cape Town	021-797-1400
Stikland Hospital	Cape Town	021-940-4400
Stikland Drug Unit	Cape Town	021-919-1110
Libertas Hosp Alcohol and Substance Rehab Centre	Cape Town	021-591-6111
Kenilworth Place	Cape Town	021-797-0190
Tough Love	Cape Town	021-404-3056
Staanvas Stabilis Centre	Cape Town	021-333-7702
Muslim Assembly	Cape Town	021-637-4021
Pharmacists Against Drug Abuse	Cape Town	021-434-8703
Toevlug Treatment Centre	Worcester	023-342-1162
Nar-Anon Helpline		088-129-6791
Narcotics Anonymous		088-130-0327
Mossel Bay Alcohol and Drug Centre	Mossel Bay	044-691-1463
Knysna Alcohol and Drug Centre	Knysna	044-382-5260
Serenity Care Centre	Knysna	044-343-2179
Lamprecht Medi-Centre	Knysna	044-874-2785
Swartfontein (Witrivier)	White River	013-113-2235
Riverview Manor	KwaZulu-Natal	033-701-2605

THE ELDERLY

CPOA	Cape Town	021-843-3927
Heal (Halt Elder Abuse Line)		080-000-3081
Focus on Elder Abuse	Cape Town	021-713-1360

EPILEPSY

SA National Epilepsy League	Cape Town	021-447-3014

HIV/AIDS

	www.redribbon.co.za	
Aids Resource Centre	Cape Town	021-434-2017

Aticc (also does testing)	Cape Town	021-797-5327
Napwa	Cape Town	021-424-1106
Aids Help Line		080-001-2322
CACTAS City Aids Counselling, Testing and Support Centre	Cape Town	021-422-5219
Aids Counselling (Zulu-speaking)	Durban	031-202-9132
	Durban	031-300-3104
Voluntary Testing Centre at UPE	Port Elizabeth	041-504-2330

LIFELINE/CHILDLINE

	Cape Town	021-461-1111
	Johannesburg	011-728-1347
	Pretoria	012-342-2222
	Durban	031-312-2323
	Pietermaritzburg	033-394-4444
	East London	043-722-2000
	Port Elizabeth	041-585-5581

MOUNTAIN RESCUE SERVICES

	Cape Town	107 or 021-9489900

POISON INFORMATION

Tygerberg Poison Information Centre	Cape Town	021-931-6129
Red Cross Hospital Poison Line	Cape Town	021-689-5227
SA Institute for Medical Research	Johannesburg	011-489-9000
	Gauteng	080-0 11-1990
	Johannesburg	011-495-5112
	Bloemfontein	051-447-5353
Universitas Hospital	Bloemfontein	051-405-3067
		051-447-5353
		051-405-3033 (a/h)
KwaZulu-Natal		080-033-3444

RAPE AND VIOLENCE

Rape Crisis	Cape Town	021-447-1467
		021-447-9762
The Trauma Centre	Cape Town	021-465-7373
Chris Barnard Memorial Hospital	Cape Town	021-480-6271/2
The Triangle Project for Gay and Lesbian Rape Victims	Cape Town	021-442-2500
Men Against Rape	Cape Town	021-883-3050
		083-735-9907
Johannesburg General Hospital	Johannesburg	011-488-4911
Chris Hani Baragwanath Hospital	Johannesburg	011-933-8000
Sunninghill Hospital	Johannesburg	011-806-1826

Milpark Hospital	Johannesburg	011-480-5923
Adapt	Johannesburg	011-885-3305
Netcare Rape Clinic	Johannesburg	011-480-5600
Rape Crisis & Trauma Centre,		
Baragwanath	Johannesburg	011-933-2333
	Hillbrow	011-735-2811
	Florida	011-674-1200
Kalafong Hospital	Pretoria	012-318-6400
Unitas Hospital	Pretoria	012-677-8217
Lifeline Rape Counselling	Pretoria	082-340-061
Rape Crisis	Pretoria	012-342-2222
Lifeline Rape Counselling		
(Zulu-speaking)	Durban	031-202-9132
KZN Programme for Survivors		
of Violence	Durban	031-305-3497
		083-735-9907
Nkosi Albert Luthuli Hospital	Durban	031-241-000
St Augustine's Hospital	Durban	031-268-5082
Network on Violence against Women	Durban	031-261-3471
Lifeline Rape Counselling	East London	043-722-2000
Lifeline Rape Counselling	Port Elizabeth	041-585-8565
Livingstone Hospital	Port Elizabeth	041-405-9111
Greenacres Hospital	Port Elizabeth	041-390-7362
Rape Crisis	Port Elizabeth	041-484-3804
Dora Nginza Hospital Rape		
Counselling	Port Elizabeth	041-406-4111
Rape Crisis	Bloemfontein	051-444-6143

SEA RESCUE

	Cape Town	021-449-3500

SNAKEBITE AND INFORMATION

Dr Gerbus Muller, Dept		
Pharmacology, Tygerberg Hospital	Cape Town	021-931-6129
SA Vaccine Producer	Johannesburg	011-882-9940
Fitzsimmons Snake Park, Durban	Durban	073-156-9606

TEEN PREGNANCY

Pregnancy Help Centre	Cape Town	021-797-5000
Options	Cape Town	021-592-2183
Mary Stopes Clinic		080-011-7785

TERMINAL CARE/HOME CARE

St Lukes Hospice	Cape Town	021-531-2094
Joy for Life	Cape Town	021-423-7413
		021-423-7452
Eagle's Rest	Cape Town	021-988-9935

Johannesburg		011-483-9100
Pretoria		012-348-1934
KwaZulu-Natal		031-208-6110
East London		043-721-0051
Port Elizabeth		041-360-7070

TRAUMA AND EMERGENCY MANAGEMENT TRAINING

Advanced Trauma Life Support Training	http://www.atls.co.za	
Trauma Society of SA	www.traumasa.co.za	
Advanced Cardiac Life Support Training	Cape Town	021-939-8390
Advanced Paediatric Life Support Training Course	Cape Town	021-939-8390
Flight Medical Attendant Courses, UCT Dept Emergency Medicine	Cape Town	021-447-4321

TRAUMA COUNSELLING SERVICES

Rondebosch Police Station	Cape Town	021-689-9321
TraumaClinic Counselling Network	Cape Town	021-683-7603
		082-870-8926
Trauma Centre for Victims of Violence and Torture	Cape Town	021-465-7373

TRAUMA RESEARCH

National Trauma Research Programme (MRC)	Cape Town	021-938-0216

TRAUMA UNITS

Tygerberg Hospital	Cape Town	021-938-5132
Groote Schuur Hospital	Cape Town	021-404-4112
GF Jooste Hospital	Cape Town	021-690-1068
Christiaan Barnard Mem Hospital	Cape Town	021-480-6271/2
Vincent Palotti Hospital	Cape Town	021-406-4001
Milnerton Medi Clinic	Cape Town	021-529-9299
N1 City Hospital	Cape Town	021-590-4111
Johannesburg General Hospital	Johannesburg	011-488-4911
Chris Hani Baragwanath Hospital	Johannesburg	011-933-8000
Milpark Hospital	Johannesburg	011-480-5923
Sunninghill Hospital	Johannesburg	011-806-1826
Kalafong Hospital	Pretoria	012-381-6400
Pretoria-East	Pretoria	012-422-2378
Moot Algemene Hospitaal	Pretoria	012-330-2020
Nkosi Albert Luthuli Hospital	Durban	031-240-1000
King Edward Hospital	Durban	031-360-3111
St Augustine's Hospital	Durban	031-268-5178

Umhlanga Hospital	Durban	031-560-5612
Livingstone Hospital	Port Elizabeth	041-405-9111
Greenacres Hospital	Port Elizabeth	041-390-7362
Cuyler Hospital	Port Elizabeth	041-991-1331
Universitas Hospital	Bloemfontein	051-405-3911
Kroon Hospital	Bloemfontein	056-215-3266/5

Index